RD 32 .R6324 2007

Robotics in surgery

NEW ENGLAND INSTITUTE OF TECHNOLOGY
LIBRARY

Robotics in Surgery: History, Current and Future Applications

ROBOTICS IN SURGERY: HISTORY, CURRENT AND FUTURE APPLICATIONS

RUSSELL A. FAUST
EDITOR

Nova Science Publishers, Inc.
New York

Copyright © 2007 by Nova Science Publishers, Inc.

All rights reserved. No part of this book may be reproduced, stored in a retrieval system or transmitted in any form or by any means: electronic, electrostatic, magnetic, tape, mechanical photocopying, recording or otherwise without the written permission of the Publisher.

For permission to use material from this book please contact us:
Telephone 631-231-7269; Fax 631-231-8175
Web Site: http://www.novapublishers.com

NOTICE TO THE READER

The Publisher has taken reasonable care in the preparation of this book, but makes no expressed or implied warranty of any kind and assumes no responsibility for any errors or omissions. No liability is assumed for incidental or consequential damages in connection with or arising out of information contained in this book. The Publisher shall not be liable for any special, consequential, or exemplary damages resulting, in whole or in part, from the readers' use of, or reliance upon, this material.

This publication is designed to provide accurate and authoritative information with regard to the subject matter covered herein. It is sold with the clear understanding that the Publisher is not engaged in rendering legal or any other professional services. If legal or any other expert assistance is required, the services of a competent person should be sought. FROM A DECLARATION OF PARTICIPANTS JOINTLY ADOPTED BY A COMMITTEE OF THE AMERICAN BAR ASSOCIATION AND A COMMITTEE OF PUBLISHERS.

LIBRARY OF CONGRESS CATALOGING-IN-PUBLICATION DATA

Robotics in surgery : history, current, and future applications / Russell A. Faust (editor).
p. ; cm.
Includes bibliographical references and index.
ISBN 10: 1-60021-386-3   ISBN 13:978-1-60021-386-1
1. Robotics in medicine--History. 2. Surgery, Operative--Computer simulation--History. 3. Surgical instruments and apparatus--Technological innovations. 4. Robotics in medicine--Forecasting. I. Faust, Russell A.
[DNLM: 1. Robotics--methods. 2. Surgery, Computer-Assisted--methods. 3. Telemedicine--legislation & jurisprudence. 4. Telemedicine--methods. WO 505 R666 2006]
RD32.R6324 2006
617'.001'13--dc22
                         2006024152

Published by Nova Science Publishers, Inc. ✣ New York

Dedication

To Lori, Rachel and Owen, for their love, inspiration, encouragement, and support.
I am blessed to have each of them in my life.

Contents

Foreword xi

Introduction xiii

SECTION I

Chapter 1 History of Robotic Surgery 3
Christine G. Gourin and David J. Terris

Chapter 2 Anesthetic Implications of Robot Assisted Surgical Procedures 13
Zulfiqar Ahmed and Maria Zestos

Chapter 3 Telementoring and Remote Telepresence Surgery 35
Mehran Anvari

Chapter 4 Legal Perspectives on Telemedicine and Telerobotic Surgery 47
Raymund C. King

SECTION II

Chapter 5 Robots for Orthopaedic Joint Reconstruction 61
Peter Kazanzides

Chapter 6 Robotics in General Surgery 95
Jacques Marescaux, Ali Alzahrani and Francesco Rubino

Chapter 7	The Role of Robotics in Urologic Surgery *Sanjeev Kaul, Gabriel P Haas and Mani Menon*	105
Chapter 8	Female Urologic Robotic Surgery: Gynecologic Indication for Robotic-Assisted Laparoscopy - Sacrocolpopexy for the Treatment of Hight Grade Vaginal Vault Prolapse *Daniel S. Elliott, David S. DiMarco and George K. Chow*	137
Chapter 9	Robotic Applications in Neurosurgery *Lucia Zamorano, Qinghang Li and Richard Rhiew*	147
Chapter 10	Application of Robotics to Cardiothoracic Surgery *Sumit Bose and David D. Yuh*	173
Chapter 11	Robotics Technology in Pediatric General and Thoracic Surgery *Mustafa H. Kabeer, Vinh T. Lam and David L. Gibbs*	185
Chapter 12	Robotic Applications in Advanced Gynecologic Surgery *Arnold P. Advincula*	205
Chapter 13	Robotic Applications in Otolaryngology-Head and Neck Surgery *David M. Walters and David J. Terris*	223
Chapter 14	Transoral Robotic Surgery (TORS) *Neil G. Hockstein, Gregory S. Weinstein and Bert W. O'Malley*	243

SECTION III

Chapter 15	Robotic Surgery of the Upper Airways: Addressing the Challenges of Dexterity Enhancement in Confined Spaces *Nabil Simaan, Russell H. Taylor, Alecxander Hillel and Paul Flint*	261

Chapter 16	Future Developments in Robotic Surgery: An Outside-The-Box Look Into The Next Ten Years	**281**
	Gregory Auner and Abhilash Pandya	

About the Authors   **297**

Index   **305**

FOREWORD

It is a great pleasure and honor to have the opportunity to write the forward for this comprehensive and much needed text about the history, current, and future applications of robotic surgery. Dr. Faust has not only been a significant contributor to this field himself, but has successfully assembled a pioneering and knowledgeable combination of authors who understand not only the clinical aspects of how to apply robotic technology to improve and advance surgical procedures, but also how the technical, legal, commercial, and scientific aspects of this field have and will continue to evolve.

At clinical meetings the typical discussions about robotic surgery focus on the details of the clinical application of surgical robots to various procedures. Although this is the ultimate measure of the current value of robotic surgery, it does not bring awareness to all of the other aspects that are considered in order to advance the field. For example, the technical issues, the legal & business challenges, and the regulatory barriers all play a significant part in driving the field forward. This comprehensive text gives its readers a 360 degree overview of all aspects that need consideration when developing the field of robotic surgery. It is a must-read text for those considering adding the surgical robot to their surgical tools.

Although robotic surgery has been under development for decades, it is still in its formative stage. This long incubation period is due to the complexity and expense of developing the technology, the difficulty of introducing new technology into clinical applications, and the significant regulatory and commercial challenges. However, given that two decades of effort have already gone into this promising new field, those who are interested in entering the discipline at this stage will find well-established technology and clinical experience upon which to built new clinical applications. As presented in the overview presented here, the breadth of clinical applications is rapidly expanding; this is an exciting time to be a surgeon. I believe that advancements in many of the areas described in this text will elevate the importance of this technology quantum steps.

Surgery is a fundamental tool of therapeutics in our healthcare system. Robotic surgery is now considered a new but important technology, that will play an integral role in further improvements in surgical care. I would encourage anyone who is interested in learning about, and hopefully contributing to, this exciting field to read this text. It will be of value to clinicians, hospital administrators, medical engineers, healthcare business leaders, and entrepreneurs.

Yulun Wang, PhD
CEO, InTouch Health

INTRODUCTION

It is my great privilege to introduce this collection of work from some of the most progressive surgeons of our time – those who have embraced the robot as a surgical tool. I appreciate Dr. Wang's articulate Forward – his role as one of the founders of the field of robotic surgery lends great authority to his comments.

Minimally-invasive surgical techniques are rapidly becoming the desired standard, in keeping with our "first do no harm" mandate. The consensus of these authors has been that surgical robots offer an excellent tool in our minimally-invasive repertoire. Increasingly, those of us who use these surgical robotic systems are discovering that surgical robots can augment and extend our human abilities. They enable us to operate in increasingly smaller spaces, through increasingly smaller incisions, resulting in more rapid recovery times and, in some well-documented examples, to operate with lower complication rates. Due to miniaturization and addition of the "wrist" to the robotic endoscopic instruments, these systems enable some endoscopic procedures to be performed that are otherwise not possible with manually-controlled endoscopic instruments.

The text is grouped roughly into 3 Sections. The first section begins with "The History of Robotic Surgery," in which Drs. Gorin and Terris trace the origins of surgical robots to modifications of early industrial robots whose progeny are now pervasive in manufacturing, in the auto industry for example; these authors work with one of a few groups in the area of otolaryngology – head and neck surgery who are exploring new robotic applications in surgery of the head and neck. Their experiences are reviewed in the chapter, "Robotic Surgery in the Head and Neck" by Drs. Walters and Terris, (in Section 2). Drs. Ahmed and Zestos provide a look at robotic surgery from the perspective of the anesthesiologist, and also briefly review the breadth of surgical applications of robotics in general surgery, cardiovascular surgery, gynecological surgery, and urological surgery. Also in this section, Dr. Anvari reviews the role of robotics in tele-mentoring and tele-presence medicine, or how this technology allows us to oversee and assist surgeons at a distance, and to potentially treat patients at a distance.

This section concludes with some thoughts on the unique legal, regulatory, and licensing issues that are introduced into the already-complex world of medical licensure by surgical robotics, in "Legal Perspectives on Telemedicine and Telerobotic Surgery," by Dr. King. Dr. King, who holds both the M.D. and J.D. degrees, is an authority in medical litigation and regulation.

From there, Section 2 provides a tour through several surgical fields guided by pioneers of robotic surgery in each of these surgical specialties. Several of these include descriptions of original research or clinical results. Note that Dr. Zamorano provides an interesting market analysis of robotic surgery in the chapter on "Robotic Applications in Neurosurgery."

The 3rd and final Section provides some insight into the sort of multidisciplinary research effort that has led to adapting the surgical robot to new areas of surgery. The example provided is the chapter entitled "Robotic Surgery of the Upper Airway," where Drs. Simaan, Taylor, Hillel, and Flint describe the research behind developing robotic instruments that are optimized for surgery through a laryngoscope. The text concludes with a look into the very near future of robotic surgery. In "Future Developments – An Outside-the-box Look Into the Next Ten Years of Robotic Surgery," Drs. Auner and Pandya discuss the notions of macro-, micro-, and nano-robotic systems; they discuss the addition of various sensors (such as touch, or "haptics") to these systems to relieve current limitations, and to extend our senses beyond human limitations (such as through the addition of various imaging or diagnostic sensors), as well as the evolution of robotic vision and image-guidance systems. Although seemingly speculative and futuristic in nature, their discussion is firmly based on applied research and technology *that is currently available*. These 2 chapters inspire our imagination, and challenge us to think beyond our species-centric tendency to model surgical instruments after the human hand. As we see in these 2 chapters, robotic instruments of the future are limited only by our imagination.

This text is an attempt to review how we got to this early, indeed embryonal, stage in robotic-assisted surgery, to sample some of the current surgical applications of robots in the various surgical fields, and to consider where we are rapidly going with this astonishing technology. Based on what I have seen, we can look forward to a fantastic voyage.

It has been my honor and privilege to be associated with this amazing group of author-surgeons. In their efforts to bring the very best minimally-invasive techniques to their patients, this group has demonstrated extraordinary imagination, perseverance in the face of costly equipment, burdensome regulatory oversight, prolonged training on robots, as well as enormous commitment of time to develop methods in the laboratory and in animal models. It is my hope that their experiences will inspire wider acceptance and application of this versatile surgical tool – the robot.

I gratefully acknowledge the superb organizational and editing skills of my assistant, Gene Seiter, without whom this project may never have been completed. I am also grateful to Dr. Michael Klein for introducing me to the Zeus surgical robot and supporting my own work, and to Dr. Attila Lorincz, who inspired me with his extraordinary surgical abilities with the surgical robot. Finally, I am most grateful to the William and Marie Carls Foundation, whose support has made my own foray into robotic surgery, and other research, possible.

Russell A. Faust, PhD, MD, FAAP
Carls Foundation Endowed Chair,
and Chief, Otolaryngology
Children's Hospital of Michigan
Bloomfield Hills, MI
March, 2006

SECTION I

Chapter 1

HISTORY OF ROBOTIC SURGERY

Christine G. Gourin and David J. Terris
Department of Otolaryngology-Head and Neck Surgery,
Medical College of Georgia, Augusta, GA

INTRODUCTION

Robot: "*A mechanical device that can be programmed to carry out instructions and perform complicated tasks usually done by people*". *(World English Dictionary)* [1]

The term "robot" is derived from the Czechoslovakian word "robata", which is defined as forced labor or servitude. In 1921, Karel Capek first coined the term "robot" in his play, "Rossum's Universal Robots", a satirical work written to protest the industrialization of Europe.[2] (**Figure 1**) Robots as depicted by Capek were automatons that replaced humans for the performance of mechanical tasks, and were designed to be able to remember everything but were incapable of independent thought. However, Rossum's robots developed self awareness and attempted to overthrow their human masters. Capek's play was intended as a protest against the increasing application of modern technology in Western civilization, which he considered as having a dehumanizing effect, and indeed "Rossum's Universal Robots" generated considerable controversy when it was first presented at St. Martin's Theater in England in 1922. Ironically, an unintended effect of Capek's work was public fascination with his depiction of robots, leading him to respond one year later that "…as the author I was much more interested in men than in Robots."[3] However inadvertently, Capek introduced the term robot into modern language and lighted the initial spark of public interest in the concept of robots.

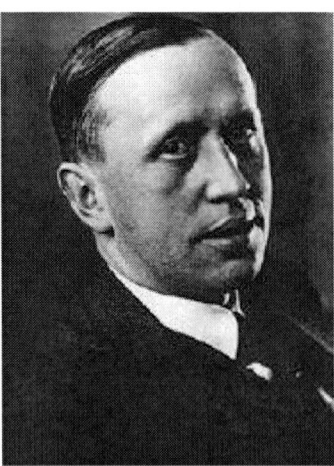

Figure 1. Carel Kapek (1890-1938).

Isaac Asimov first coined the term "robotics" in 1938 in the short story "Runaround" for *Super Science Stories* Magazine, followed by a collection of short stories describing robots coming into conflict with their human masters which was published as a collection called "I, Robot" in 1942. (**Figure 2**) Asimov used the term robotics to describe 3 laws governing robot behavior:[4]

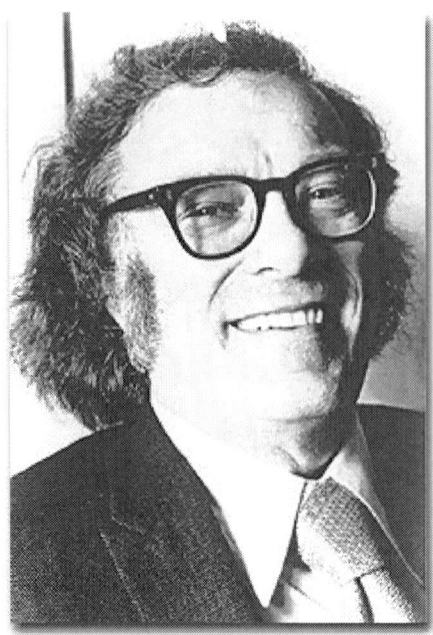

Figure 2. Isaac Asimov (1920-1992).

1) A robot may not injure a human being or through inaction allow a human to come to harm.

2) A robot must obey orders given it by humans except when doing so conflicts with the first law.

3) A robot must protect its own existence as long as this does not conflict with the first or second law.

Asimov's laws of robotics were conceived of to impose order on the free will of fictional robots. Robots have since been depicted widely in literary and cinematic fiction, sometimes as man's friend (*Star Wars*), but more often as man's enemy (*The Terminator*) when the laws of robotics are broken to dramatic effect. In actuality, the robots first envisioned by Capek have become a reality in the past 5 decades and have been increasingly utilized to perform mechanical labor in factories, in an effort to minimize human error and injury while increasing production efficiency.

The first robot successfully designed for commercial use was the Unimate (short for universal automation), built in 1958 for General Motors for use with heated die casting machines and welding. (**Figure 3**) Unimate inventors Joseph Devol and Joseph Engelberger were inspired by Asimov's science fiction stories to create machines to replace human workers in the performance of dangerous tasks. In 1961 General Motors installed the first Unimate in one of its factories. The Unimate was so successful that by 1968 multiple factories were employing Unimate robots. Robots have since been used for a variety of purposes including deep sea exploration and recovery efforts, military use in launching guided missiles, and interplanetary exploration as in the recent Rover mission to Mars, where the robots *Opportunity* and *Spirit* were employed to explore a climate inhospitable to humans and relay information back to earth about surface conditions.

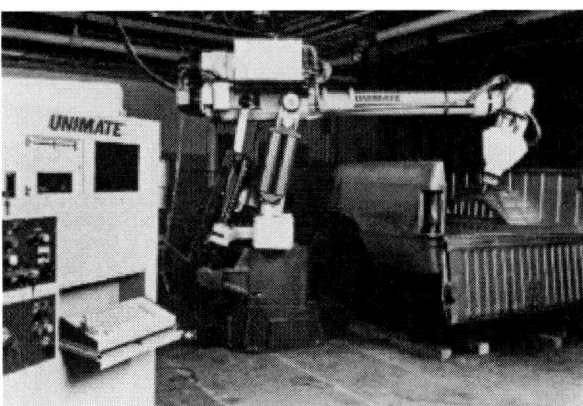

Figure 3. The early Unimate robot.

Perhaps the ultimate marriage of fiction and reality was realized with the introduction of the Honda robot ASIMO (an acronym for Advanced Step in Innovative Mobility) in 2000 (Honda Motor Co., Ltd., Tokyo, Japan).[5] With its appealing, humanoid design and ability to walk and climb stairs, ASIMO is promoted as "people-friendly" and is able to perform basic tasks such as opening doors and turning on light switches. (**Figure 4**) The Honda ASIMO is capable of interpreting the postures and gestures of humans and moving independently in response. ASIMO rang the opening bell at the New York Stock exchange on February 14, 2002 and is currently used by several corporations and museums to greet people at offices and events. In 2005, ASIMO was featured at Disneyland in a show that demonstrated the robot functioning in a home environment, suggesting a future role for such technology in assisting humans in their homes.

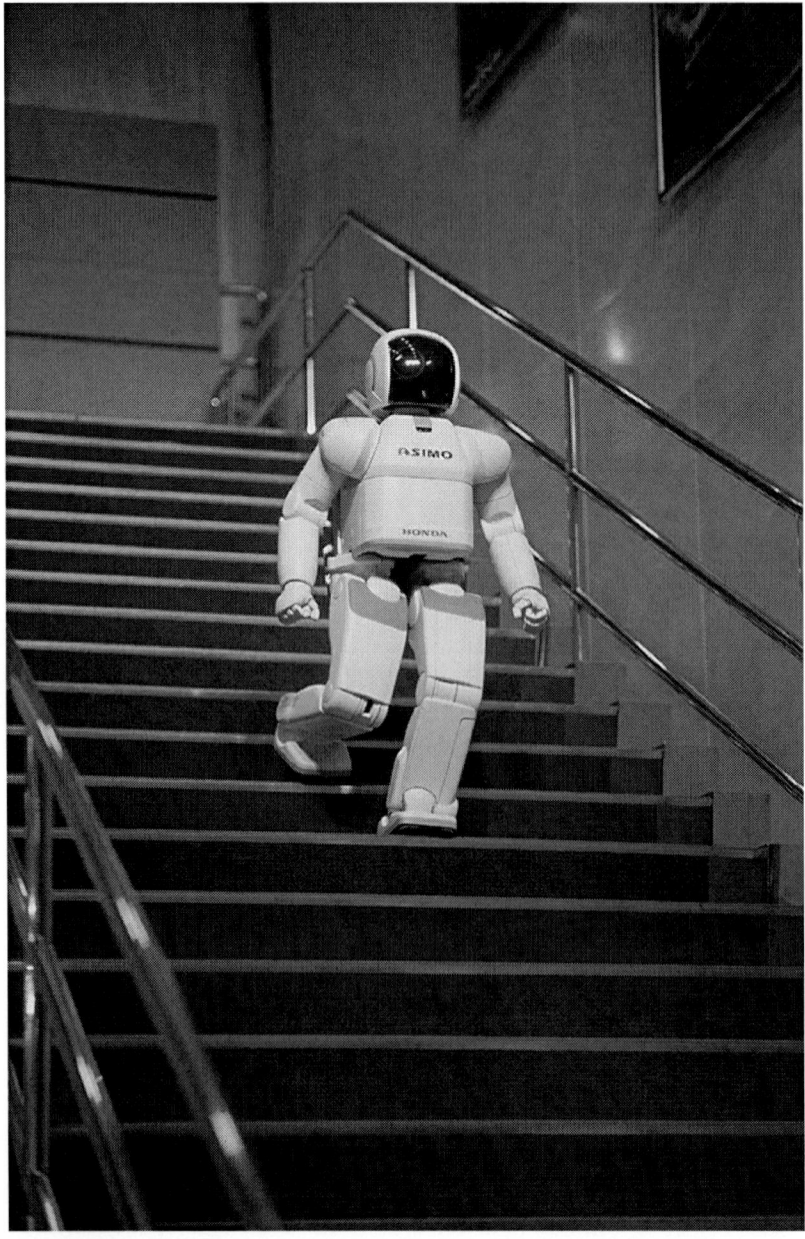

Figure 4.The Honda ASIMO robot.

ROBOTIC SURGERY

The first surgical application of industrial robotic technology was described in 1985, when a modified industrial robot was used to guide a needle for brain biopsy with 0.05 mm accuracy.[6] This served as the prototype for the Neuromate (Integrated Surgical Systems, Sacramento, CA) which received FDA approval in 1999 for passive use in image guidance stereotactic brain surgery under surgeon control. In 1992, the Robodoc (Integrated Surgical Systems) was introduced for use in hip replacement surgery in coring out the femoral shaft to accept a hip replacement prosthesis. In clinical trials, the Robodoc has been found to have greater accuracy than conventional techniques, and has been used in more than 5000 human hip replacement procedures in Europe, where it has gained wide acceptance, but is not yet FDA approved for use in the United States where it remains investigational.[7] Variations on such programmable robotic technology include the Acrobot (The Acrobot Company, Ltd., London, UK), designed for use in total knee replacement, which is currently in clinical trials, and the RX-130 robot (Stäubli Unimation Inc., Faverges, France) which has been experimentally used to drill temporal bone wells prior to cochlear implant insertion.[8] While programmable robotic surgical applications show promise, by far the greatest growth and acceptance of robotic technology has been in the area of telerobotic surgery.

TELEPRESENCE SURGERY CONCEPT

In the 1980's, researchers at the National Aeronautics and Space Administration (NASA) conceived of a head mounted virtual reality display to depict and interpret the large amounts of information transmitted from NASA's planetary exploration missions, and joined forces with researchers from the Ames Research Center (Palo Alto, CA) to develop this concept.[9] Scott Fisher, PhD of NASA coined the term *telepresence* to describe the projection of the self into a virtual world, which was a possibility afforded by virtual reality displays. Fisher and Joe Rosen, MD of the Department of Plastic Surgery at Stanford University were part of the NASA-Ames team engaged in developing virtual reality environments. The addition of 3-dimensional (3D) stereoscopic vision and the DataGlove (VPL Research, Inc., Redwood City, CA), a wired glove worn by the user that uses fiber optics to determine hand and finger position in space making it possible to grasp virtual objects, resulted in the first virtual reality system that allowed the user to interact manually with virtual objects and feel immersed in the scene.

Fisher and Rosen recognized the surgical potential of telepresence technology to enhance surgeon dexterity in microsurgery. Their vision of telepresence surgery involved surgeon manipulation of remote robotic arms, and they collaborated with Phil Green, PhD of the Stanford Research Institute (now SRI International, Menlo Park, CA)) for assistance with robotic arm development. A surgical telemanipulator designed for hand surgery was the result, with a virtual reality intuitive interface that afforded the surgeon the visual sensation of operating on a hand directly positioned in front of them, when in reality the surgeon controlled robotic hands that worked in a field located across the room.[9] When general surgeon Richard Savata, MD joined the NASA-Ames group, he recognized that this telepresence surgery prototype was uniquely suited for clinical use in the new field of laparoscopic surgery, using robotic arms to control laparoscopic instrumentation.

Subsequent development of telepresence surgery systems focused on laparoscopic applications. When a videotape of the telepresence surgery system was demonstrated at Walter Reed Army Medical Center, the Pentagon's Defense Advanced Research Projects Agency (DARPA) became interested in the idea of telepresence and robotic surgery and its potential military applications. Specifically, DARPA envisioned the application of telecommunication and robotic technology to the battlefield, allowing a surgeon to operate on a wounded soldier in the field from a virtual reality workstation at a remote location, with robotic arms in the field duplicating the motion of the surgeon's hands.[7] **(Figure 5)**

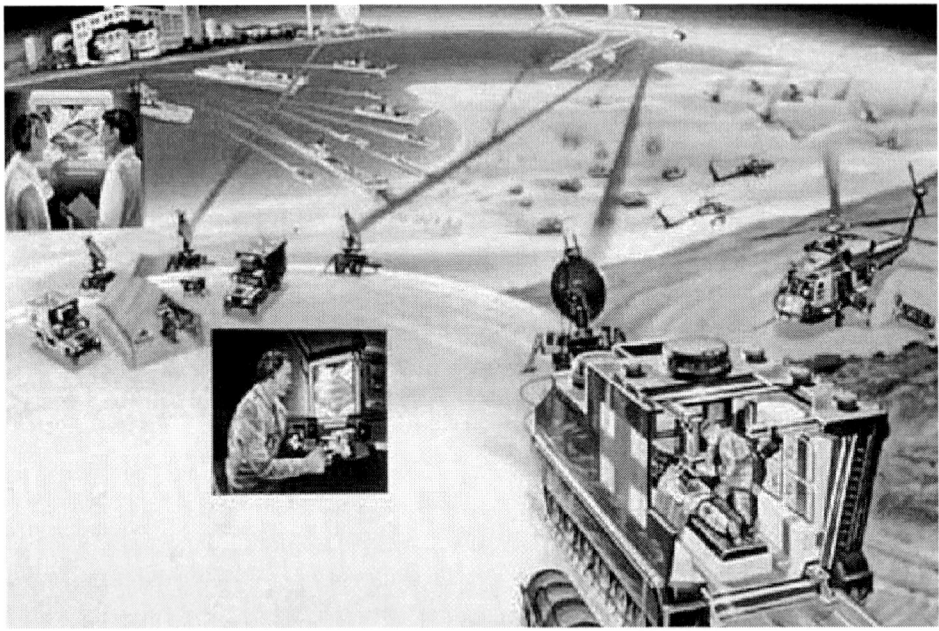

Figure 5. The DARPA vision for telepresence surgery.

With initial funding by DARPA, Yulan Wang, PhD developed the first voice activated robotic camera for laparoscopic surgery that replaced a surgical assistant, called AESOP (Automated Endoscopic System for Optimal Positioning) for his new company, Computer Motion, Inc. (Goleta, CA). AESOP consisted of a robotic arm modified to hold a laparoscopic camera, whose movement was controlled by the surgeon.[10] Subsequent modifications using the Hermes voice-activation system allow control of movement by voice commands. The success of AESOP as an assistive device resulted in FDA approval in 1994 for use in humans for laparoscopic surgery.

Haptics, or the sense of touch was an important component of surgery that was missing from early robotic applications. In the early 1990s, Kenneth Salisbury, PhD at MIT and his graduate student Akhil Madhani were experimenting with touch-guided grasping robots. In 1995, a presentation at MIT by Richard Savata about DARPA's vision for telesurgery in the battlefield inspired Madhani to focus his PhD efforts on development of the first teleoperated surgical instrument with force feedback sensors. He specifically became interested in applying this technology to minimally invasive surgery. With the assistance of Gunter

Neimeyer, PhD, force feedback programming was incorporated to provide tactile feedback. Madhani developed the "Black Falcon", the first teleoperated surgical instrument for minimally invasive surgery, with funding from DARPA. [11](**Figure 6**) The surgical operator manipulated the surgical instrument from a remote location using a hand piece that directly controlled the instrument. Images of the surgical field were viewed on a monitor transmitted by a separate camera. This technology won Madhani his PhD thesis as well as 4 patents and numerous awards, and became the industry standard for providing haptics to virtual reality environments.

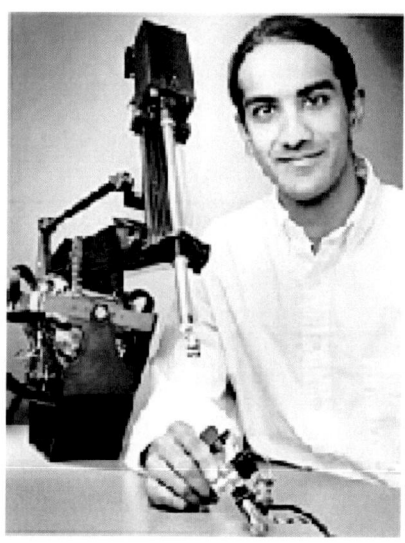

Figure 6. Akhil Madhani and the "Black Falcon".

TELEROBOTIC COMMERCIAL APPLICATIONS

While the original telepresence surgery concept was designed with the battlefield in mind, the success of AESOP as an assistive device and the potential clinical applications realized by Madhani's teleoperated surgical instrument resulted in commercial interest in robotic surgical applications. Frederick Moll MD, Robert Younge and John Freund, MD licensed the original Stanford Research Institute telepresence surgery system rights and started Intuitive Surgical, Inc. (Sunnyvale, CA) in 1995 to develop robotically controlled instruments for minimally invasive surgery. The patent for Madhani's "Black Falcon" robotic instrument arm was sold to Intuitive Surgical Inc., who brought in Salisbury and Madhani as consultants. Together they developed the da Vinci telerobotic surgical system, which was first used in 1997 in Brussels, Belgium to perform a laparoscopic cholecystectomy. The robotically controlled endoscopic instrumentation is controlled by the surgeon located at a remote console. (**Figure 7**)Two of the robotic arms manipulate operative instruments and the 3rd arm controls a video endoscope. The arms allow use of a full range of articulated instruments. The surgeon's console has 2 control handles and a virtual 3D vision projection system. (**Figure 8**) Alignment of the visual axis with the surgeon's hands in the console enhances hand-eye coordination and gives the surgeon the illusion that the patient is directly in front of him or her. The 3D vision system improves depth perception and has the ability to magnify images by a factor of 10. The articulating endowrist permits a large range of motion and rotation that follows the natural range of articulation of the human wrist and allows 6 degrees of freedom plus grip, 2 more than conventional endoscopic instrumentation. The da Vinci instruments directly follow the movement of the surgeon's hands and track the surgeon's hand movements 1300 times per second. Gross movements at the surgeon's console are translated to much finer movements of the instruments tips at the operative site. Through motion scaling, surgeon tremor may be dampened or filtered out, improving surgical technique.

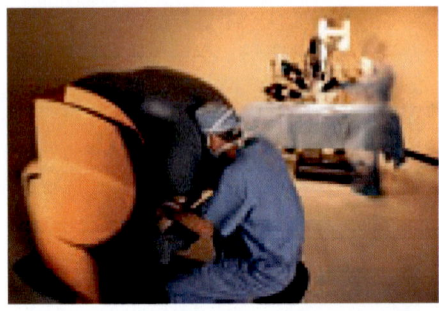

Figure 7. The da Vinci telerobotic surgical system.

Computer Motion Inc. introduced a similar system, Zeus, in 1999, differing from the da Vinci only in the design of the surgeon's workstation. The Zeus workstation is designed so that the surgeon is seated in front of a video monitor and wears polarized 3D glasses to view the projected image from the operative field in 3D. As a result, the surgeon does not have the illusion of being directly in front of the patient, unlike the da Vinci design.

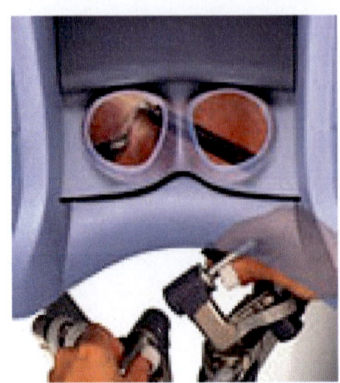

Figure 8. The da Vinci surgeon's console.

The da Vinci was the first operative surgical robotic system to receive FDA approval and has since been approved for use in mitral valve repair, prostatectomy, Nissen fundoplication, gastric bypass surgery, hysterectomy and uterine myomectomy, and is currently in clinical trials to evaluate its utility in coronary artery bypass grafting. Most of the clinical data generated from the use of both the da Vinci and Zeus systems is derived from minimally invasive coronary artery bypass surgery, as the original robotic instrumentation was designed for microvascular surgery. Currently, instrumentation is being developed for a variety of intra-abdominal and soft-tissue procedures, as additional applications for the use of robotic technology are explored.

Fisher's initial concept of telepresence surgery was most famously realized in 2001 when the journal *Nature* reported the first transatlantic use of telerobotic technology.[12] The patient, located in Strasbourg, France, underwent laparoscopic cholecystectomy performed by surgeons seated 3800 miles away in New York City, using the Zeus system with a fiberoptic bandwidth of 155 msec to minimize time delay between surgeon hand movement and robotic response. Code named "Operation Lindbergh" the procedure was successful and realized the initial military vision of telepresence surgery as well as the concept of telementoring, an extension of telepresence that allows dissemination of new techniques virtually anywhere by allowing one surgeon to demonstrate or teach a technique to surgeons at a remote location.[7] Using telementoring, an expert can be seated at a console at one location and supervise a procedure done by a surgeon in training at a remote site. The teaching surgeon has the ability to see the same 3D field of view as the operating surgeon and can seize control of the operation when needed.

In 2001, the FDA approved the Socrates telecollaborative system developed by Computer Motion, Inc. as the first robotic telemedicine device designed for telementoring in real time. The Socrates system networked shared telecommunication equipment, medical devices and robotics and was originally designed to work with the AESOP, Hermes, and Zeus systems, and allowed surgeons to collaborate using audio and video conferencing and to share control of robotic devices. In 2003, Intuitive Surgical, Inc. purchased Computer Motion, Inc., ending legal battles between the 2 companies over patent rights. Intuitive Surgical Inc. now owns and markets the da Vinci robot as well as the original Computer Motion Inc. products Zeus, Hermes, AESOP and Socrates: at present, the Zeus surgical robotic system is no longer commercially available.

THE FUTURE

In less than a century since the term "robot" was coined, robotic surgery has found an increasingly growing niche in medicine and is here to stay. No longer experimental, robotic surgery systems are safe and may result in improved patient satisfaction and quality of care when accuracy is improved and a minimally invasive alternative to conventional surgery is possible with the use of robotic technology. The costs associated with robotic surgery systems are significant: the da Vinci surgical system costs $1,000,000 with physician training costs of $250,000, annual maintenance costs of $100,000 and the cost of robotic surgical instruments, which must be replaced after 10 uses.[13] When robotic surgery is associated with decreased length of hospitalization, as has been suggested for cardiac and prostate surgery, an overall cost benefit may be realized. The success of commercial systems has led to a renewed interest by the military in battlefield applications, and in 2005, SRI International, Inc. (Menlo Park, CA) won a 2 year, 12 million dollar contract from DARPA to develop a telerobotic surgical system for use in the battlefield that would allow medical personnel to treat wounded patients from a remote location.[14] In the future, more widespread use of robotic systems, with greater applications in both the commercial and military sectors can be expected.

REFERENCES

1. Encarta® World English Dictionary [North American Edition], Microsoft Corporation, Bloomsbury Publishing Plc, 2005.

2. Capek K. R.U.R. (Rossum's Universal Robots). New York, NY; Penguin Group USA, 2004.

3. Capek K. The Meaning of R.U.R. *Saturday Review* July 21, 1923; 136: 79.

4. Asimov I. "Runaround" In: *Astounding Science Fiction* March 1942.

5. Honda Motor Co., Ltd. 2005. Available at http://world.honda.com/ASIMO/. Accessed July 7, 2005.

6. Guyton SW. Robotic surgery: the computer-enhanced control of surgical instruments. *Otolaryngologic Clinics of North America*, 2002 Dec; 35(6):1303-1316.

7. Gourin CG, Terris DJ. Surgical robotics in otolaryngology: expanding the technology envelope. *Current Opinion in Otolaryngology & Head and Neck Surgery*. 2004 Jun; 12(3):204-208.

8. Federspil PA, Geisthoff UW, Henrich D, Plinkert PK. Development of the first force-controlled robot for otoneurosurgery. *Laryngoscope*. 2003 Mar; 113(3): 465-471.

9. Satava RM. Surgical robotics: the early chronicles. *Surgical Laparoscopy, Endoscopy, and Percutaneous Techniques*. 2002; 12(1):6-16.

10. Ballantyne GH. Robotic surgery, telerobotic surgery, telepresence, and telementoring. *Surgical Endoscopy*, 2002 Oct; 16(10):1389-1402.

11. Madhani AJ, Niemeyer G, Salisbury JK. The Black Falcon: A teleoperated surgical instrument for minimally invasive surgery. *Proceedings IEEE/Robotics Society of Japan International Conference on Intelligent Robotic Systems*, 1998; 2: 936-944.

12. Marescaux J, Leroy J, Gagner M, Rubino F, Mutter D, Vix M, Butenr SE, Smith MK. Transatlantic robot-assisted telesurgery. *Nature*, 2001 Sep 27; 413(6854):379-380.

13. Gerhardus D. Robot-assisted surgery: the future is here. *Journal of Healthcare Management*, 2003 Jul-Aug; 48(4):242-251.

14. Gerin, R. "SRI to develop robotics for battlefield care". Washington Post, April 4, 2005: page E04. Available at: http://www.washingtonpost.com/wp-dyn/articles/A23899-2005Apr3.html.

Chapter 2

ANESTHETIC IMPLICATIONS OF ROBOT ASSISTED SURGICAL PROCEDURES

Zulfiqar Ahmed and Maria Zestos
Department of Anesthesiology
Children's Hospital of Michigan
3901 Beaubien, Detroit, MI, USA

From inability to leave well alone;
From too much zeal for what is new and contempt for what is old;
From putting knowledge before wisdom, science before art, cleverness before commonsense;
From treating patients as cases; and
From making the cure of a disease more grievous than its endurance,
Good Lord, deliver us.

Sir Robert Hutchison 1871-1960 (London, England)

Abstract

Advances in surgical sciences are intimately correlated with advances in perioperative medicine. For the anesthesiologist: the ability to safely keep the patient anesthetized in the presence of a robot presents a new challenge. These include preoperative optimization, airway management, surgical stress, blood and blood component transfusion, intraoperative and post operative pain management, temperature maintenance, organ preservation, prevention of nerve injury and study of differences in adult and pediatric physiology are some of the biggest achievements in this area. The advances in robotics are among the most fascinating and technologically oriented achievements. The potential advantages and disadvantages to the patient in terms of the minimally invasive approach will be elucidated in this chapter. Our role as an anesthesiologist is to carefully examine the technique, its impact on the patient and establish the safest approach to best manage patients.

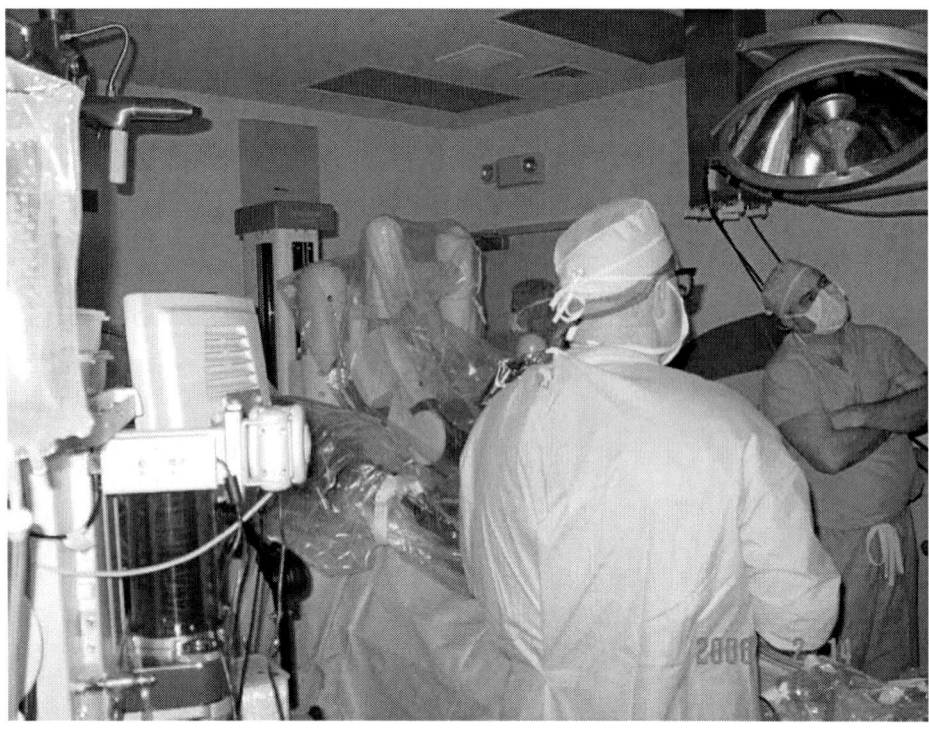

Picture 1. A robotic procedure at Detroit Medical Center in Detroit, MI. The presence of a robotic tower has decreased the available operating room space and the robotic tower is located by the patient's head side and to the patient's airway (arrow).

INTRODUCTION

The primary role of an anesthesiologist as a perioperative physician is to create analgesia, amnesia and akinesia in a safe environment for the patient. Perioperative optimization of physiology, organ protection, and pain management are among some of the goals of an anesthesiologist. New technologies like robot assistance to the surgical procedure endow even more responsibility on the shoulders of the anesthesiologist. The above mentioned quote only leads us to be scientific and methodical about our inquiry for new scientific developments. As with any new technological improvement, questions arise regarding the advantages and disadvantages of these techniques. In general, the advantages in the minimally invasive procedure have shown smaller incision size, decreased postoperative pain, earlier return to normal diet, and shorter hospital stay{Raiser, 1995 #107}. Areas where the improved outcome is still debated or in fact may be more deleterious are; hernia surgery, or in laparoscopic resection of colon cancer where trocar site recurrence of tumor has been reported [27]. The marriage of rocket science and advanced medicine has given rise to the era of master-slave tele-manipulations with extreme accuracy of movements and positions. For example, the surgeon can operate on a live patient across the Atlantic Ocean with a magnified 3-D vision, tremor filtration and a scaled motion with precision and accuracy [31; 32].

Minimally invasive surgical techniques like laparoscopic procedures have posed multiple new challenges regarding the safety and effectiveness of the techniques, which are being answered over time. The most common problems include a limited space, a 2-dimensional image on a TV screen, only 2 degrees of freedom of motion inside the body cavity, increased length of the procedure, carbon dioxide insufflation for long hours, and single lung ventilation and fulcrum effect among others. Table 1 lists a glossary of terms, which is commonly used in association with the robotic technology. Robot assisted surgery techniques have attempted to significantly minimize most of these disadvantages. Though this has been done at a certain bargain for example increased duration of the procedure and addition of complex machines in the small operating rooms.

Table 1

AESOP	Automated Endoscopic System for Optimal positioning African slave in ancient Greece. 620-560 B.C
Telepresence	The connection between the patient and the surgeon through virtual reality
Latency	Time taken from a hand motion to the actual visualization of the action
Fulcrum Effect	A non intuitive motion of the tip of the instrument in the opposite direction usually at the skin entrance site
Slave	The electronic device to be controlled
Master	The remote location from which the slave is controlled. Usually the surgical console
Robot	A mechanical device which performs automated physical tasks, either according to direct human supervision, a pre-defined program, or a set of general guidelines
Registration	A process of transforming the different sets of data into one coordinate system
Zeus	The leader of the gods and god of the sky and thunder in Greek mythology Brand name for a surgical robot
DaVinci	Italian Renaissance architect, musician, anatomist, inventor, engineer, sculptor, geometer, and painter
Degree of Freedom	flexibility of motion
Pitch	tilting up and down
Yaw	turning left and right
Grip	Grasping the object
Heaving	Moving up and down
Surging	moving forward and back

Table 2

Adrenalectomy
Anti-reflux surgery
Bowel section
Heller's Myotomy
Pyloromyotomy
Splenectomy

As anesthesiologists, we are an intimate part of these advancements in surgical techniques. Our aim is to closely understand the nature of techniques and their effects on the patient's physiology and to ensure that the risk benefit ratio is on the side of the patient's safety.

In this chapter, we will first discuss the effects of various factors that are involved in robot assist surgery. These include carbon dioxide insufflations, long duration of the procedures, non-physiologic positions, operating room hazards and presence of huge machines. Most importantly, intraoperative airway complications may occur in a patient whose airway may not be readily accessible in the perioperative settings (see photo 1). We will then follow with a discussion on the unique considerations for individual surgical areas. Finally, a separate section on pediatric anesthetic considerations will be presented.

PHYSIOLOGICAL EFFECTS OF LAPROSCOPY IN ADULTS

Most robotic procedures involve an introduction of robotic arms, a camera, and a number of retractors in a body cavity. Carbon dioxide (CO_2) insufflation is maintained at a variable pressure of 4-20 mm Hg. The amount of time spent to do the procedure, especially during the early stages of the learning curve, may be significantly longer and may contribute to the perioperative stress. The procedure involves insufflation of CO_2 in the abdomen or chest cavities and confers a number of changes on the physiology. In addition a gasless technique has been described where the abdominal wall is suspended to create the space needed to work.

Ventilatory Change

CO_2 insufflation into the peritoneal cavity causes abdominal distention and cephalad displacement of the diaphragm. This may result in 30% to 50% reduction in thoracopulmonary compliance [6; 23; 28; 41]. Despite the increase in the compliance curve, the shape of the pressure volume curve does not change [26; 40; 43]. Hence, intraoperative monitoring of pressure volume curve and pulmonary compliance can help diagnose certain conditions like bronchospasm, endobronchial intubation, pneumothorax or changes in the degree of muscle relaxation. Increase in the airway pressure leads to ventilation perfusion mismatch and reduction for functional residual capacity due to an elevated diaphragm. However, the abdominal pressures up to 14 mm Hg in a patient with up to 20° tilt, whether head up or down, does not significantly change physiologic shunt or dead space in healthy patients or pressure volume curve[11; 26; 47].

Increased arterial CO_2 (PaCO_2)

The introduction of CO_2 in the peritoneal cavity at induction leads to a rise of arterial CO_2 (PaCO_2) which plateaus in 20 to 30 minutes[38]. A number of factors affect this increase in arterial CO_2, such as the degree of abdominal distention, patient positioning, volume control ventilation, and anesthetic induced respiratory depression in a spontaneously ventilating patient. These mechanical factors affect pulmonary ventilation-perfusion ratio[3], and cause an increasing PaCO_2 secondary to increased absorption of CO_2 from the body cavity[2; 3]. In an awake patient undergoing CO_2 insufflation under local anesthetic, PaCO_2 remains normal secondary to a compensatory increase in minute ventilation. In an anesthetized patient, impaired ventilation causes a rise in PaCO_2. End tidal carbon dioxide (ETCO_2) and transcutaneous CO_2 can be used to detect the increase in PaCO_2 [23]. This may not be reliable in patients with cardiopulmonary disturbances such as congenital heart disease or chronic obstructive pulmonary disease or other. A high index of suspicion should be maintained whenever clinical signs and symptoms of hypercarbia are seen even in the absence of high ETCO_2 which may include CO_2 subcutaneous emphysema. The rate of rise of CO_2 diffusion into the body spaces depends on the duration and location of CO_2 insufflation[38] and is exaggerated in sicker patients[52].

In cases of prolonged procedure, large amount of absorbed CO_2 can be buffered into muscles, bone and tissues giving rise to additional load of CO_2 to be eliminated via lungs during the early postoperative period.

Hemodynamic Problems

A variety of hemodynamic changes are seen with peritoneal CO_2 insufflation. These include decreased cardiac output (CO), increased arterial pressure, increased systemic vascular resistance (SVR), and increased pulmonary vascular resistance (PVR). Heart rate (HR) is usually unchanged or slightly increased. The decrease in CO is usually proportional to intra abdominal pressures, especially above 10 mm of Hg. This is independent of either head up or head down positions. These changes are accompanied by normal mixed venous oxygen saturation (V$_{CO2}$) and lactate levels. Joris at el showed increased vasopressin levels during peritoneal insufflation. Increased intra-abdominal pressures (IAP) lead to increased cardiac pressures and paradoxical decrease in venous return. This is due to increase intra thoracic pressures associated with increased IAP. This leads to pooling of blood in the lower extremities and increased venous return due to vena caval compression. Methods to attenuate these changes include slight head down before insufflation, fluid boluses, elastic bandages on the leg, and intermittent sequential compression devices.

The above changes are well tolerated by healthy patients, but can result in significant hemodynamic upset in patients with impaired oxygen delivery or cardiopulmonary derangements. These patients have very low preoperative cardiac output and central venous pressure. Treatment of these patients should be individualized and under expert care. Some of these patients may be candidates for judicious use of volume expansion, nitroglycerine, nicardipine, lower IAPs and slower rate of insufflation. Arrhythmias may develop, but unlikely to be due to high $PACO_2$ as they develop earlier during insufflation. The major complications expected during laparoscopy are subcutaneous CO_2 emphysema, pneumothorax, capnothorax, endobronchial intubation and gas embolism[51]. For a more detailed discussion please refer to the bibliography[13].

Patient Positioning

Patient positioning during the perioperative period may have significant effects on patient's physiology, cardiovascular, respiratory as well as peripheral nerves. Part of the reason may be presence of a robotic arms or tower in close proximity to the patient either next to him or her or positioned in between the legs with patient in steep Trendelenburg positions.

Cardiovascular
Trendelenburg (TR) and reverse Trendelenburg (rTR) positions are commonly used in laparoscopy surgery to improve vision. These non-physiologic positions effect hemodynamics in multiple ways. TR causes an increase in CVP and CO which is compensated by systemic vasodilatation and bradycardia mediated by a baroreceptor reflex. This reflex maybe impaired by general anesthesia, but in healthy patients these changes may not be hemodynamically significant. Increased intraocular pressure (IOP) and cerebral perfusion pressure (CPP) may result as well. rTR positions bring in opposite effects which may not be significant in healthy patients as well[36].

Respiratory
Reverse Trendelenburg (rTR) position favors improved ventilatory functions by increased functional residual capacity (FRC), total lung volume (TLV) and pulmonary compliance. TR leads to opposite changes in perioperative pulmonary functions.

Nerve injury
A number of factors, including overextension of the arms to accommodate surgeons standing on patient's side or shoulder braces for long hours, may cause nerve injury.
Common peroneal nerve and other lower extremity nerve injuries are among the most common problems in lithotomy positions.

Physiologic effects of Thoracoscopy

Since Jacobaeus introduced thoracoscopy in 1910[10], the technique has evolved to its current form of video assisted thoracoscopic surgery (VATS) as a safe and accurate technique. Advantages described for VATS include (1) less postoperative pain, (2) improve

Table 3

Video Assisted Thoracic Surgery
Lungs
Pneumonectomy
Lobectomy
Wedge, subsegmental, segmental resection
Resection of pulmonary metastasis
Excision of blebs and bullae
Heart
Pericardiocentesis
Pericardiectomy
Insertion of implantable cardioverter-Defibrillator
Esophagus
Esophagectomy
Repair of esophageal perforation
Fundoplication
Mediastinum
Excision of tumors and cysts
Sympathetic nervous system
Truncal vagotomy
Thoracic Spine
Anterior release for posterior spine fusion
Disc herniation
Deformity correction
Abscess drainage

pulmonary functions, (3) shorter hospital stay, and (4) earlier return to work[13]. There is a long list of indications for the procedure of VATS in Table 3. Over time more of these maybe performed by robotic assistance. Single lung ventilation is used to facilitate the VATS and to improve visualization. However it also gives rise to an obligatory right to left transpulmonary shunt through the non-dependent lung. Hypoxic pulmonary vasoconstriction, which would help to decrease the shunt fraction, is also impaired in the presence of certain anesthetics. This shunt creation is influenced by factors like lateral decubitus position, presence of anesthetics, presence of paralysis, and closed versus open chest conditions. Insufflation of carbon dioxide for creation of pneumothorax is advocated[13]. Animal experiments have shown that creation of this pneumothorax has caused a 36% decrease in cardiac index, 34% decrease in stroke volume, and a 49% decrease in left ventricular stroke volume index at an insufflation pressure of 5 mm of Hg[25]. Increasing the pressure to 15 mm of mercury leads to a 64% decrease in mean arterial blood pressure, 81% decrease in cardiac index, and a 95%

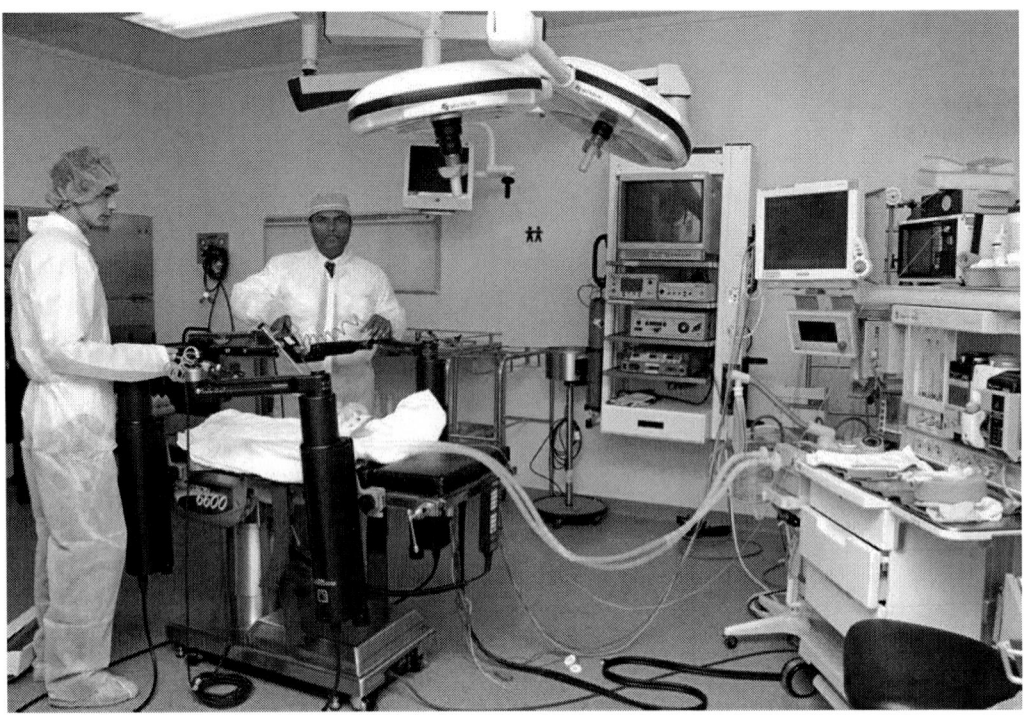

Picture 2. This picture illustrates the three Zeus arms and the location of the patient (arrow) at the operating table. Picture taken in the operating room of Children's Hospital of Michigan, Detroit, MI

decrease in left ventricular stroke volume index compared to base line. These changes are easily reversed after restoration of intrapleural pressures. Good candidates for VATS are the patients with significant bilateral pulmonary disease, who are not candidates for thoracotomy. Barker describes 22 patients with significant disease who underwent VATS ablation of emphysematous bullae[8]. These patients tolerated 170 minutes of single lung ventilation, with the exception of one. Elective postoperative ventilation was utilized. Complications reported post VATS are prolonged air leak, atelectasis, dysrhythmias, bleeding requiring transfusion and pneumonia[13].

ANESTHETIC IMPLICATIONS OF ROBOTIC SURGERY

General Surgery

Laparoscopic robot assisted gastrointestinal surgery is the most established field in the area. A number of procedures have been carried out by robot assistance, described in Table 2:

The FDA and European Union have approved these procedures and in the future, more procedures are expected to be approved.

Anesthetic Plan

Patients should be physiologically optimized according to the indications. An example of this may be a Hb F of less than 40% in a patient with sickle cell disease for minimally invasive splenectomy and fluid resuscitation for a patient presenting for pyloric stenosis. Patients should have bilateral intravenous access as the one side of the body may be inaccessible to the perioperative team because of the robotic tower. Patients may be anesthetized with an intravenous anesthetic like sodium thiopental and a rapid sequence intubation may be performed when indicated along with cricoid pressure as in the patients with gastroesophageal reflux (GERD). An appropriate combination of intravenous agents, opioids and muscle relaxants may be used. Upon securing the airway with a single lumen endotracheal tube, the patient should be prepared and draped accordingly. Monitors include EKG, non-invasive blood pressure cuff, pulse oximetry, capnography, and a Foley catheter. An orogastric tube should be passed to empty the stomach as well. Arterial and central lines would be appropriate in patients with significant cardiopulmonary compromise. Degree of invasiveness in monitors is variable and should be tailored to individual patients. Patients may be placed in TR positions for pelvic or rTR procedures for upper abdominal procedures, lateral or semi-lateral for renal or adrenal procedures. Usually 3 to 4 trocars are inserted in the abdominal cavity. With the Zeus system, the robotic arms are mounted on the operating table (as shown in Photo 2) but this system is no longer serviced by the company. In DaVinci system the mechanical arms are mounted on a separate tower and then the cart is moved to an appropriate place and then locked. The location of the robot arms or the tower may be too close to the patient's body and care should be taken to prevent contact between them. Once the robotic arms are engaged and the trocars are introduced in the body cavity, the patient cannot be moved. Hence it is of the paramount importance that a plan by the surgical and the anesthesia team is in place in case of an airway, anesthetic or surgical emergency. The plan should include disengaging the robotic arms, moving the tower away from the patient, taking the patient out of the surgical position and approaching the patient[34]. These actions cannot be initiated until the robot arms are disengaged, and the tower is moved away from the patient. Practice runs are recommended and should be rehearsed.

Abdomen is then prepped and draped in the usual fashion, insufflating needle inserted and abdominal cavity is insufflated with CO_2 up to pressures of 10-20 mm Hg. The anesthesiologist need to pay close attention to the insufflation pressures as overzealous insulation may cause hemodynamic compromise. The trocars, camera and endo wrist are introduced and then engaged with the robotic arms. Once the arms are engaged and all is in place, the patient cannot be moved. Hence muscle relaxants are of vital importance. Long acting relaxants like pancuronium should be considered if appropriate. Rise in $ETCO_2$ should be counter balanced by ventilator adjustments. Patients with significant volume deficit should have the deficit corrected before the insufflation begins as increased intraperitoneal pressures may decrease venous return resulting in decreased cardiac output and decreased blood pressure.

Complications of laparoscopic carbon dioxide insufflation include CO_2 subcutaneous emphysema, pneumothorax, pneumomediastinum and pneumopericardium. These problems should be anticipated and aggressively managed[51]. Endobronchial intubation, and gas embolism should also be expected to occur and should be prepared for. A detailed discussion of diagnosing and managing complications during laparoscopy is mentioned elsewhere[26].

Cardiac Surgery

The inflammatory response and morbidity post operatively from sternotomy and cardiopulmonary bypass (CPB) is well described[4; 12]. Minimally invasive surgery can significantly reduce of IL-6, IL-8, C3a and troponin I in the postoperative period which translates to better patient outcome. The incidence of postoperative infection also decreases. Improved post operative outcome along with other benefits of endoscopic and robot assisted surgery, have led to a dramatic change in the surgical world of cardiovascular diseases. This has evolved from thoracoscopic harvesting of internal mammary artery to total endoscopic beating heart CABG. The first robot assisted CABG was reported in 1998 by Loulmet et al.[29].

With the recent advances in techniques, total endoscopic CABG has led to beating heart procedures. These procedures have evolved from classic sternotomies and use of heart lung machines to mini-incisions (10-12 cm) working under direct vision, video assisted vision using micro-incision (4-6 cm), port incision (1-2 cm) to current status of port incisions using robotic instruments[20].

The new challenge that the anesthesiologists are facing is prolonged periods of CO_2 insufflation in thoracic cavity and SLV. This will significantly alter patient physiology. A number of patients are either not eligible for the potentially beneficial procedure or may experience significant metabolic abnormalities as previously discussed. The extent of the physiologic changes depends on the age, duration of the procedure, PIPs and the ability of the ventilators.

Mitral valve surgery

Although mitral valve surgery can be performed via thoracoscopy and endovascular bypass, the patients need to be carefully selected. Patients excluded currently include those with increased left atrial pressure (LAP), pulmonary hypertension (PHTN), chronic obstructive pulmonary disease (COPD) and coronary artery disease (CAD).

Patients on oral anticoagulant such as coumadin should be changed to short acting intravenous agents such as Heparin. Some patients may be on peripheral vasodilators preoperatively to reduce afterload in cases of hypertension. Chronically elevated LAP may result in pulmonary hypertension that may coexist with COPD. These patients are not currently a candidate for robotic surgery.

Anesthetic intervention starts on the day of pre anesthetic visit with a detailed history and physical exam. Pertinent investigations like hematologic and chemistry values, coagulation studies along with relevant pulmonary and cardiac studies are evaluated. Detailed discussion of the relevant anesthetic plan is done as well. Patient is evaluated for his or her ability to withstand prolonged single lung ventilation, regional anesthetic technique, airway assessment for double lumen endotracheal tube placement, presence of major scoliosis and presence of large emphysematous bullae. Patient's skin in the thoracic region is also examined for possible neuroaxial or thoracic paravertebral block for the surgery. On the day of the operation with appropriately optimized patient, two large peripheral intravenous lines are started and mild sedation may be given with midazolam before placement of invasive lines. Perioperatively, patients are monitored with EKG leads II and V5 with automated ST segment analyzers, pulse oximetry, capnograph, and Foley catheter. Invasive lines, such as central line, and pulmonary arterial catheter should be individualized including radial arterial lines, which may be bilateral depending on the protocol. Anesthesia is induced after adequate preoxygenation and cardio stable technique which may include a mixture of fentanyl, vecuronium, and isoflurane. Upon attainment of adequate anesthetic depth, tracheal intubation is performed with a double lumen endotracheal tube, whose position can be confirmed by fiberoptic bronchoscopy. Tans-esophageal echocardiography (TEE) can be used to confirm central line placement along with assessment of valve function. The details of intra aortic balloon occlusion and femoral-femoral cardiopulmonary perfusion are discussed elsewhere in this book. Previously, patients with diseased femoral vessels were not a candidate for femoral-femoral cannulation. They can now be operated upon with Heartport Straight shot™ (Heartport, Inc., Redwood city, CA) via anterior chest wall.

After induction the patient is placed in a left lateral position with chest tilted at 30 degrees. The left arm may be suspended over the head or upper torso with support to improve the exposure of the chest with care to prevent brachial plexus injury [36]. Sometimes the left arm may be draped also for surgical access and hence only right arm will be available to the anesthesiologist. External defibrillator pads and transcutaneous pacing pads are applied over the chest before anesthetic induction for any unexpected cardiac event.

After adequate positioning the right lung is collapsed and single lung ventilation (SLV) is instituted. If the lung is not adequately collapsed, the position to bronchial blocker or double lumen tube should be checked for misplacement and appropriately adjusted. Excessive intrapulmonary shunting may give rise to hypoxia and should be addressed by application of continuous positive air pressure (CPAP) or positive end expiratory pressure (PEEP). Failure to achieve adequate oxygenation may result in abandoning the robotic assist or modification of the technique. As described before prolonged SLV may give rise to hypercarbia and hypoxia. Although effects of mild to moderate hypercarbia have been studied, effects of severe prolonged hypercarbia on the patients have not yet been fully elucidated. Severe hypercarbia and hypoxia can elevate pulmonary artery pressure and pulmonary vascular resistance and decrease cardiac output simultaneously.

Perioperatively a vigilant care towards adverse cardiac events like arrhythmias due to hypercarbia, hypoxia, acidosis and preexisting conditions is needed. Placement of transcutaneous pacing (TCP) and defibrillating pads, boluses of lidocaine and magnesium to decrease myocardial irritability, nitroglycerine for ST segment changes are to be considered. The resulting pneumothorax from CO_2 insufflation needs vigilant monitoring as it may become a tension pneumothorax if the insufflating pressure rises too high or too fast. Continued communication between the anesthesiologist and the surgeon, careful monitoring of tidal volumes, peak airway pressures, insufflation pressures and central venous pressures are a must. The mean duration of these SLV has been reported to be 196±67 minutes [39].

Regional anesthetic technique has been described in these patients to control pain which has been described to last about 48 hours. Continuous thoracic or low lumber epidural analgesia or continuous thoracic paravertebral block may be utilized in appropriately selected patients and according to the local expertise. As these patients receive a relatively smaller amount of heparin perioperatively (10,000-20,000 U) [16], the regional techniques may be suited for these patients [39]. These patients should be followed very closely and any suspicion of neurological compromise should be evaluated aggressively. Hence these patients may be managed with a light general anesthetic with regional analgesic and guaranteed paralysis as small movements by the patient can lead to catastrophic results like hemorrhage and myocardial injury. Prevention of the intraoperative recall should not be neglected.

Prevention of perioperative hypothermia can be of advantage in a number of ways. It may expedite extubation postoperatively and decrease the risk of shivering and hence prevent excessive oxygen utilization during a critical period of the perioperative events. It has been reported that forced air warmer around the head only and intravenous fluid warmers are usually sufficient to prevent intraoperative hypothermia and maintain body temperature at the desirable levels. Fluid administration must be carefully balanced and can be titrated with the pulmonary capillary wedge pressure (PCWP), which may be maintained close to the desired value. Postoperative complications to anticipate are anastomotic patency, myocardial ischemia and infarction, arrhythmias, bleeding and hypothermia. These patients may be extubated in the operating rooms (OR) or in the ICU as per local protocol and patient condition.

Coronary Artery Bypass Grafting (CABG)

The benefits of endoscopic repair have led enthusiasts to venture into performing CABG with the robot assist. Minimally invasive surgical procedures in cardiac patients have so far shown comparable results on intermediate term, acceptable revascularization and an acceptable clinical outcome [49]. The mean time to harvest internal mammary artery (IMA) was 59 minutes and the mean total operating time was 162 minutes (118-282 minutes). The graft patency rate was 99.3% in the overall outcome at 6-month results. Average ICU stay was 11.5 hours and mean stay in the hospital was 2.2 days. In 88% patients, the trachea was extubated in the operating room. To date minimally invasive technique has shown a remarkable improvement in post operative recovery and may soon be deriving the consumer market towards more minimally invasive techniques.

Patients are appropriately selected and preoperative preparation should be optimized. TEE is utilized to rule out Patent Foramen Ovale (PFO) or persistent superior vena cava (SVC). Mild sedation is performed intravenously and invasive lines like arterial lines are inserted. Bilateral arterial lines are often placed to monitor internal mammary artery dissection. These also help monitor the endovascular occlusion balloon placement when endovascular CPB is to be utilized. Central lines along with the pulmonary artery catheter are inserted as indicated. Femoral lines are placed when endovascular CPB is expected to be performed and is mentioned else where in the book. Of note the aortic cannula has a separate lumen for cardioplegia to be delivered into the aortic root to perform diastolic arrest. To position the aortic occlusion balloon guidance by TEE is essential. TEE also monitors the residual flow around the balloon. The patient may then be anesthetized with cardio stable technique. This is achieved by avoiding tachycardia; blood pressure swings secondary to vasodilation, sympathomimetic response to laryngoscopy and avoidance of myocardial depression hence maintaining myocardial oxygen delivery. The trachea is intubated with a double lumen endotracheal tube, a Univent tube or a bronchial blocker, the position of which can then be confirmed by fiber optic bronchoscopy. Inspired oxygen and $ETCO_2$ are monitored along with expired anesthetic agents when utilized. Defibrillation and transcutaneous pacing pads can also be placed at this time. Intraoperative TEE is also utilized to monitor intraoperative cardiac function, confirming catheter placement and volume status.

Appropriate positioning may involve supine, right lateral position and suspension of the arm over the body or the face, to facilitate the introduction of the trocars. This position thins the skin overlying the chest wall area to be operated on. The left chest can be prepped if left or both internal mammary arteries are to be dissected. For right internal mammary artery only, both sides of the chest are prepped. Insufflation of the carbon dioxide on the left side also exposes the RIMA due to leftward shift of the heart and movement of the mediastinal fat pad medially, all of which improve the angle of vision. Intrathoracic pressure is maintained at 5-10 mm Hg and is raised slowly in 2-4 mm Hg increments. The patient's volume status should be optimized prior to insufflation especially in patients with CVP below 5 mm Hg. Single lung ventilation and CO_2 insufflation at low pressures decrease PAP and increase CVP slightly. Bilateral pneumothoraces may be produced if required and have been shown to be tolerated well. If CPB is to be performed, lung is deflated after the cannulation. The other lung is ventilated with peak pressures of 35-40 mm Hg. Ports are then placed on the collapsed side and CO_2 is insufflated to further facilitate lung collapse. Larger tidal volumes may prevent mediastinal shift towards the ventilated side. The surgeons may use sternal hooks to increase the retrosternal space in order to improve visualization. In cases where CPB is not utilized and surgery is performed on the beating heart, articulating stabilizers are placed on the heart through a sub-xiphoid port. These stabilize the surface of anterolateral heart and ease the anastomoses. Coronary arteries are occluded and anastomosis is performed. Bilateral internal mammary artery grafting has also been performed as well[26]. Stabilization devices have been designed to make off pump CABG common place and their miniaturization have made it easy to be used endoscopically. Problems currently being faced are the limitations of view through the scope where smaller vessels may be mistaken for the target vessels[19]. Absence of tactile sensation, hidden vessels in the epicardial fat, vessels buried in the myocardium, calcified vessels will pose a challenge for the creation of the anastomosis. Epicardial Doppler ultrasound has been used to help. Motion gating technology now allows the heart to appear still by using a strobe light that synchronizes with the heart rate and facilitating the working on a moving target.

Atrial Septal Defects (ASD) Repair

The surgical technique and instrumental requirements for ASD are similar to that for mitral valve repair/replacement. However the need for mini thoracotomy is not there. The surgical manipulation can be done entirely through the scopes and hence need prolonged period of SLV. Endovascular methods for CPB are needed and are described in other chapters. The mean duration of CPB and Aortic occlusion is described to be 102±40 and 64±22minutes respectively[48].

Thoracic Surgery

Video Assisted Thoracoscopic Surgery (VATS) is now considered standard of care when indicated. A larger thoracotomy incision is utilized when needed. Hence robotic assistance is only an extension of the current technique. Currently lung tumor resections and esophagectomies are being evaluated for possible robotic assistance. Although potentially useful, trials have yet to be conducted to evaluate the efficacy and benefit.

Appropriately selected patients may undergo robot assisted thoracoscopic surgery. For thoracic and cardiac procedures, preoperative pulmonary functions are essential for optimum intraoperative care. Continuous intraoperative assessment of cardiac functions with TEE is appropriate. The usual indication is for resection for esophageal carcinoma. Criteria for lung tumor resectability via thoracoscopic or robot assisted VATS are summarized in Table 3. Robot assisted esophagectomy can replace the thoracotomy part of the traditional three point approach to an esophagostomy where after laparotomy for initial mobilization of esophagus and the stomach, a thoracotomy is performed for the release of the organ. A neck dissection is performed to mobilize the cervical esophagus and proximal anastomosis between the stomach and the cervical esophagus is then performed. Monitors may include EKG, pulse oximetry, capnography, non invasive blood pressure measurements, Foley catheter, arterial line and invasive monitoring as indicated. Postoperative pain can be managed with neuroaxial opioids or thoracic paravertebral blockade.

Urologic Surgery

Transurethral resection of the prostate (TURP) is the most common surgical procedure among the robot assisted surgeries in the U.S. at present. There are a number of methods described for prostatectomy. Earlier methods such as suprapubic retropubic or trans vesicular prostatectomy followed by the description of transurethral resection of prostate, robot assisted transurethral evaporation of the prostate[30] and now the laparoscopic robot assisted prostatectomy. Its indications include benign prostatic hyperplasia and carcinoma of the prostate.

After appropriate screening of patients assessing surgical indications and anesthetic pre-evaluation, patients are anesthetized with appropriate technique. The patient is placed in supine position with adequate padding. Legs are placed in lithotomy position with robotic system placed in between the legs for patient 6 feet tall or more. For shorter patients, the legs are placed in frog leg position with ankles padded. Patient is placed in a steep Trendelenburg position. Monitors should be individualized for the patient. In a healthy patient monitors include intravenous lines, pulse oximetry, capnography, mechanical ventilation, blood pressure monitor and Foley catheter. Invasive lines should be reserved for expected large blood loss or patients with cardiopulmonary problems but with relatively less blood loss are probably not indicated. The procedure is performed under general anesthetic and patient may be treated like a robot assisted laparoscopic cholecystotomy including ensuring paralysis.

Gynecologic Surgery

The surgical specialty which started the saga of minimally invasive surgery has been less affected by its use. Its primary interest is in robot assisted microsurgical reversal of fallopian tube ligation [15; 18; 33]. Vasectomy is another area which is being currently evaluated currently in animals[44].

After anesthetic induction patient is placed in a modified lithotomy position in Trendelenburg position. The uterus should be easily accessible with legs apart and pneumoperitoneum is obtained by CO_2 insufflation. At the end of the procedure methylene blue is used to assess the patency of the fallopian tubes.

Orthopedic Surgery

Among the earliest applications of robotic surgery was collaboration between IBM and some Sacramento, CA orthopedic surgeons. This resulted in Robodoc® (Integrated Surgical System, Sacramento, CA). Despite increased cost to the hospitals and possibly increased trauma to the patients, use of robot in the orthopedic systems is increasing due to better patient outcome[46]. The objective of Robodoc® system in hip surgery is to create a femoral canal for insertion of the femoral prosthesis with a high degree of accuracy in a cementless total hips replacement (THA). This will enable significantly better adhesion of the femoral implants in the proximal femur and prevent crackling, loosening and producing osteolysis[7]. The cavity created is 10 times more accurate then the one created by manual methods and hence has less chances of failure for the prosthesis. The cementless system needs a smoother surface in an accurately created canal. This allows better fitting of the prosthesis and better adhesion of the implant and the femur surfaces. In the operating room, after the initial dissection and removal of the native femoral head, the robot fixator is allowed to firmly clamp the femur. The robot then compares the data from the CT scan and the registration data from three titanium pins on the femur. This allows precision milling of the femoral canal. Surgery is then finished manually. Intraoperative movements are to be prevented as it will cause misalignment and the registration needs to be repeated. A bone motion monitor continuously monitors the relative motion between bone of the patient and the Robodoc®. The other aspects of using a robot in the procedure are decreased blood loss and increased duration of the procedure.

Robotic surgical assistance is also used to increase the accuracy of prosthetic knee replacement. It improves the jig system used to align bone sawing. The jig system uses the surgeon's visual assessment but resulted in the patello-femoral pain and limited movements in 40% of the patients[1]. Small misalignments as much as 2.5 mm can cause 20 degrees alteration in the range of motion of the prosthetic joint[35].

Anesthetic implications may include a general anesthetic with endotracheal intubation and guaranteed paralysis with an epidural catheter placement for postoperative pain control.

Neurosurgery

Neurosurgery had its share in advances and developments in robotic assist procedures. NeuroMate™ (Integrated Surgical Systems, Sacramento, CA) and Programmable Universal Machine for Assembly industrial robot PUMA™ (Advanced Research & Robotics, Oxford, CT) are two systems used. Most of the thrust is currently on precise positioning and guidance of the instruments through the neural parenchyma. NeuroMate™ was the first such machine approved by FDA. In these procedures the surgeon plans the procedure and the data in integrated with the robot. Then the robotic arm is used to perform limited task during the procedures. Fiducial markers are utilized to guide the arm which allows accurate localization. NeuRobot™ (Shinshu University School of Medicine, Matsumoto, Japan) is the first robot that performed tele controlled surgery through an endoscope[42].

Opthalmic Surgery

The true test for robotic skill was found in this area of ophthalmic surgery. The ability to manipulate distances of 10 μm in an area where the distance between blood vessels in 25 μm is the real adventure involved. RAMS™ (Robot-Assit Microsurgery System) was developed at NASA's Jet Propulsion Laboratory[45]. The current projects address important aspects of ocular surgery with novel ideas: precise intercorneal inlay insertion for treating presbyopia, computer-assisted laser photocoagulation and development of untethered MEMS robotic devices for minimally invasive retinal surgeries. The picture of these extremely tiny robotic instruments is available to be seen on the web: http://co-me.ch/projects/phase2/p08/index.en.html. Nowhere else can the tremor filtration and motion scaling of 100:1 be as useful as inside the eye. The ability to cannulate retinal vein for the treatment of retinal vein thrombosis is another fine example[5; 9; 24; 50].

Physiologic Aspects of Pediatric/Newborn Patients

Although many adults act like small children infants are not small adults. They have a different physiology from adults and even older children[17]. Below is a brief description of these differences. Oxygen consumption is 6 ml/kg in neonates as compared to the adult levels of 3 ml/kg. This leads to a higher rate of alveolar ventilation. The neonates' cardiovascular status is characterized by a functionally closed foramen ovale, possible reopening of ductus arteriosus in response to severe hypoxia, and high degree of dependence on heart rate to maintain cardiac output and blood pressure. Newborns also have a decreased ability to produce vasoconstriction in response to volume depletion. They have a higher ratio of extra cellular fluid of about 40% of total body water as compared to 20% in adults. Neonates are obligate losers of sodium and are unable to concentrate urine and paradoxically excrete volume load slower than adults. Since birth their glomerular filtration rate (GFR) is very low and has to increase four fold by the age of 3 to 5 weeks to reach adult levels. The presence of Hb F causes a leftward shift in the oxygen-hemoglobin dissociation curve. Increased hemoglobin concentration compensates the decreasing oxygen delivery by hemoglobin F. Physiologic anemia occurs at age 2 to 3 months with a hematocrit of 35. Neonates lack shivering mechanism of thermogenesis and rely on brown fat for heat production. They lose body heat more quickly due to higher body surface area. Radiation is the most important mechanism to lose body heat and is minimized by humidifying and warming inspired gases, transporting in heated modules, heating of intravenous lines and increasing the ambient temperature of the operating rooms.

Laparoscopy in Pediatrics

The physiologic effects of an artificial pneumoperitoneum depend on age and insufflation pressure. These are further exacerbated by the position of the head relative to the body, either TR or rTR positions. Like adults, respiratory physiology is affected with abdominal distention leading to decreased diaphragmatic excursion, ventilation perfusion mismatches, and potential hypoxia. Ventilation is severely affected by abdominal pressures of 15 mm of Hg or higher which leads to hypercarbia and hypoxia. Also, risks of pneumo mediastinum increase. Cerebral perfusion is decreased, especially in TR positions. The resultant decreases in FRC, TLC, and lung compliance, leads to an increase in the work of breathing. Venous return from lower extremities in TR increases, which also increases the cardiac output, while venous return from SVC decreases. This contributes to decreased cerebral perfusion pressure. TR causes cephalad movement of carina and predisposes to endobronchial intubation. Carbon dioxide insufflation leads to increase arterial CO_2 which results in a number of cardiac and pulmonary changes, including increased sympathetic tone, increased heart rate, and increased blood pressure. These changes are most pronounced at low insufflation pressures. At high insufflation pressures, the risk of reversal of left to right shunt and opening of ductus arteriosus exists. Venous return from inferior vena cava decreases, leading to decreased cardiac output. External compression on the heart from the insufflation pressure also leads to decreased cardiac compliance and ionotropy. These children may undergo significant variations in IAPs leading to variable levels in anesthetic depth.

Formation of carbon monoxide as a result of electrocautery is a risk, but its significance is not yet known. Positioning is another challenge in pediatric patients, as the risk of positional injury is proportional to duration of the procedure. There is a rare risk of injury to large vessels by the insufflating needles, which may result in CO_2 embolism or hemorrhagic shock. Postoperative respiratory function in children, especially newborns is likely to be impaired in immediate postoperative period and should be watched carefully.

Carbon dioxide excretion during CO_2 insufflation is age dependent. McHoney et al. has shown that younger children absorb carbon dioxide more than older patients[37]. The transient post desulfation increase in CO_2 is related to an increased venous return from the lower extremity after the release of abdominal pressure.

In lateral decubitus position, the dependent lung collapses relatively more secondary to more compliant chest wall along with the decreased FRC. This may lead to worsened V/Q mismatch. Heaf and Davies have shown that in contrast to adult patients, in infants ventilation is preferentially distributed to the non-dependent lungs[14; 22].

Anesthetic Implications for Robotic Surgery in Children

Robotic surgery is considered an extension of laparoscopic surgery, with added advantages. These include the ability to filter for tremors, added degrees of freedom (ability to reduplicate wrist movements inside a very small space), ability to create a virtual 3D vision, capacity to use lower insufflation pressure which results in smaller working space and less surgical stress. Endotracheal tube size, ability to ventilate at high pressures and minimal leak around the ET tube may lead to consider cuffed E.T. tubes. Reliable iv access for rapid infusion of intravenous fluids is essential for a safe outcome. Invasive monitoring needs to be individualized. Minimally invasive technique may require the infant to be placed at the center of the operating table which may translate to minimally access anesthetic (Dr.Francis Veyckemans Brussels, Belgium). Hence a plan to unmount the robotic arms after withdrawing the scopes and trocars from the body cavity, lifting the drapes and approaching the patient should be planned and rehearsed. For thoracoscopic procedures pediatric single lung ventilation techniques may be utilized[21].

SUMMARY

By the time this book publishes, there will be new indications and applications of robot assist procedures and there will be new issues to resolve. The famous chinese proverb "May you live in interesting times" certainly applies to today's technology driven and market oriented medical world. The ever growing challenge for an anesthesiologist is to set the pace and lead the way towards a safe perioperative environment and especially for pediatric anesthesiologist as they care for the most vulnerable and precious segment of patient population.

ACKNOWLEDGEMENTS

I would like to sincerely thank Drs. Christina Shanti, Michael Klien and Scott Langenberg of Children's Hospital of Michigan Detroit, MI (Maxine and Stewart Frankell Foundation Computer Assisted Robot Enhanced Surgery Program), Dr. Hans Stricker of Department of Urology at Henry Ford Hospital in Detroit, MI and Alex Cao of Department of Surgery Children's Hospital of Michigan Detroit, MI for their help and technical advice in the area of robotic surgery.

REFERENCES

1. Aglietti P, Buzzi R, Gaudenzi A. Patellofemoral functional results and complications with the posterior stabilized total condylar knee prosthesis. *Journal of Arthroplasty* 1998; 3(1): 17-25.

2. Andersson L, Lagerstrand L, Thorne A, Sollevi A, Brodin LA, Odeberg-Wernerman, S. Effect of CO(2) pneumoperitoneum on ventilation-perfusion relationships during laparoscopic cholecystectomy. *Acta Anaesthesiologica Scandinavica* 2002 May; 46(5): 552-60.

3. Andersson LE, Baath M, Thorne A, Aspelin P, Odeberg-Wernerman, S. (2005). Effect of carbon dioxide pneumoperitoneum on development of atelectasis during anesthesia, examined by spiral computed tomography. *Anesthesiology* 2005; 102(2): 293-9.

4. Ascione R, Lloyd CT, Underwood MJ, Lotto AA, Pitsis AA, Angelini GD. Inflammatory response after coronary revascularization with or without cardiopulmonary bypass. *Annals of Thoracic Surgery* 2000 Apr; 69(4): 1198-204.

5. Attariwala R, Jensen PS, Glucksberg MR. The effect of acute experimental retinal vein occlusion on cat retinal vein pressures. *Investigative Ophthalmology and Visual Science* 1997; 38(13): 2742-9.

6. Bardoczky GI, Engelman E, Levarlet M, Simon P. Ventilatory effects of pneumoperitoneum monitored with continuous spirometry. *Anaesthesia* 1993; 48(4): 309-11.

7. Bargar WL, Bauer A, Borner M. Primary and revision total hip replacement using the Robodoc system. *Clinical Orthopaedics and Related Research* 1998 Sep; (354): 82-91.

8. Barker SJ, Clarke C, Trivedi N, Hyatt J, Fynes M, Roessler P. Anesthesia for thoracoscopic laser ablation of bullous emphysema. *Anesthesiology* 1993 Jan; 78(1): 44-50.

9. Bek T, Jensen PK. Three-dimensional structure of human retinal vessels studied by vascular casting. *Acta Ophthalmologica (Copenh)* 1993 Aug; 71(4): 506-13.

10. Braimbridge MV. The history of thoracoscopic surgery. *Annals of Thoracic Surgery* 1993 Sep; 56(3): 610-4.

11. Bures E, Fusciardi J, Lanquetot H, Dhoste K, Richer JP, Lacoste L. Ventilatory effects of laparoscopic cholecystectomy. *Acta Anaesthesiologica Scandinavica* 1996 May; 40(5): 566-73.

12. Caputo M, Yeatman M, Narayan P, Marchetto G, Ascione R, Reeves BC, Angelini GD. Effect of off-pump coronary surgery with right ventricular assist device on organ function and inflammatory response: a randomized controlled trial. *Annnals of Thoracic Surgery* 2002 Dec; 74(6): 2088-95; discussion 2095-6.

13. Cunningham AJ, Dowd, N. Anesthesia for Minimally Invasive Surgery. In: Barash PG, Cullen BF, Stoelting RK, editors. *Clinical Anesthesia,* 4th Edition. Philadelphia, Pennsylvania: Lippincot Williams & Willkins.2001.

14. Davies H, Kitchman R, Gordon I, Helms P. Regional ventilation in infancy. Reversal of adult pattern. *New England Journal of Medicine*1985 Dec; 313(26): 1626-8.

15. Degueldre M, Vandromme J, Huong PT, Cadiere GB Robotically assisted laparoscopic microsurgical tubal reanastomosis: a feasibility study. *Fertility and Sterility* 2000 Nov; 74(5): 1020-3.

16. Diegeler A, Matin M, Falk V, Battellini R, Walther T, Autschbach R, Mohr FW. Coronary bypass grafting without cardiopulmonary bypass--technical considerations, clinical results, and follow-up. *Thoracic and Cardiovascular Surgeon* 1999; 47(1): 14-8.

17. Stoelting RK, Dierdorf SF. Diseases Presenting in Pediatric Patients. In: Stoelting RK, Dierdorf, editors. *Anesthesia and Coexisting Diseases*. Indianapolis, Indiana: Churchill Livingstone;2002.

18. Falcone T, Goldberg JM, Margossian H, Stevens L. Robotic-assisted laparoscopic microsurgical tubal anastomosis: a human pilot study. *Fertility and Sterility* 2000; 73(5): 1040-2.

19. Falk V, Fann JI, Grunenfelder J, Burdon TA. Endoscopic Doppler for detecting vessels in closed chest bypass grafting. *Heart Surgery Forum* 2000; 3(4): 331-3.

20. Felger JE, Nifong LW, Chitwood WR Jr. The evolution of and early experience with robot-assisted mitral valve surgery. *Surgical Laparoscopy Endoscopy & Percutaneous Techniques* 2002 Feb; 12(1): 58-63.

21. Hammer GB. Single-lung ventilation in infants and children. *Paediatric Anaesthesia* 2004 Jan; 14(1): 98-102.

22. Heaf DP, Helms P, Gordon I, Turner HM. Postural effects on gas exchange in infants. *New England Journal of Medicine* 1983 Jun; 308(25): 1505-8.

23. Hirvonen EA, Nuutinen LS, Kauko M. Ventilatory effects, blood gas changes, and oxygen consumption during laparoscopic hysterectomy. *Anesthesia and Analgesia* 1995; 80(5): 961-6.

24. Jensen PK Scherfig E. Resolution of retinal digital colour images. *Acta Ophthalmologica Scandinavica* 1999 Oct; 77(5): 526-9.

25. Jones DR, Graeber GM, Tanguilig GG, Hobbs G, Murray GF. Effects of insufflation on hemodynamics during thoracoscopy. *Annals of Thoracic Surgery* 1993 June; 55(6): 1379-82.

26. Joris, JL Anesthesia for Laproscopic Surgery. In: Miller RD, editor. *Miller's Anesthesiology*: Churchill Livingston; 2004: Chapter 57.

27. Joris JL, Chiche JD, Canivet JL, Jacquet NJ, Legros JJ, Lamy ML. Hemodynamic changes induced by laparoscopy and their endocrine correlates: effects of clonidine. *Journal of the American College of Cardiology* 1998 Nov; 32(5): 1389-96.

28. Kendall AP, Bhatt S, Oh TE. Pulmonary consequences of carbon dioxide insufflation for laparoscopic cholecystectomies. *Anaesthesia* 1995 Apr; 50(4): 286-9.

29. Loulmet D, Carpentier A, d'Attellis N, Berrebi A, Cardon C, Ponzio O, Aupecle B, Relland JY. Endoscopic coronary artery bypass grafting with the aid of robotic assisted instruments. *Journal of Thoracic and Cardiovascular Surgery* 1999 Jul; 118(1): 4-10.

30. Nathan MS, Wickham JEA. Robotic Transurethral Electrovapourization of the Prostate. *Minimally Invasive Therapy* (1995) 4, 283-287.

31. Marescaux J, Leroy J, Gagner M, Rubino F, Mutter D, Vix M, Butner SE, Smith MK. Transatlantic robot-assisted telesurgery. *Nature* 2001; 413(6854): 379-80.

32. Marescaux J, Leroy J, Rubino F, Smith,M, Vix M, Simone M, Mutter D. Transcontinental robot-assisted remote telesurgery: feasibility and potential applications. *Annals of Surgery* 2002 Apr; 235(4): 487-92.

33. Margossian H, Garcia-Ruiz A, Falcone T, Goldberg JM, Attaran M, Miller JH, Gagner M. Robotically assisted laparoscopic tubal anastomosis in a porcine model: a pilot study. *Journal of Laparoendoscopic & Advanced Surgical Techniques* 1998; 8(2): 69-73.

34. Mariano ER, Furukawa L, Woo RK, Albanese CT, Brock-Utne JG. Anesthetic concerns for robot-assisted laparoscopy in an infant. *Anesthesia and Analgesia* 2004 Dec; 99(6): 1665-7, table of contents.

35. Martelli M, Marcacci M, Nofrini L, LA Palombara F, Malvisi A, Iacono F, Vendruscolo P, Pierantoni M. Computer- and robot-assisted total knee replacement: analysis of a new surgical procedure. *Annals of Biomedical Engineering* 2000 Sep; 28(9), 1146-53.

36. Warner, MA, Martin JT. Patient Positioning. In Barash PG, Cullen BF, Stoelting RK, editors. *Clinical Anesthesia*. Philadelphia: Lippincott Williams & Wilkins; 2002; 639-55.

37. McHoney M., Corizia L, Eaton S, Kiely EM, Drake DP, Tan HL, Spitz L, Pierro A. Carbon dioxide elimination during laparoscopy in children is age dependent. *Journal of Pediatric Surgery* 2003 Jan; 38(1): 105-10; discussion 105-10.

38. Mullett CE, Viale JP, Sagnard PE, Miellet CC, Ruynat LG, Counioux HC, Motin JP, Boulez JP, Dargent DM, Annat GJ. Pulmonary CO2 elimination during surgical procedures using intra- or extraperitoneal CO2 insufflation. *Anesthesia and Analgesia* 1993 Mar; 76(3): 622-6.

39. Murkin JM, Ganapathy S. Anesthesia for robotic heart surgery: an overview. *Heart Surgery Forum* 2001; 4(4), 311-4.

40. Mutoh T, Lamm,WJ, Embree LJ, Hildebrandt J, Albert RK. Volume infusion produces abdominal distension, lung compression, and chest wall stiffening in pigs. *Journal of Applied Physiology* 1992 Feb; 72(2): 575-82.

41. Oikkonen M, Tallgren M. Changes in respiratory compliance at laparoscopy: measurements using side stream spirometry. *Canadian Journal of Anaesthesia* 1995 Jun; 42(6): 495-7.

42. McBeth PB, Louw DF, Rizun PR, Sutherland GR. Robotics in neurosurgery. *American Journal of Surgery* 2004 Oct; 188 (4A Suppl): 68S-75S.

43. Rauh R, Hemmerling TM, Rist M, Jacobi KE. Influence of pneumoperitoneum and patient positioning on respiratory system compliance. *Journal of Clinical Anesthesia* 2001 Aug; 13(5), 361-5.

44. Schiff J, Li PS, Goldstein M. Robotic microsurgical vasovasostomy and vasoepididymostomy: a prospective randomized study in a rat model. *Journal of Urology* 2004 Apr; 171(4), 1720-5.

45. Siemionow M, Ozer K, Siemionow W, Lister G. Robotic assistance in microsurgery. *Journal of Reconstructive Microsurgery* 2000 Nov; 16(8), 643-9.

46. Sparmann, M., Wolke, B. Value of navigation and robot-guided surgery in total knee arthroplasty. *Orthopade*, 32(6), 498-505.German.

47. Tan PL, Lee TL, Tweed WA. Carbon dioxide absorption and gas exchange during pelvic laparoscopy. *Canadian Journal of Anaesthesia* 1992 Sep; 39(7): 677-81.

48. Torracca L, Ismeno G, Quarti A, Alfieri O. Totally endoscopic atrial septal defect closure with a robotic system: experience with seven cases. *Heart Surgery Forum* 2002; 5(2): 125-7.

49. Vassiliades TA Jr, Rogers EW, Nielsen JL, Lonquist JL. Minimally invasive direct coronary artery bypass grafting: intermediate-term results. *Annals of Thoracic Surgery* 2000 Sep; 70(3): 1063-5.

50. Vucetic M, Jensen PK, Jansen EC. Diameter variations of retinal blood vessels during and after treatment with hyperbaric oxygen. *British Journal of Ophthalmology* 2004 Jun; 88(6): 771-5.

51. Wahba RW, Tessler MJ, Kleiman SJ. Acute ventilatory complications during laparoscopic upper abdominal surgery. *Canadian Journal of Anaesthesia* 1996 Jan; 43(1): 77-83.

52. Wittgen CM, Andrus CH, Fitzgerald SD, Baudendistel LJ, Dahms TE, Kaminski DL. Analysis of the hemodynamic and ventilatory effects of laparoscopic cholecystectomy. *Archives of Surgery* 1991 Aug; 126(8): 997-1000; discussion 1000-1.

Chapter 3

TELEMENTORING AND REMOTE TELEPRESENCE SURGERY

Mehran Anvari
McMaster Institute for Surgical Innovation, Invention and Education, Faculty of Health Sciences, McMaster University

INTRODUCTION

While telemedicine has been in practice for several decades [1], the complexity of the medical interventions that are possible has increased dramatically as telecommunications and computer technologies advance. In the field of surgery, telementoring – real-time interactive teaching of a student by an expert surgeon not at the same location [2] – now offers the potential for surgeons to safely and confidently acquire new techniques with the assistance of an experienced mentor without leaving their local hospital. With the development and commercialization of a number of remotely controlled robotic surgical devices during the later 1990's, surgeons at last gained true telepresence, allowing the visualization and manipulation of tissues and instruments at a distance from the patient. Robotic devices that have been controlled from a distance via telecommunications link include single-armed robotic devices such as the AESOP® arm for remote endoscopic manipulation [3] and PAKY, a device for positioning the needle during percutaneous renal access [4], as well as the three-armed Zeus TS telesurgery system [5,6].

Both telementoring and telepresence surgery offer the potential to enhance surgical training and education, and raise the standard of healthcare by offering improved access to expert surgeons and advanced surgical techniques. As access to modern telecommunications networks expands, these techniques may help provide access to advanced surgical care to those living in remote and traditionally under serviced regions. However, there are a number of technological and medico-legal issues that will need to be addressed in order for these technologies to reach their full potential.

HISTORY AND DEVELOPMENT OF TELEMENTORING

The concept of telementoring is not new. In fact, Dr. Michael DeBakey used a broadband satellite connection to perform real-time surgical teaching between Europe and the United States in 1965 [7]. But, widespread interest in evaluating the feasibility and safety of telementoring developed in the late 1990's, in part due to the rapid advances in telecommunications and videoconferencing technology, and due to a reduction in the time delay between the two sites, allowing for more efficient interaction.

In 1994, Kavoussi et al. [8] successfully performed three telementored surgeries in which the instructing surgeon was in an adjacent room. The remote surgeon controlled the AESOP® arm (Computer Motion, Santa Barbara, CA), which manipulated the laparoscope. In further studies at the Baltimore Medical School, 22 of 23 basic and advanced laparoscopic urologic procedures were successfully completed by a junior surgeon with mentoring from an expert surgeon located in a separate building using telecommunications systems connected via fibre-optic and copper cables. The operative times and clinical outcomes in this series were comparable to those for live instruction [3].

Rosser et al. further explored the utility of telementoring for teaching advanced laparoscopic procedures in a two-phase study that compared traditional on-site mentoring with telementoring [9]. In phase 1, 4 colon resections were performed by a novice surgeon with the mentor within the OR, and an additional 4 were performed with the mentor located in a control centre on the hospital grounds. Phase 2 involved 2 Nissen fundoplications mentored from within the OR and 2 during which the mentor was located 5 miles away and in communication with the OR via video and two-way audio over ISDN lines. The authors found no significant differences between the telementored procedures and those in which the mentor was physically present. In 1997, Schulam et al. reported the creation of a telesurgical system that allowed an experienced laparoscopic surgeon to guide a trainee with limited laparoscopic experience from a location approximately 3.5 miles away [10]. The system used a T1 line to provide two-way video, duplex audio, telestration, and control of the endoscope and electrocautery by the remote surgeon. 7 procedures, including an orchiopexy, an internal spermatic vein ligation, two pelvic node dissections, two radical nephrectomies, and a renal biopsy were all completed without complications. The success of these early investigations led to studies of telementoring over substantially longer distances. Early reports of transcontinental telementoring include performance of an adrenalectomy between the United States and Austria [11] and a series of 5 laparoscopic inguinal herniorrhaphies completed on board a US aircraft carrier by the ship surgeon under the guidance of an experienced laparoscopic surgeon at a land-based location in the U.S. [12]. The surgeons were linked via the Battle Group Telemedicine System (BGTM), which provided real-time audio and visual connection via ship to ship and ship to shore communications. Since this time, numerous groups have reported the successful use of telementoring for education and surgical assistance in a wide range of procedures and over substantial distances. Telestration devices, which allow the expert surgeon to make annotations over live video, have frequently been used to enhance the telementoring experience [3,9]. In addition, several studies have reported on remote control of other devices by the expert surgeon, including a robotic arm that guides needle placement for percutaneous renal access [13].

TELEMENTORING IN REMOTE AND RURAL AREAS

One of the most promising applications of telementoring is the potential for expert surgeons to share their knowledge with surgeons in rural and remote areas where access to advanced laparoscopic procedures is not currently available. While the benefits of laparoscopic surgery are well demonstrated, there is a substantial learning curve for these procedures, and the skills required cannot be mastered in a classroom setting. See et al. conducted a survey of surgeons who had completed a laparoscopic training course and reported that surgeons who performed laparoscopic procedures without further training had higher complication rates than those who pursued additional training [14]. While completing a preceptorship with an experienced laparoscopic surgeon is strongly recommended [15], traveling to a distant tertiary care facility is simply not a feasible option for most surgeons practicing in rural or remote areas. However, telementoring offers the possibility for a novice surgeon to safely gain experience in new techniques through real-time instruction from an expert surgeon in a distant locale.

In 1999, Rosser et al. demonstrated the use of telementoring in a remote region in Ecuador [16]. A laparoscopic cholecystectomy was performed by a surgical resident in a mobile surgical unit with guidance from an expert surgeon in the U.S. Plain old telephone service (POTS) provided the telecommunication link for this procedure, necessitating slow movements and minimal camera motion in order to compensate for the low bandwidth.

In Canada, telementoring was put into routine clinical use in 2002, providing surgeons in two rural communities with access to real-time guidance from a distant laparoscopic surgeon [. 1]. An expert surgeon from the Centre for Minimal Access Surgery (CMAS), located at St. Joseph's Healthcare in Hamilton, Ontario has guided community surgeons with minimal experience in laparoscopic surgery during the performance of a variety of advanced laparoscopic procedures. In a series of 19 telementored procedures, including 10 colon resections, 5 Nissen fundoplications, 2 splenectomies, 1 reversal of Hartmann's and 1 hernia repair, 2 anterior resections were converted to open when the mentee was unable to locate the correct plane of mesorectal dissection [17]. There were no intraoperative complications and 2 post-operative complications (11%), including a hemoperitoneum requiring laparotomy and a small bowel obstruction requiring reoperation.

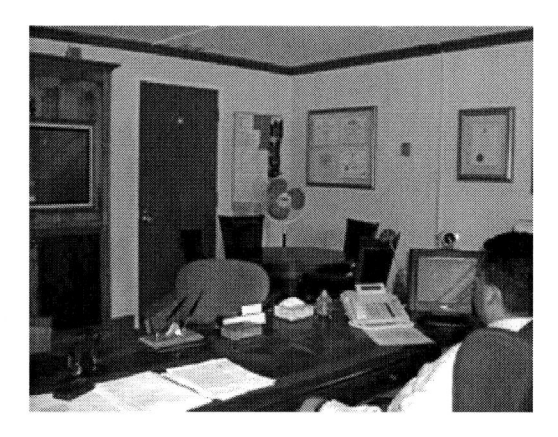

Fig 1: Telementoring between Hamilton and North Bay. The video display in the mentor's office can be split to show both the operative field and a view of the OR

Two different telecommunications networks were used to link the two facilities, providing two-way audio and visual connections. The first network was a combination of ISDN (Integrated Services Digital Network) and IP (Internet Protocol), and the second was a dedicated IP connection with surgical grade virtual private network (IP/VPN). This second configuration provided a significantly higher bandwidth and lower latency, resulting in better quality video images and reduced background noise. Evaluations completed following each telementoring session showed that the mentor was consistently satisfied with the quality of the surgery and that the mentees felt that the virtual presence of an experienced surgeon was most beneficial. As a result of this program, the mentored surgeons have succeeded in adopting advanced laparoscopic techniques with clinical outcomes comparable to those of tertiary care centres [17]. Due to the success of this program, the Centre for Minimal Access Surgery plans to expand this telementoring network to include over 30 rural communities within the next few years.

Enabling community surgeons to safely offer advanced laparoscopic techniques will provide patients in rural areas with access to the latest in surgical care without the need to leave their communities and the support of family and friends. Furthermore, such programs may aid in the recruitment and retention of community surgeons by offering them opportunities for continuing education and access to the expertise of mentors that are currently only available to those who practice in major urban centres.

TELEMENTORING IN EXTREME ENVIRONMENTS – THE NEEMO 7 MISSION

The development of telemedicine is very closely linked to the growth of the space program and the resulting need to monitor and maintain the health of astronauts. Research by NASA and the Soviet Union space program fueled the development of much of the technology behind modern telemedicine programs. The United States military has also had a keen interest in the development of telemedicine and telepresence surgery applications in order to provide emergency medical treatment to soldiers on the battlefield or in other locations inaccessible to medical specialists.

In October 2003, surgeons from the Centre for Minimal Access Surgery (CMAS) collaborated with NASA, the Canadian Space Agency and TATRC, the telemedicine research division of the U.S. military, to investigate the ability of telementoring to enable non-surgeons to deliver emergency medical and surgical care to patients in extreme environments. The NEEMO 7 mission took place off the coast of Florida aboard Aquarius, an underwater habitat operated by the University of North Carolina at Wilmington for the National Oceanographic and Atmospheric Administration (NOAA). The Aquarius habitat provides an excellent simulation of the confined quarters and extreme environment encountered in space and has been used by NASA for a number of previous space analogue research missions.

During the NEEMO 7 mission, expert surgeons from CMAS successfully used telementoring to guide non-surgeon Aquarius aquanauts through simulations of diagnostic and surgical procedures. Real-time videoconferencing provided two-way audio and video between the telerobotic room at St. Joseph's Healthcare and the Aquarius habitat. The telecommunications link was via Internet Protocol (IP) connection with virtual private network (VPN) technology as well as broadband microwave technology. Using this system, expert surgeons and radiologists were able to guide non-surgeon aquanauts through a range of simulated procedures selected to represent typical medical emergencies that might be encountered on a space mission. The procedures, performed on artificial cadavers, included laparoscopic cholecystectomy, arterial anastomosis, cystoscopy and removal of a kidney stone, and ultrasound-guided percutaneous drainage of a cyst. Aquanauts were also guided through an ultrasound examination on a fellow crewmember. While some of the Aquarius crewmembers participating in these experiments had a non-surgical medical background, others were astronauts or aquanauts with no prior medical training. Regardless of background, all crewmembers were able to successfully complete each of the procedures with real-time instruction from the expert mentors.

The NEEMO 7 mission showed that telementoring is an incredibly powerful tool in knowledge translation, and has demonstrated the potential for expert surgeons to use telementoring to guide even non-medical personnel through the steps of life saving emergency medical care in an extreme environment where there is no access to a trained surgeon. Development of this technology could bring life-saving emergency medical care not only to astronauts in space and soldiers on the battlefield, but also to people living in remote or isolated areas here on earth as well.

REMOTE TELEPRESENCE SURGERY

Despite showing great potential in the areas of surgical education and dissemination of new techniques, telementoring has major limitations as well. First and foremost, since the mentoring surgeon does not have true telepresence, it is not possible to either take over or even offer physical assistance to the novice surgeon if complications arise. However, remote telepresence surgery has the potential to overcome this weakness by allowing the distant surgeon to assist or even perform an entire procedure as necessary.

Virtually all current uses of the multi-armed surgical robotic systems developed to date involve control from a surgical console located near the patient. While the potential has theoretically existed to control such master-slave systems over greater distances using telecommunications links, in the past it was widely believed that time delay issues would severely limit their use in remote applications [18]. However, recent developments in telecommunications have led to the emergence of high bandwith, low latency networks that can transfer the large amounts of data necessary required for remote telepresence surgery.

On September 7, 2001 Dr. Jacques Marescaux performed the first true remote telepresence surgical procedure - a laparoscopic cholecystectomy performed on a woman in Strasbourg, France from a surgical console located in New York [5]. This groundbreaking procedure was performed using the Zeus TS robotic system (Computer Motion, CA) and a private dedicated ATM (asynchronous transfer mode) fibre-optic network. The surgery was completed without any complications or technical difficulties in 54 minutes, demonstrating for the first time the feasibility of remote telepresence surgery.

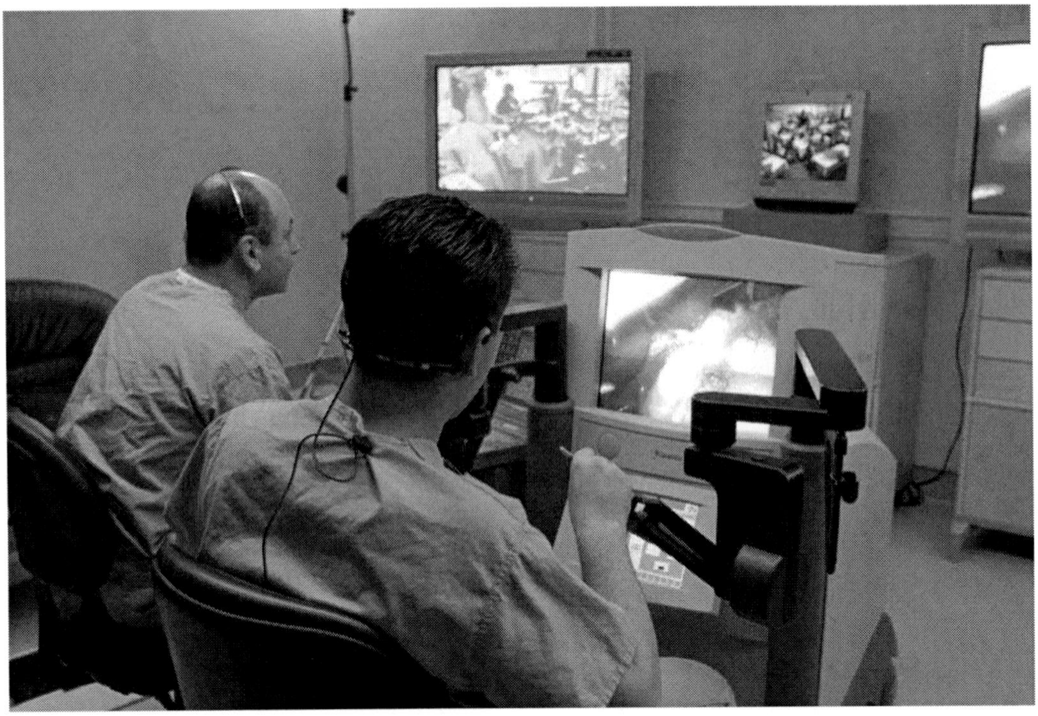

Fig 2a: Operative console in the telerobotic room at St. Joseph's Healthcare in Hamilton

CANADA'S REMOTE TELESURGICAL SERVICE

In February 2002, the world's first remote telesurgical service was established at the Centre for Minimal Access Surgery [6]. The program was developed to enhance the Centre's pre-existing telementoring program, thus enabling community surgeons to offer advanced laparoscopic procedures to patients in a rural community. The service linked a teaching hospital (St. Joseph's Healthcare, Hamilton, Ontario) with a community hospital (North Bay District Hospital) located over 400 km away. The service utilized the Zeus TS microjoint system, consisting of three robotic arms, which were placed by the local surgeon and controlled by the remote surgeon from a console located in the telerobotic room at St. Joseph's Healthcare. Two-way audio and large video displays showing both the operative field and views of the OR allowed remote surgeon to become immersed in the operative setting. The telecommunication link used was a virtual private network (VPN), which utilizes a public telecommunication infrastructure to connect regional hospitals with those in major urban centres. The network operated at a bandwidth of 15 Mbps, and provided the security, redundancy and Quality of Service required for telesurgical applications. Figure 2 shows views of the telerobotic room at St. Joseph's Healthcare and the OR in North Bay during a telerobotic procedure.

Using this system, a series of 22 remote procedures have taken place with no major complications, no conversions to open procedures, and clinical outcomes comparable to those of procedures performed at a tertiary care centre [6]. Procedures performed include

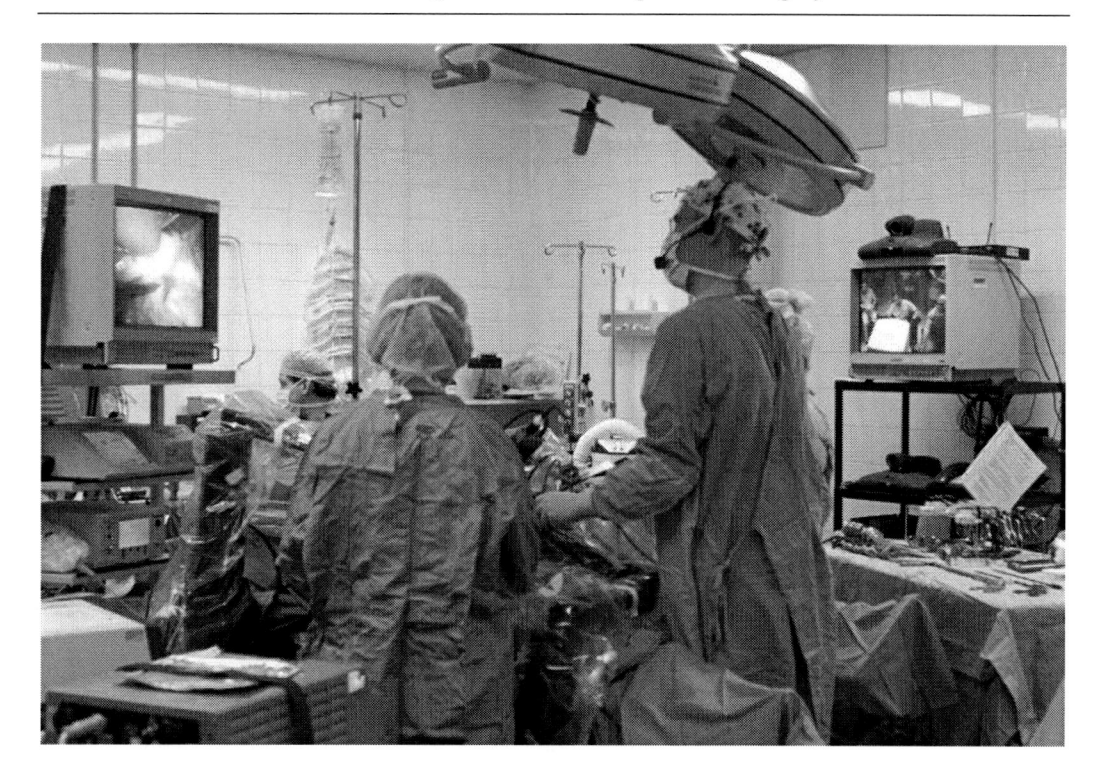

Fig 2b: The OR in North Bay during a remote telesurgical procedure

laparoscopic colon resections, Nissen fundoplications, and inguinal hernia repairs. The configuration of the robotic arms allowed either the remote or the local surgeon to perform all aspects of the procedures and to switch roles seamlessly. This allowed the expert surgeon at the remote site to act as the primary surgeon for some cases and as the first assistant for others, providing guidance and demonstrating correct planes of dissection to the local surgeon, who had minimal previous experience with laparoscopic techniques.

This initial experience has demonstrated that remote telepresence surgery can be safely and effectively used to provide advanced laparoscopic procedures in a rural hospital, and can enable community surgeons to safely acquire new skills without taking time away from their practices to work with a preceptor at a distant teaching hospital.

LIMITATIONS OF TELEMENTORING AND TELEPRESENCE SURGERY

Despite their potential to disseminate surgical knowledge and improve the quality of care for patients in rural or remote areas, telementoring and remote telepresence surgery face a number of barriers to widespread use. These include both medico-legal issues, which are discussed in another chapter, as well as a number of technical challenges [19-21].

One of the major limitations of telementoring is the inability of the mentoring surgeon to offer physical assistance to the novice surgeon, or to take over the procedure if complications arise. Consequently, the novice surgeon must always have the technical ability and the required support staff present to convert to an open procedure if necessary. Although remote telepresence surgery does permit the mentoring surgeon to either demonstrate specific aspects of a procedure or assume the role of primary surgeon, a number of safety concerns still remain. While the availability of a redundant second communication line minimizes the chance of a telecommunication failure, the potential still exists for failure of the telemanipulation system or some other technical component. In the event of an equipment failure or intraoperative complication such as bleeding or cardiac arrest, the local surgeon must be capable of taking the required action and completing the procedure, converting to open if required.

Telesurgical applications require rapid and secure transmission of large quantities of data, including audio, video, and robotic control signals. Both telementoring and remote telepresence surgery rely on high quality video images, necessitating high bandwidth connections for optimal performance. Network latency is also an important consideration. While some data suggests that surgeons may be able to adapt to latencies of 500 ms or greater [22,23], increasing latencies require a conscious effort by the remote surgeon to slow all movements, thus increasing stress and fatigue levels. The majority of the latency in current networks is a result of the need for compression and decompression of video signals using CODEC devices. Development of new compression/decompression technology designed specifically to address the requirements of telesurgery would reduce latency and significantly improve system performance.

ISDN, ATM and IP networks have become increasingly affordable and consequently increasingly available. However, there are still many remote regions and areas in the developing world in which reliable land-based telecommunications still do not exist. Thus, telepresence surgery is not currently feasible in regions that are most urgently in need of such services. While satellite technology can be used for other telemedicine applications, the latency of current systems (in excess of 1 second) makes them unsuitable for telepresence surgery.

Initial experiences with remote telepresence surgery have also demonstrated the need for new and innovative robotic surgical platforms. Of the two multi-armed robotic surgical systems to receive approval for clinical use (the Zeus and Da Vinci systems), only the Zeus system was designed to allow control via a telecommunications link. However, following the acquisition of Computer Motion by Intuitive Surgical, manufacturer of the Da Vinci system, the Zeus system is no longer commercially available. Furthermore, current systems are expensive, bulky, time consuming to set up and not designed to interact effectively with human operators. The next generation of robotic surgical devices will need to be portable, compact, flexible for use in varying procedures, and will need to interact more effectively with both surgical staff and other devices in the OR. Another critical feature that must be integrated into future systems is haptic feedback. Providing remote surgeons with tactic sensation and force feedback would reduce the remote surgeon's reliance on visual cues, thus increasing ease of use and decreasing operator fatigue.

CONCLUSION

The information age, together with the advent of laparoscopic techniques, has connected the once-isolated OR to the outside world. Advances in telecommunications have enabled real-time collaboration between surgeons in distant locales, and the development of surgical devices that can be remotely manipulated has allowed a distant surgeon to gain true telepresence. Investigations to date have shown that telementoring and telepresence surgery are safe and technically feasible when performed by an expert surgeon. Future developments in telecommunication and robotic technology, together with the development of much-needed guidelines and policies will enable telementoring and telepresence surgery to significantly improve surgical education and health care delivery around the world.

REFERENCES

1. DeBakey ME. Telemedicine has now come of age. *Telemedicine Journal* 1995; 1(1):3-4.

2. Board of Governors of Society of American Gastrointestinal Endoscopic Surgeons. Guidelines for the surgical practice of telemedicine. *Surgical Endoscopy* 1997; 11(7): 789-92.

3. Moore RG, Adams JB, Partin AW, Docimo SG, Kavoussi LR. Telementoring of laparoscopic procedures: initial clinical experience. *Surgical Endoscopy* 1996; 10(2): 107-10.

4. Micali S, Virgili G, Vannozzi E, Grassi N, Jarrett TW, Bauer JJ, Vespasiani G, Kavoussi LR. Feasibility of telementoring between Baltimore (USA) and Rome (Italy): the first five cases. *Journal of Endourology* 2000; 14(6): 493-6.

5. Marescaux J, Leroy J, Gagner M, Rubino F, Mutter D, Vix M, Butner SE, Smith MK. Transatlantic robot-assisted telesurgery. *Nature* 2001 Sep 27; 413(6854): 379-80.

6. Anvari M, McKinley C, Stein H. Establishment of the world's first telerobotic remote surgical service: for provision of advanced laparoscopic surgery in a rural community. *Annals of Surgery* 2005; 241(3):460-4.

7. Allen D, Bowersox J, Jones GG. Telesurgery. Telepresence. Telementoring. Telerobotics. *Telemedicine Today* 1997; 5(3):18-20, 25.

8. Kavoussi LR, Moore RG, Partin AW, Bender JS, Zenilman ME, Satava RM. Telerobotic assisted laparoscopic surgery: initial laboratory and clinical experience. *Urology* 1994 Jul; 44(1): 15-9.

9. Rosser JC, Wood M, Payne JH, Fullum TM, Lisehora GB, Rosser LE, Barcia PJ, Savalgi RS. Telementoring. A practical option in surgical training. *Surgical Endoscopy* 1997; 11(8): 852-5.

10. Schulam PG, Docimo SG, Saleh W, Breitenbach C, Moore RG, Kavoussi L. Telesurgical mentoring. Initial clinical experience. *Surgical Endoscopy* 1997 Oct; 11(10): 1001-5.

11. Janetschek G, Bartsch G, Kavoussi LR. Transcontinental interactive laparoscopic telesurgery between the United States and Europe. *Journal of Urology* 1998 Oct; 160(4): 1413.

12. Cubano M, Poulose BK, Talamini MA, Stewart R, Antosek LE, Lentz R, Nibe R, Kutka MF, Mendoza-Sagaon M. Long distance telementoring. A novel tool for laparoscopy aboard the USS Abraham Lincoln. *Surgical Endoscopy* 1999 Jul; 13(7): 673-8.

13. Bove P, Stoianovici D, Micali S, Patriciu A, Grassi N, Jarrett TW, Vespasiani G, Kavoussi LR. Is telesurgery a new reality? Our experience with laparoscopic and percutaneous procedures. *Journal of Endourology* 2003 Apr; 17(3): 137-42.

14. See WA, Cooper CS, Fisher RJ. Predictors of laparoscopic complications after formal training in laparoscopic surgery. *JAMA: Journal of the American Medical Association.* 1993 Dec 8; 270(22): 2689-92.

15. Society of American Gastrointestinal Endoscopic Surgeons. Framework for post-residency surgical education and training. *Surgical Endoscopy* 1994; 8(9): 1137-42.

16. Rosser JC Jr, Bell RL, Harnett B, Rodas E, Murayama M, Merrell R. Use of mobile low-bandwith telemedical techniques for extreme telemedicine applications. *Journal of the American College of Surgeons* 1999 Oct; 189(4): 397-404.

17. Sebajang H, Trudeau P, Dougall A, Hegge S, McKinley C, Anvari M. Telementoring: An important enabling tool for the community surgeon. *Surgical Endoscopy* 2004; 18 Suppl.: S284.

18. Mack MJ. Minimally invasive and robotic surgery. *JAMA: Journal of the American Medical Association* 2001 Feb 7; 285(5): 568-72.

19. Eadie LH, Seifalian AM, Davidson BR. Telemedicine in Surgery. *British Journal of Surgery* 2003; 90(6): 647-58.

20. Link R, Schulam P, Kavoussi L. Telesurgery: Remote monitoring and assistance during laparoscopy. *Urology Clinics of North America* 2001; 28(1): 177-88.

21. Ballantyne G.H. Robotic surgery, telerobotic surgery, telepresence and telementoring. Review of early clinical results. *Surgical Endsocopy* 2002 Oct; 16(10): 1389-1402.

22. Fabrizio MD, Lee BR, Chan DY, Stoianovici D, Jarrett TW, Yang C, Kavoussi LR. Effect of time delay on surgical performance during telesurgical manipulation. *Journal of Endourology* 2000 Mar; 14(2): 133-8.

23. Anvari M, Broderick T, Stein H, Chapman T, Ghodoussi J, Birch DW, McKinley C, Trudeau P, Dutta S, Goldsmith CH. The impact of latency on surgical precision and

task completion during robotic assisted remote telepresence surgery. *Computer Aided Surgery* 2005 Mar; 10(2): 93-9.

In: Robotics in Surgery: History, Current and Future Applications ISBN 1-60021-386-3
Editor: Russell A. Faust, pp. 47-57 © 2007 Nova Science Publishers, Inc.

Chapter 4

LEGAL PERSPECTIVES ON TELEMEDICINE AND TELEROBOTIC SURGERY

Raymund C. King
Kings Park Business Center
Plano, TX, USA

Abstract

Advances in telemedicine and telerobotic surgery have compelled us to redefine and confront many new legal issues such as those involving the Food and Drug Administration, physician licensing, the physician patient relationship, medical negligence, the standard of care, medical liability, jurisdictional concerns, patient confidentiality, privacy, security, informed consent, physician competence, physician advertising, telementoring, and continuing medical education (CME). Indeed, the interface between telemedicine, telerobotic surgery and the law will always result in the genesis of challenging new legal frontiers. Existing laws may need to be reinterpreted, modified, or changed in order to accommodate the ever-expanding boundaries of our scientific knowledge. Along this journey, man must continue to discover ways to overcome the medical, ethical, and legal hurdles that confront him.

INTRODUCTION

Legal issues associated with health care become more complex as healthcare technology advances. To understand the legal context of the issues inherent in telemedicine and telerobotics, it is important to articulate basic principles and definitions. Telemedicine is specifically defined as the application of telecommunications to the care of the individual.[1] The terms "telemedicine" and "telehealth" have generally come to mean the convergence of the technology of the telecommunications industry with the health care professions. At its core, telemedicine is the electronic transfer of health care information from one site to another.[2]

Teleoperation means "doing work at a distance." In the context of this chapter, "work" encompasses a broad range of telehealth services ranging from basic visual examination to surgery. "Distance" can refer to a physical distance, where the operator is separated from the robot by a large distance, but it can also refer to a change in scale, where a surgeon, for example, may use micro-manipulator technology to perform microsurgery. Devices designed to allow an operator to control a robot at a distance are sometimes called telecheric robotics.

R.C. Geortz developed the first teleoperator, or telecheric, a device that allows an operator to perform a task at a distance, isolated from the environment that the task is performed in.[3] The telecheric was designed to manipulate radioactive materials. The operator was separated from the radioactive task by a concrete wall with viewing ports. Two handles on the "master" side allowed the operator to manipulate a pair of tongs on the "slave" side. Tongs and handles were coupled by multi-degree of freedom mechanisms allowing the operator the ability to manipulate the tongs with dexterity.

The Robotics Institute of America defines a robot as "a reprogrammable multifunctional manipulator designed to move material, parts, or tools or specialized devices through variable programmed motions for the performance of a variety of tasks." Interestingly, the term "robot" originates from the Czech word "robotnik," which means worker or serf. It was first introduced in a play by playwright Carl Kapek in 1920, then became popularized in the late 1940's and early 1950's by Isaac Asimov in science fiction novels, followed by Hollywood productions.

Telemedicine can probably trace its historic roots back to the Civil War when Union Army physicians telegraphed for medical supplies. Many also believe the term "telemedicine" was introduced at least half a century ago when the Bureau of Indian Affairs used telephone and video programs to train paramedics on the reservations. Today, Telemedicine includes all aspects of practicing medicine at a distance, including but not limited to: Diagnoses (including remote monitoring), Treatment (including telesurgery), Physician education, Patient education, medical administration, video conferencing between healthcare providers, telementoring, and continuing medical education.

Probably nothing has contributed to the advances in telemedicine more than digital imaging. Digital photographs work with light sensitivity just like standard film captured on a chip instead of on film and the digital image can capture millions of colors and multiple shades of gray. When digital imaging is coupled with image enhancement, the electronic image produced can be clearer and sharper than what the on-site observer can see with the naked eye. In addition, the development of fiberoptic transmission and data compression techniques has aided the speed of transmission and helped prevent contamination of the signals. Virtual reality techniques have added the possibility of a three-dimensional image evaluation, and satellite transmissions have added an international, intercontinental, and even an interplanetary scope to telemedicine.[4]

With the many advances in telemedicine and telerobotics, perhaps the most significant challenge before us is the application of laws and/or legal principles to modern situations that may not even have been contemplated when the laws were enacted.

THE FOOD AND DRUG ADMINISTRATION

The Food and Drug Administration (FDA) was given the authority to regulate medical devices in 1976 under the Medical Device Amendments of 1976.[5] The Safe Medical Device Act of 1990 built upon the 1976 foundation and created an extensive FDA regulatory scheme to ensure the safety of medical devices. The scheme is cumbersome, and one requires registration, premarketing notification, inspection of the manufacturing facility, warnings to purchasers, and reporting of adverse events for all devices and premarket approval of all new devices.

Premarket approval is a lengthy process requiring proof of the safety and efficacy of the device. Section 321(h) of the Food, Drug, and Cosmetics Act defines a medical device very broadly. In fact, 21 U.S.C. §321(h) defines a medical device as: an instrument, apparatus, implement, machine, contrivance, implant, in vitro reagent, or other similar or related article including any component part or accessory, which is (1) recognized in the official National Formulary, or in the United States Pharmacopeia, or any supplement to them, (2) intended for use in the diagnosis of disease or other conditions, or in the cure, mitigation, treatment or prevention of disease in man or other animals, or (3) intended to affect the structure or function of the body of man or other animals, and which does not achieve its primary intended purpose through chemical actions within or on the body of man or other animals and (4) which is not dependent upon being metabolized for the achievement of its primary intended purpose. Only one of the three elements must be met to classify the object as a medical device. Undoubtedly, the FDA will likely assume a regulatory role in telemedicine in the future.

The FDA has also shown great interest in teleradiology and is already regulating the hardware of teleradiology systems and the software connected with medical imaging systems.[6] Currently, FDA regulation influences whether a device is promoted as a medical device or not. Equipment marketed for general communication purposes has escaped FDA attention. The FDA's approach has been thoughtful and helpful. However, if the FDA acts as most administrative regulatory agencies are so inclined, it will gradually extend its authority over all aspects of telemedicine. If the FDA tries to regulate telemedicine systems as a whole, it could potentially impede the development and use of telemedicine. Theoretically, the FDA approval system could wreak havoc on upgrading systems, as well as discouraging manufacturers of communications hardware and software from entering the telemedicine field. One can envision the rapidly evolving telemedicine technology suddenly brought to the glacial pace that only an administrative agency may invoke. Only time will tell.

LICENSING

In the United States, the current law is generally that "each state has plenary power to regulate the practice of medicine."[7] Technology outpaces the law at every turn. This is particularly true with telemedicine and medical licensing. Medical license requirements vary in different states. Unlike law, the practice of medicine should not be substantially different in every state. Even though all states now require the United States Medical Licensing Exam (USMLE) as a national standard for medical competence, state medical boards are holding tight to licensing powers.

In its 1996 meeting, the American Medical Association rejected a proposal for an interstate license. This adherence to tradition and a reluctance to relinquish power is making the practice of telemedicine difficult. Furthermore, state medical licensure is tightly linked with payment. Some insurance companies will only pay a physician if he or she is licensed to practice in the state where treatment occurs. The legitimate fear of state medical boards and insurance companies is that telemedicine physicians are not aware of local resources. This could lead to poor utilization of existing resources and overestimating others.

The most conservative step proposed allows state medical boards to keep their licensing power and requirements. The proposal merely asks that states consider expedited reciprocity agreements with other states that do not have less stringent licensing requirements than the home state. In contrast, some propose national licensure, which is prompted by the growing feeling of a "national standard of care." The main advantage of this method would be to reduce the bureaucracy involved with duplicating forms associated with seeking multi-state licensure. It may also resolve the inconsistencies in state telemedicine law and the burden of insuring compliance with these different systems. Alternatively, some propose a national license just for practicing telemedicine. Regular face-to-face medicine would require a standard medical license.

Interstate licensure is a compromise between full licensure rights within a state and a national license. An interstate license would be a special license for practicing telemedicine across state lines. This type of license would be a limited license that would allow state medical boards to retain their power over full state licensure, but would protect telemedicine physicians from being labeled as "unlicensed physicians."

State licensing laws are highly individual and set up a barrier to the practice of telemedicine across state lines. Each state has the right to license physicians to practice medicine as part of the state's police power to protect the health and safety of its citizens. This police power is granted to the states by the U.S. Constitution.[8] Two U.S. Supreme Court cases also endow this power to the states.[9,10] Therefore, there is a presumption that the state will find anyone examining, diagnosing, or treating a state resident practicing medicine within that state. The Federation of State Medical Boards (FSMB) has maintained the necessity of individual state licensure in its Model Act to Regulate the Practice of Medicine by Other Means Across State Lines.[11]

THE PHYSICIAN PATIENT RELATIONSHIP

Traditionally, the physician-patient relationship has been considered a contractual relationship. The contract is implied by the actions of the parties in seeking and providing advice and care.[12,13] Unless the physician has made any specific warranties, he or she is deemed to have promised that professionally acceptable care will be provided — with no guarantee. Courts will not infer that a physician has guaranteed treatment success. The fact that a patient does not pay for services does not affect the existence of the contract or lessen the physician's duties, responsibilities, obligations, or liabilities.

In the absence of a physician-patient relationship or some other special relationship, physicians are not legally compelled to treat strangers, even during an emergency, in almost all jurisdictions.[14] Whenever an individual seeks the services of a physician for the purposes of medical or surgical treatment, that person becomes a patient, and the traditional physician-patient relationship forms. A contract is implied by the mutuality of the relationship. The physician is not an employee of the patient, and the patient has consciously sought out a physician who as agreed affirmatively to provide care. The mutuality of the relationship is independent of who solicits the relationship or who pays for the services provided.[15] The physician who discusses a patient with the treating physician does not ordinarily establish a physician-patient relationship with that patient.[16]

In the traditional medical malpractice case, the plaintiff must establish the existence of a physician-patient relationship. Telemedicine provides a challenge to this traditional model, however: it is difficult to define exactly when and where the physician-patient relationship begins. It is possible to compare the establishment of a telemedical physician-patient relationship with the establishment of a physician-patient relationship via telephone.

A number of factors must be present to form a physician-patient relationship based on telephone contact: the physician must agree, directly or indirectly, to see or counsel the patient.[17] The content of the interaction must include some evaluation by the physician as to the patient's complaint.[18] Finally, the patient must rely on the physician's determination.[19] Applying these principles to telemedicine, it seems likely that when a physician enters into a dialogue with a patient using the Internet or email, complies with a patient's request for evaluation and proffers medical advice that the patient then relies on, a provider-patient relationship is formed.

NEGLIGENCE AND THE STANDARD OF CARE

For a person to be professionally liable to another, four conditions must be met: 1) the plaintiff (or individual claiming compensation for malpractice) must show that the professional owed a duty of care to that person; 2) the duty was not met (i.e., an accepted standard of care was not breached); 3) the breach of duty resulted in the damages or injury (i.e., causation); and 4) Injury to the plaintiff (i.e., damages). Commonly, duties arise from hospital-patient relationships, which impose duties upon the physician. Whenever a physician becomes entangled in a medical malpractice lawsuit involving the hospital-patient relationship, it is usually because of the special relationship between the hospital and the physician.

At the time of this writing, no cases of telemedical malpractice have been reported, but the potential nevertheless exists. The standard of care for medical encounters and that which constitutes a physician-patient relationship has yet to be determined by the courts. The medical community has been highly critical of the prescription of medications over the Internet after only a patient questionnaire has been completed. In response to this practice, the American Medical Association (AMA) has taken the position that whereas the practice of online medicine is not illegal per se, it is considered unethical and not "good medicine" when physicians prescribe medications to a person they have not personally examined.

Though the practice of Internet medicine represents just one extreme aspect of the field of telemedicine, the medical community remains skeptical that any computer-based examination, even with the assistance of audio and video real-time interactions, is suitable for making medical decisions. This skepticism is partly due to the fear of malpractice claims based on the negligence of the physician practicing telemedicine or the failure of the technology used by the physician.

Once the existence of a physician-patient relationship is established, the patient-plaintiff in a malpractice suit must prove that the physician breached the standard of care. The duty of care a physician owes to his patient turns on situational criteria which courts analyze case-by-case. For example, in Greenberg v. Perkins, 845 P.2d 530 (Colo. 1993), the court held that even if a traditional doctor-patient relationship is not present, a physician who examines a non-patient still has a duty to not cause harm to the person being examined. The duty of care turns on "fairness under contemporary standards - that is, would reasonable persons recognize and agree that a duty of care exists." The *Greenberg* case illustrates the tendency of courts to examine the surrounding circumstances in deciding the duty of care definition. Whereas the duty of care determines the court's interpretation of surrounding circumstances, two contradicting schools of thought are foreseeable regarding courts' treatment of the duty of care in relation to telemedicine.

Some authors believe the duty of care would be greater for physicians practicing telemedicine than for doctors limiting their practice to traditional methods. Courts could reach this conclusion by determining that telemedicine providers assume the risk of possible misdiagnosis by relying on information provided by their patients. In addition, the decision to conduct medicine over the Internet is left to the doctor's discretion. Thus, courts could reason that telemedicine providers need to proceed with a level of skill and care necessary to obtain the information needed to accurately treat the patient. Failure to do so may be viewed by courts as a breach of the physician's professional duty of care.

On the other hand, the courts may also conclude that the duty of care telemedicine providers owe their patients is *less* than the duty of care for traditional doctors. This view could be adopted by courts placing the assumption of risk with the patients rather than the telemedicine providers. When a patient seeks telemedical treatment, it could be argued that patients are necessarily assuming the risk of misdiagnosis or mistreatment since they are choosing not to be physically examined. In the same way, courts may also be hesitant to find a telemedicine provider liable in a situation where a patient misrepresented his ailments or neglected to seek follow-up care.

Many telemedicine and telelaw websites issue disclaimers as to the liability of the physicians and lawyers who are giving advice on those sites. It has yet to be determined whether those disclaimers would be given any weight in a malpractice claim.

LIABILITY

Liability for practicing telemedicine can be divided into three basic categories: low level liability for information dissemination and patient education via electronic devices, moderate level liability for the practice of consultation and communication of medical advice over electronic mediums, and high level liability for the actual practice of medicine, diagnosis, and treatment of patients on the Internet. Generally, as the level of involvement between patient and physician increases, so does the likelihood that a court would find that the physician owes the patient the duty of care.

The technology utilized by telemedicine also poses a malpractice risk for telemedicine practitioners. When a physician fails to use a piece of equipment in a reasonable and diligent manner, he will be liable for the harm caused to the patient, even if the hospital or health care facility owns the equipment. In Mahfouz v. Xanar, Inc., 646 So. 2d 1152 (La. Ct. App. 1994), for example, while a dermatologic surgeon used a laser to remove a lesion, the patient suffered a burn. The court held that although the physician had no duty to inspect the equipment prior to the surgery, he did have a duty to stop the surgery on experiencing technical difficulties and to ascertain the problem and correct it if possible. Because telemedicine is so dependent on technology, telemedicine practitioners run the risk of being held liable for malpractice if that technology fails. Moreover, the liability for technology failures is apt to be shared among all involved parties, including the manufacturer of the technology.

Theories of direct and vicarious liability would likely still apply to the practice of telemedicine. For example, small rural hospitals with telemedicine capacity currently staff their emergency departments with physician extenders (e.g., advanced nurse practitioners, physician assistants or specially trained registered nurses) rather than emergency physicians. The physician extender performs an initial evaluation of the patient and faxes the evaluation and any diagnostic test results to the telemedicine emergency physician. The patient, physician extender and emergency physician then engage in a two-way, interactive videoconferencing. The physician and physician extender discuss the diagnosis with the patient, prescribe treatment and discharge the patient. If one link in this chain were to fail, it is conceivable that all of the parties would be subject to a malpractice suit, including both the rural hospital that employs the physician extenders and the distant hospital that employs the emergency physician.

JURISDICTION

Another issue related to telemedical malpractice involves the applicable jurisdiction in which a lawsuit should be filed. The practice of medicine includes at a minimum any attempt to diagnose or treat a person for any illness. Under this definition, telemedical treatment might be considered to take place at the patient's location. In *Wright v. Yackley*, 459 F.2d 287 (9th Cir. 1972), for example, a malpractice action involving an Idaho patient and a South Dakota doctor resulted in a ruling that proper jurisdiction lay in South Dakota because all diagnoses and prescriptions were made in that state.

The patient, a former South Dakota resident, could not claim Idaho jurisdiction because the malpractice action arose from the confirmation of an old prescription. However, the court noted that had it been a new treatment rather than the continuance of a prior visit, the jurisdiction of the patient's state might also be controlling. The court ultimately ruled that the focus must be on the place where services are rendered. Based on rulings like *Yackley*, a physician practicing telemedicine may need to be aware of laws and regulations in other states that may have jurisdiction over his activities.

CONFIDENTIALITY, PRIVACY, SECURITY

Confidentiality is more difficult to achieve in cyberspace than it is to achieve in a standard office visit. There are billions of medical records in the United States and these records contain some the most personal of information. This information includes records of alcoholism, domestic abuse, sexual assault, sexually transmitted disease, pregnancy, and abortion records. By definition telemedicine will require the transmission of some or all of this information over a great distance. At some time in that transmission, patient confidentially surrounding this information may be breached.

There are at least three ways confidentiality can be broken with telemedicine. Records can be viewed and disseminated before they are sent, records can be intercepted while they are being sent, or they can be improperly used once they are received at the site of treatment. With the passage of the Health Insurance Portability and Accountability Act of 1996, we see further restrictions and regulations governing electronic as well as non-electronic data. The Department of Health and Human Services (HHS) announced the adoption of final security standards for protecting individually identifiable health information when it is maintained or transmitted electronically.[20]

The security standards work in tandem with the final privacy standards adopted by HHS in 2002.[21] The privacy standards went into effect for most covered entities on April 14, 2003.[22] On February 20, 2003, the security standards were published as a final rule, with the effective date of April 21, 2003. Most covered entities will have until April 21, 2005 to comply with these standards.[23] The Center for Medicare and Medicaid Services (CMS) is responsible for implementing and enforcing the security standards, the transaction standards, and other HIPAA administrative simplification provisions, except for the privacy standards. On the other hand, the Office for Civil Rights is responsible for implementing and enforcing the privacy rule.[24]

HHS has emphasized the tight link between security and privacy. Privacy protection depends largely upon the existence of security measures to protect that information. Important to note, however, is the fact that there are some important distinctions between the privacy rule and the Security Rule: 1) The Privacy Rule sets standards for how Protected Health Information (PHI) should be controlled by establishing guidelines for what uses and disclosures are authorized or required, and what rights patients have with respect to their health information;[25] 2) The information covered by the Security Rule is consistent with the privacy rule, which addresses privacy protections for PHI, but the scope of the Security Rule is more limited than that of the privacy rule. The privacy rule applies only to PHI in any form, whereas the Security Rule applies only to PHI in electronic form.

There are certain safeguards set forth under the Security Rule.[26] Physicians' offices that maintain or transmit health information are required to maintain reasonable and appropriate administrative, physical and technical safeguards for ensuring the integrity and confidentiality of the information in order to protect against any reasonably anticipated threats or hazards to the security or integrity of the information and/or unauthorized use or disclosure of the information.[26] There are nine administrative standards, four physical standards, and five technical standards.[26]

HHS has adopted "required" and "addressable" implementation specifications. Required specifications are mandatory. Addressable specifications provide covered entities with additional flexibility with regard to compliance. The flexibility depends upon factors such as the covered entity's risk analysis, risk mitigation strategy, and current implemented security measures, as well as the cost of implementation.

INFORMED CONSENT

Many tests, procedures, and examinations require that the patient give informed consent. Informed consent requires the physician to tell the patient everything a reasonable patient would want to know about a procedure or test. The patient is then able to make the most informed decision about medical treatment. Telemedicine has opened up new possibilities and complexity to informed consent. The physician and staff interpreting or even performing certain procedures may not even be on the same continent as the patient. In addition, the information required in the test or procedure will likely be transmitted over countless interchanges. The distance and complexity associated with telemedicine may stress the physician's ability to adequately explain all the possible risks associated with a procedure.

COMPETENCE

Ethically, physicians should not treat a patient that has a disease beyond the physician's competence. Even if the physician is properly licensed, some diseases may be out of her depth. Competence is difficult to gauge in person or at a distance. Furthermore, a great deal of medicine is related to a physical exam which may not be done adequately over the Internet. Internet questionnaires are limited, and they do not convey any of a patient's demeanor. The Internet al.lows anyone to come into the physician's virtual office. It may be difficult to completely gather the entire relevant medical history at a distance. A seemingly simple case or prescription might prove more complex, moving beyond the skill of the telemedicine physician. In short, the traditional medical interview made is easier for a physician to know when to refer a patient to a specialist.

ADVERTISING

The medical profession has advertising regulations that are regulated through legislation and ethical norms. The Internet crosses these boundaries and may present ethically unacceptable advertising in some markets. Standards for ethical advertising on the Internet vary from profession to profession, as well as from state to state. To avoid potential ethical violations, professionals may use various safeguards, including disclosures and disclaimers. Professionals should disclose the states in which the professional is currently licensed, as well as the qualifications of each professional named on the website.

To maintain the integrity and quality of professional websites, one proposal encourages the establishment of a cyberprofessional data bank that the public could access to confirm information disclosed on the website. One idea might be the institution of a data bank that could contain information to authenticate the disclosed credentials. Additionally, a data bank could contain information indicating disciplinary actions taken by the professional association. However, it is likely that public dissemination of such information would meet with great resistance from professionals.

TELEMENTORING

Online medical education is used now more than ever before. This includes both the graduate and undergraduate medical education levels. This is particularly valuable because physicians and students in rural training areas can have access to the latest possible medical information. Today, almost every portion of the medical curriculum is now available online at many medical schools. In class forums student and professors continue to discuss class material. Some classes such as medical informatics are taught almost entirely online. Others, such as anatomy have supplemental multimedia presentations available.

In the final years of medical school, students have different needs that are also met online. First, almost every form needed in patient care is also available to medical students online. Second, webpages like www.mdconsult.com are also available to help with any diagnostic or therapeutic decision. In addition, many of these resources are available through handheld computing devices and cell phones.

CONTINUING MEDICAL EDUCATION (CME)

Continuing graduate medical education or CME is also available online. Online medical education has allowed any practicing physician access to the best possible education. Furthermore, the physician does not have to leave his home or office to attend. Many online CME courses are inexpensive or free because the production costs associated with online CME are much lower than traditional CME courses. Previously, a substantial cost was incurred by organizations offering CME because of food, venue rental, and speaker fees. One can find a fairly comprehensive list of CME opportunities at http://www.cmelist.com/list.htm. In addition, the National Institutes of Health also offers online CME at http://consensus.nih.gov/cme/cme.htm.

CONCLUSION

The interface between telemedicine, telerobotic surgery and the law will always result in the genesis of challenging new legal frontiers as long as our technology continues to advance. Existing laws may need to be reinterpreted, modified, or changed in order to accommodate the ever-expanding boundaries of our scientific knowledge. Indeed, the physician-patient relationship will also continue to evolve with technology, and man will continue to discover ways to overcome the medical, ethical, and legal hurdles along the way.

REFERENCES

1. U.S. Federal Food and Drug Administration, Center for Devices and Radiological Health, White Paper on Telemedicine Related Activities (1996); Joint Working Group on Telemedicine, Executive Summary: Telemedicine Report to Congress (Jan. 1997), available from: http://www.ntia.doc.gov/reports/telemed.

2. California Telemedicine Development Act of 1996, 1996 Cal. Statute 864 Section 1(d).

3. Goertz, RC. Manipulators Used for Handling Radioactive Materials. In: Bennet, EM, editor. *Human Factors in Technology*, Chicago, IL: McGraw-Hill; 1963; Chapter 27.

4. Campbell, MR. Surgical Care in Space. *Aviation, Space and Environmental Medicine,* 1999 70(2); 170-181.

5. 21 United States Code. Sections 360c-360k..

6. FDA (Federal Drug Administration), Center for Devices and Radiological Health, *Guidance for the Content and Review of 501(K) Notifications for Picture Archiving and Communications Systems and Related Devices* (1997).

7. *Gibbons v. Ogden*, 22 U.S.1, 3 (1824).

8. United States Constitutional Amendment X. *Powers of the States and People;* ratified 12-15-1791

9. *Dent v. West Virginia*, 129 U.S. 114 (1889).

10. *Hawker v. New York*, 170 U.S. 189 (1898).

11. Federation of State Medical Boards. (Proposed, 1996). An Act to Regulate the Practice of Medicine across State Lines.

12. *Pike v. Honsinger*, 155 N.Y.201, 49 N.E. 760 (1898).

13. *Greenstein v. Fornell*, 275 N.Y.S.673 (1932).

14. *Childs v. Weis*, 440 S.W.2d 104 (Texas 1969) (physician may arbitrarily refuse to render care to a non-patient.

15. *Hoover v. Williamson*, 236 Md. 258, 203 A. 2d 861 (1964) (services paid for by employer but duty to employee).

16. *Lopez v. Aziz,* 852 S.W.2d 303 (1993).

17. *Bovara v. St. Francis Hospital*, 700 N.E.2d 143, 145 (Illinois Appeals Court 1998).

18. *Bienz v. Central Suffolk Hospital*, 557 N.Y.S.2d 139, 139-40 (1990).

19. *Clanton v. Von Haam*, 340 S.E.2d 627, 629-30 (Georgia Court of Appeals 1986).

20. Title 45, Code of Federal Regulations, Sections 160, 162, and 164.

21. Title 45, Code of Federal Regulations, Sections 160 and 164.

22. Title 45, Code of Federal Regulations, Section 164.534.

23. Title 45, Code of Federal Regulations, Sections 160, 162, and 164.

24. Title 45, Code of Federal Regulations, Section160.304.

25. Title 45, Code of Federal Regulations, Section 164.502.

26. Title 45, Code of Federal Regulations, Section164.308 *et seq.*

SECTION II

Chapter 5

ROBOTS FOR ORTHOPAEDIC JOINT RECONSTRUCTION

*Peter Kazanzides**
Johns Hopkins University Center for Computer Integrated Surgical Systems
and Technology, Baltimore, MD 21218

Abstract

Orthopaedic procedures have motivated the development of many medical robot systems for research and clinical use. The first commercially-available[1] active medical robot in any surgical discipline was ROBODOC®, initially developed for total hip arthroplasty (THA) and later extended to total knee arthroplasty (TKA). This chapter first reviews the rationale for applying robotic technology to common joint reconstructive procedures such as THA and TKA. Although other procedures, such as spine surgery, osteotomies, and fracture reduction, can and do benefit from robotic assistance, they are beyond the scope of this chapter. A historical review of the different robot systems that have been developed over the last twenty years is then presented. These systems are subsequently grouped into five categories, based on the system size (or method of attachment) and whether or not the robot operates actively (autonomously) during key stages of the surgical procedure. One representative system from each of the five categories is described in detail. The chapter concludes with a review of the in-vitro experiments and clinical studies that were performed for the two robot systems, ROBODOC and CASPAR, that achieved modest market penetration, especially in Europe, but also stirred controversy within the medical community and the general public. The results of the experiments and clinical trials have fueled this controversy, but also indicate issues that must be resolved for future success in the field.

1. Introduction

The specialty of orthopaedics has provided fertile ground for the development of medical robots, as evidenced by the number of research systems and commercial offerings in this

---

*E-mail address: pkaz@cs.jhu.edu
[1] In Europe, CE Marking in 1996

area. A recent survery article [1] reports that nearly 20% of all medical robots are in orthopaedics. This has been motivated by the large number of orthopaedic procedures that are performed annually, especially in the areas of joint reconstruction (e.g., hip and knee arthroplasty) and spine surgery, and by several technical advantages that are obtained by working with bony structures. These advantages include excellent contrast in X-ray/CT images and high rigidity. The excellent image contrast allows robot systems to utilize preoperative images and/or intraoperative images. Preoperative images can be used to construct precise models of the patient's anatomy for planning purposes. Intraoperative images can also be used for this purpose, or they can be used to orient (register) the robot to the anatomical target. Bone rigidity ensures that preoperative or intraoperative models and plans remain valid under most conditions, especially if rigid fixation between the robot and bone can be established.

This chapter will review the motivation for, and history of, orthopaedic robots for joint reconstructive procedures, such as hip and knee surgery. Although robot systems have been developed for other orthopaedic procedures, such as spine surgery, fracture reduction, osteotomies, ligament repair, and femoral nailing, those topics are beyond the scope of this chapter. In addition, this chapter does not describe other types of computer-assisted technology for orthopaedic surgery, such as navigation systems and patient-specific templates. The interested reader should consult other books [2–5] and survey articles [1, 6] for a broader perspective.

2. Orthopaedic Joint Reconstruction

This section describes the orthopaedic joint reconstructive procedures (in the hip and knee) that have been addressed by the majority of robot systems in this field.

2.1. Total Hip Arthroplasty (THA)

The following subsections describe the conventional technique and the rationale for robotic assistance for THA. This surgery is also called total hip replacement (THR).

2.1.1. Conventional technique for THA

THA surgery involves preparing an elongated cavity in the femur (thigh bone) and a rounded cavity in the acetabulum (hip socket) to accommodate the two components of a hip prosthesis: the femoral stem (Fig. 1, top) and acetabular cup. There are two basic types of prostheses–cemented and uncemented (or cementless)–which correspond to the methods for affixing the prostheses to the bones. Cemented prostheses are held in place by the application of bone cement, whereas cementless prostheses rely on bone ingrowth. As a result, a typical cementless prosthesis will contain either a porous surface (Fig. 1, top) or a special coating, such as hydroxyapatite, over the desired ingrowth regions. When bone cement is used, the precise shape of the cavity is not critical because the cement will fill most gaps. On the other hand, for cementless prostheses, studies have shown that bone ingrowth cannot occur across gaps, which are present when the femoral canal is not precisely shaped and positioned to accommodate the prosthesis.

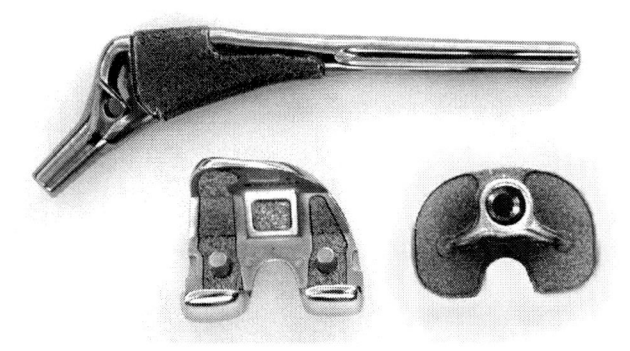

Figure 1. Cementless prostheses: femoral component of hip joint (top), femoral and tibial components of knee joint (bottom).

Prostheses can also be classified according to their geometric design. In some cases, the design consists of well-defined lines and arcs whereas in other cases, the design appears to be hand-sculpted (and sometimes actually was). The latter set of prostheses are often called "anatomic" because they are intended to better match the anatomy of a typical patient. The extreme case is a custom prosthesis, which is designed to fit a specific patient. In this case, a CT scan of the patient is used during the prosthesis design phase. Custom prostheses are rarely used, compared to "off-the-shelf" prostheses, due to the higher expense associated with the CT scan and the manufacturing of both the prosthesis and associated instrumentation.

In the conventional technique, with "off-the-shelf" prostheses, preoperative planning is performed by overlaying templates (outlines) and making measurements on two-dimensional X-rays. Templates are available at different magnification factors so that errors due to X-ray magnification can be minimized. In general, the preoperative plan is limited to bracketing the prosthesis size and identifying an approximate prosthesis position.

Intraoperative bone preparation is performed using reamers (hand-held drills) and broaches (serrated cutting tools) to create the desired cavities. Proper execution relies on a significant amount of experience and "surgical feel," especially when preparing the femoral cavity, because most of the anatomy is not visible. In this case, the surgeon typically begins with the reamer and broach corresponding to the smallest prosthesis in the bracket. If the cavity feels "loose" (i.e., insufficient contact with hard cortical bone), the surgeon switches to the next larger size until he/she feels that there is sufficient, but not excessive, cortical contact. If the surgeon chooses a prosthesis that is too large, the femur can fracture either during cavity preparation or during prosthesis insertion. This is one of the most common intraoperative complications associated with THA. Similarly, although the surgeon can plan any desired prosthesis position, the actual position is determined mostly by anatomical constraints because the hand-held instruments tend to follow the path of least resistance.

2.1.2. Motivation for robotic assistance for THA

Laboratory tests have shown that the conventional method for cavity preparation is inherently inaccurate [7]. In particular, cavities prepared in femur bones by reaming and broaching were irregular, with large gaps between the bone and the prosthesis. These gaps indicated that broaches may tear out chunks of trabecular bone instead of making a smooth cut. The tendency of a broach to bounce when it contacts dense trabecular or cortical bone may also produce gaps. Difficulty in properly orienting the broach during femoral canal preparation is another problem with the traditional technique. Even when the surgeon accurately aligns the broach at the beginning of a procedure, the interior surface of the bone can exert forces that may redirect the path of the broach before the process is complete. In addition to promoting bone ingrowth, accurate shape and placement of the femoral cavity is necessary to ensure adequate stress transfer from prosthesis to femur. A poorly positioned implant will create non-uniform stress and could potentially cause dislocation from the acetabular component of the prosthesis. Sizing errors in selecting a prosthesis can cause a variety of complications. Undersized prostheses are unstable and oversized prostheses often cause complications such as femoral fracture and thigh pain.

Accurate fit, placement, and prosthesis selection are all intended benefits of the robot's ability to execute the preoperative plan. The intended clinical outcomes would include adequate and uniform bone ingrowth, uniform stress transfer, reduced stress shielding, less thigh pain, and the elimination of femoral fractures as an intraoperative complication.

Although this discussion focused on preparation of the femur, it is also important to consider installation of the acetabular cup. In this case, the conventional hemispherical reamer does an acceptable job creating the cavity, but proper positioning of that cavity is critical to avoid problems such as recurring dislocations. Furthermore, obtaining the correct geometrical relationship between the femoral stem and the acetabular component is important for restoring the joint biomechanics and maintaining parameters such as leg length.

2.2. Revision Total Hip Arthroplasty (RTHA)

Revision THA refers to the surgical procedure that is performed to repair or replace a failing hip prosthesis. This surgery is typically more challenging than the original (primary) hip replacement due to anatomical changes, such as remodeling of bone, and/or to the need to remove bone cement if a cemented prosthesis was originally used.

A robot assistant could provide a benefit by removing the bone cement, especially in the distal portion of the cavity where visibility is limited and intraoperative X-ray is often necessary to identify the cement. The robot could also ensure that the new prosthesis cavity is created in the correct location. This can be challenging with the manual technique in cases where the remodeled bone tends to incorrectly guide the reamer/broach. For example, if the original prosthesis is not aligned with the femoral canal, the remodeled bone may guide the reamer/broach along the axis defined by the original prosthesis, rather than along the femoral canal.

2.3. Total Knee Arthroplasty (TKA)

The following subsections describe the conventional technique and the rationale for robotic assistance for TKA. This surgery is also called total knee replacement (TKR).

2.3.1. Conventional technique for TKA

Modern knee prostheses consist of three components that fit the bones of the knee joint: femur, tibia and patella (for a brief history of knee prostheses, see [8]). Since current orthopaedic robot systems ignore the patellar component, it will not be discussed in this chapter. Representative femoral and tibial prosthesis components are shown in Fig. 1, bottom. The critical factors that affect clinical outcome are component alignment, to preserve the proper mechanical axis, and soft tissue (or ligament) balancing, to ensure smooth motion and stability in both flexion and extension.

In the conventional (manual) technique, preoperative radiographs (in particular, standing leg X-rays) are used to estimate component size and to determine some of the parameters that affect component alignment. Due to the requirement for soft tissue balancing, much of the information is obtained intraoperatively. An intramedullary rod is often used to measure the femoral axis, from which the mechanical axis can be estimated. Conventional TKA instrumentation includes various jigs and fixtures that are used to sequentially cut the five resection planes for the femoral component and the single resection plane for the tibial component.

2.3.2. Motivation for robotic assistance for TKA

The complexity of the instrumentation for conventional TKA has motivated the development of a number of computer-assisted surgery systems, especially in the area of surgical navigation. Navigation systems are particularly useful for intraoperative measurements, including determining the mechanical axis (i.e., the line connecting the hip, knee and ankle joints) as well as assessing the joint motion.

Although navigation systems can drastically improve the TKA procedure, there is room for robotic assistance to improve the accuracy of bone preparation. As in the hip, both proper component fit and placement are important. Because the conventional TKA procedure relies on sequentially performed bone resections (e.g., where the position of one resection depends on the result of the previous resections), it is prone to cumulative errors, which can lead to problems with component fit. Similarly, even if the ideal placement can be identified, it can be challenging to get the prosthesis components into exactly the right position.

2.4. Partial Knee Arthroplasty

In recent years, partial reconstructions of the knee joint have gained popularity. Two partial reconstruction techniques that have been addressed by robotic assistance are Unicondylar Knee Arthroplasty (UKA) and Patello-Femoral Arthroplasty (PFA). In UKA, only one side of the knee joint (usually, the medial side) is replaced by prosthetic components. In PFA, only the trochlea (distal part of femur between the condyles) and the patella are replaced by prosthetic components.

As with other procedures, the motivation for robot assistance includes the desire for higher dimensional and placement accuracy (i.e., cutting the correct shape in the correct location). Another possible motivation is to enable minimally-invasive surgical approaches. For example, an image-guided robot can overcome problems due to limited visibility, and a small, dextrous robot can operate through smaller incisions than are currently possible with (straight) manual instrumentation.

3. Historical Review of Orthopaedic Robots

This section presents an approximately chronological review of the robot systems that have been developed for orthopaedic joint reconstructions (see Table 1).

The first application of a robot to orthopaedic surgery was reported by the University of Washington [9, 10]. In this system, the robot was used to accurately position the saw and drill guides used to prepare the bone for the femoral component of TKA. This system did not require any preoperative or intraoperative imaging; planning was accomplished intraoperatively by using the robot to position specially constructed three-dimensional templates, corresponding to each supported prosthesis, on the distal femur. The robot system automatically recognized each template and determined the position and orientation of all necessary holes and cuts from the position and orientation of the selected template.

Development of the ROBODOC® System began shortly afterwards at IBM Research and the University of California, Davis [7, 11–13]. ROBODOC was the first system developed for THA and was designed to automatically mill the bone cavity for the femoral component. Another fundamental difference is that it required a CT scan to create a preoperative plan on the ORTHODOC workstation that was supplied with the system. After a short period of veterinary (canine) use, it was commercialized by Integrated Surgical Systems, Inc. (ISS), which incorporated in 1990. Although initially developed for custom prostheses, regulatory and marketing constraints restricted ROBODOC to supporting standard (off-the-shelf) prostheses. Further details about ROBODOC are presented in Section 4.1.1.

Other pioneering TKA research systems were developed at Northwestern University in Chicago [14] and at the Rizzoli Clinic and its partner Universities in Italy [15, 16]. The Northwestern system, like ROBODOC, relied on a preoperative CT scan and plan, but like the University of Washington system, used the robot to position the guides used with the manual cutting instruments. Development of this system seems to have ceased in the late 1990's. In contrast, the robotics work at the Rizzoli Clinic and its partners has progressed through several iterations, starting with an industrial robot [15] and more recently introducing a custom-designed medical robot [16]. Furthermore, these robot systems were designed to directly machine the bone based on a preoperative plan, as ROBODOC did for the hip.

The Acrobot® System [17], developed at the Imperial College in London and subsequently commercialized by the Acrobot Company, introduced a new approach for robot-assisted TKA. In particular, although Acrobot is an active (motorized) robot, it is designed to move only in response to the surgeon's input. This is often referred to as a semi-active mode. Acrobot uses Active Constraint Control™ to keep the cutting tool within the region of bone that must be removed to accomodate the prosthesis. Acrobot was initially applied to TKA and has more recently been used for UKA [18]. Additional information about Acrobot is presented in section 4.2.1.

The early commercial success of ROBODOC, especially in Germany, prompted competition from Orto Maquet, a subsidiary of the German company Maquet. Orto Maquet introduced the CASPAR (Computer Assisted Surgical Planning and Robotics) System for

THA [19] and installed it in a number of hospitals in Europe. Competition spurred Orto Maquet and ISS to develop TKA modules for their respective systems, which were both used clinically in 2000. Orto Maquet also adapted the CASPAR system to assist with anterior cruciate ligament (ACL) reconstruction [20].

A robot and navigation system have been combined at Frankfurt University Hospital to assist with minimally-invasive preparation of the acetabulum in THA [21]. The robot positions a linear carriage that supports the surgical instrument (in this case, an acetabular reamer) and the surgeon manually advances the tool. The navigation system is used for registration and for real-time compensation of patient motion. Other instruments, such as drills and saws, could be attached to the linear carriage to enable this robot to assist with preparation of the femur or with other orthopaedic procedures.

All of the systems mentioned above consist of fairly large robots, mostly derived from industrial robots. CRIGOS (Compact Robot for Image-Guided Orthopaedic Surgery) was proposed in the mid-1990's as a more compact alternative [22]. Unlike previous systems, which used robots with serial linkages, CRIGOS is based on a parallel design, also known as a Stewart platform or hexapod.

In the last five years, a number of compact orthopaedic robots have been introduced, several of them using a parallel kinematic structure (like CRIGOS). This trend was possibly fueled by the common consensus that systems such as ROBODOC and CASPAR were too bulky. These new systems went even further than CRIGOS in that they were designed to be bone-mounted. Examples include Arthrobot, developed at KAIST, Korea [23], MARS, developed at the Technion, Israel [24] and being commercialized (as SpineAssist) by Mazor Surgical Technologies, and MBARS, developed at Carnegie-Mellon University [25] and described further in Section 4.3.1.

Another recent approach has been to develop bone-mounted mini-robots, with few active degrees of freedom (typically 2) that position instrument guides for TKA. Examples include Praxiteles [26] (described in Section 4.4.1.), Galileo [27] and GP System [28]. In general, these robots are coupled with a commercially-available navigation system.

The small robot concept is taken to the extreme by the development of hand-held robots, such as ITD (Intelligent Tool Drive) [1, 29], a prototype two-axis tool [30], and PFS (Precision Freehand Sculptor) [31, 32]. The ITD is a 6-axis parallel robot intended to compensate for hand tremor and motion of the target anatomy. It uses a specially developed optical tracking system (MOSCOT) to obtain position measurements of the ITD and target anatomy. The first clinical application is planned to be pedical screw placement. A simpler concept is presented in [30], which describes a prototype 2-axis hand-held tool intended for TKA. In this system, the two axes maintain a rotary cutter in the desired resection plane, based on position feedback from an external tracking system. The authors raise the concern that commercially available tracking systems may not have sufficient bandwidth for this task. The PFS [31, 32] also consists of a hand-held cutting tool and an optical tracking system, but represents an even simpler approach. The tracking system monitors the position of the cutting tool with respect to the target anatomy and enables the cutter only when the tool is in a region where bone should be cut. Further details of the PFS System are presented in Section 4.5.1.

Despite the recent interest in compact robots, development of large orthopaedic robot systems has not ceased. A 9-axis robot system weighing 900 kg has been developed at the

University of Tokyo for TKA [33]. This system executes a preoperative plan, but allows the surgeon to make intraoperative modifications to reduce the likelihood of soft tissue damage.

The BRIGIT system (Bone Resection Instrument Guidance by Intelligent Telemanipulator) [34] is a small 6-axis robot, mounted on a wheeled trolley, that was initially developed for High Tibial Osteotomy (HTO), with future plans for THA and TKA procedures. High Tibial Osteotomy (HTO) is a procedure to correct the alignment of the femur and tibia by removing a wedge of bone from the tibia in order to reposition it. BRIGIT does not require preoperative or intraoperative images, but rather relies on the surgeon to manually guide the robot to collect several anatomical points (similar to image-free navigation systems). Once the anatomy and plan parameters are identified, the robot positions a cutting guide and the surgeon manually performs the resection. BRIGIT was originally developed by the French company MedTech, S.A., but was acquired by Zimmer, Inc. in March 2006.

A recent article describes RomEo (Robotic minimally invasive Endoprosthetics) [35], which aims to combine navigation and robotics for minimally-invasive THA (acetabulum and femur). This project appears to be in the conceptual design phase, but there are some interesting features, such as a prototype milling device designed to mill around corners (35-70 degree angle). This milling device is not described due to patent issues.

4. Classification of Orthopaedic Robots

Picard et al. [37] recently reviewed the literature of classification schemes for Computer Assisted Orthopaedic Surgery (CAOS) systems and concluded with a recommendation to classify them according to a matrix indexed by system type (active robotic, semi-active robotic, and passive) and by image guidance source (preoperative, intraoperative, or none). Note that all the systems described above use active robots. In this chapter, the distinction between active, semi-active, and passive is based on the way that the robot is used (i.e., an operational definition rather than a mechanical definition):

Active System: automatically performs an intervention, such as machining bone.

Semi-active System: performs the intervention under the direct control of the surgeon (e.g., a "hands on" or "cooperative control" mode).

Passive System: does not actively perform any part of the intervention (e.g., positions a tool guide).

In contrast, some researchers, including [37], do not distinguish between the semi-active and passive definitions and instead reserve "passive" for devices that are mechanically passive, such as navigation systems.

Considering the latest generation of bone-mounted and hand-held robot systems, it seems logical to consider another dimension that is based on the size of the robot. This can effectively be captured by the fixation of the robot relative to the patient or surgeon (externally-mounted, bone-mounted, or hand-held). This is the most static classification parameter because it is difficult for a robot system to change from one size (or fixation method) to another. In contrast, only a software change may be necessary to change an active robot system, such as ROBODOC, into a semi-active robot system, such as Acrobot,

Table 1. Summary of Robot Systems for Orthopaedic Joint Reconstruction

System	Institution	Procedures	Class[a] M | O | I			Stage[b]	Refs
	U. Washington	TKA	E	P	N	Res.	[9, 10]
ROBODOC	IBM/U.C. Davis ISS	THA,TKA	E	A	P	Comm.	[7], [11–13]
	Northwestern U.	TKA	E	P	P	Res.	[14]
	Rizzoli Clinic	TKA	E	P A	P	Res.	[15] [16]
Acrobot	Imperial College Acrobot Company	TKA,UKA	E	S	P	Comm.	[17, 18]
CRIGOS, MINARO	Aachen U. Germany	TKA,RTHA RTHA	E B	A A	I I	Res. Concept	[22], [36]
CASPAR	Orto Maquet URS	THA,TKA, ACL	E	A	P	Comm. (no longer)	[19, 20]
	Frankfurt U. Hosp.	THA	E	P	P	Res.	[21]
Arthrobot	KAIST, Korea	THA	B	A	N	Res.	[23]
MARS	Technion, Mazor	Spine	B	P	I	Comm.	[24]
MBARS	CMU, Technion	PFA	B	A	N	Res.	[25]
Galileo	Precision Implants AG, Switzerland	TKA	B	P		Comm.	[27]
GP System	Medacta	TKA	B	P	N	Comm.	[28]
Praxiteles	Praxim-Medivision	TKA	B	P	N	Res.	[26]
PFS	CMU	Various	H	S		Res.	[31, 32]
ITD	Heidelberg/ Mannheim	Spine	H	S		Res.	[1, 29]
	Paris Mines	TKA	H	S		Concept	[30]
	U. Tokyo	TKA	E	A	P	Res.	[33]
BRIGIT	MedTech, Zimmer	HTO	E	P	N	Res.	[34]
RomEo	Helmut-Schmidt-U./ BGU Hamburg	THA	E	A		Concept	[35]

[a] **Classification codes: M (mounting)**: E (external), B (bone-mounted), H (hand-held); **O (operation)**: A (active), S (semi-active), P (passive); **I (image)**: P (preoperative), I (intraoperative), N (none), blank if not known or not applicable (e.g., when provided by navigation system).

[b] **Stage of development:** Comm (already or soon to be commercially available), Res (in research phase), Concept (concept or early stage research).

or vice-versa. The same is true regarding the image guidance source. In fact, many of the bone-mounted mini-robots and hand-held robots described above are coupled with a navigation system, which could be image-free or image-based and could change in future versions.

Rather than adopting an unwieldy three-dimensional classification scheme, we focus on the method of robot fixation (externally-mounted, bone-mounted, or hand-held) and distinguish between the mode of operation (active, semi-active, or passive) when useful. Classifying the systems based on the three mounting methods and the three modes of operation would produce nine categories; some would not correspond to any current systems. It is more illustrative to group the robot systems into the five categories defined in the following sections, which include detailed descriptions of an example from each category.

4.1. Externally-mounted active robots

This group consists of robots that actively perform part of the procedure, such as milling bone. These robots are typically large industrial or modified-industrial robots [11–13, 19, 20], although some custom robots have been developed [22, 33]. The robots are mounted external to the patient (e.g., on the floor, OR table, or ceiling). They generally operate using a preoperative plan based on a three-dimensional image modality, usually CT, although some use intraoperative image guidance [22].

4.1.1. Example: ROBODOC

Development of ROBODOC began in 1986 as a joint research project between the University of California, Davis (UC Davis), and the IBM T.J. Watson Research Center in Yorktown Heights, New York. In May 1990, the UC Davis researchers performed the first clinical test of the robot in a veterinary hospital on a dog requiring a hip prosthesis. In November 1990, Integrated Surgical Systems, Inc. (ISS) was formed to develop and commercialize the technology for human clinical use. The first human surgery was performed in November 1992 at Sutter General Hospital (Sacramento, California).

The procedure for robotic joint replacement surgery is illustrated in Fig. 2. The two main components are the ORTHODOC® Preoperative Planning Workstation and the ROBODOC® Surgical Assistant. The input to ORTHODOC consists of a CT scan of the patient's anatomy, the prosthesis geometry that is supplied by the manufacturers, and clinical decisions made by the surgeon. The surgeon plans the procedure by selecting a prosthesis (or prostheses) from the database and positioning it in the CT image. ORTHODOC displays three orthographic views (i.e., orthogonal slices) of the data as well as a 3D model (see Fig. 3).

The Surgical Robot (Fig. 4) is a five-axis SCARA robot with two revolute axes (theta-1, theta-2) in the X-Y plane, a prismatic axis (Z), and two wrist rotations (roll, pitch). Each joint contains two optical encoders for redundant position feedback. The robot is mounted on a mobile base with a column that can be raised or lowered by the surgeon. This column provides a redundant Z axis, thereby extending the vertical workspace of the robot. The system includes a wrist-mounted six-axis force sensor that monitors the forces applied at the tool. This force information makes it possible to implement functionality such as manual guidance, tactile search, safety checking, and an adaptive cutter feed rate [38].

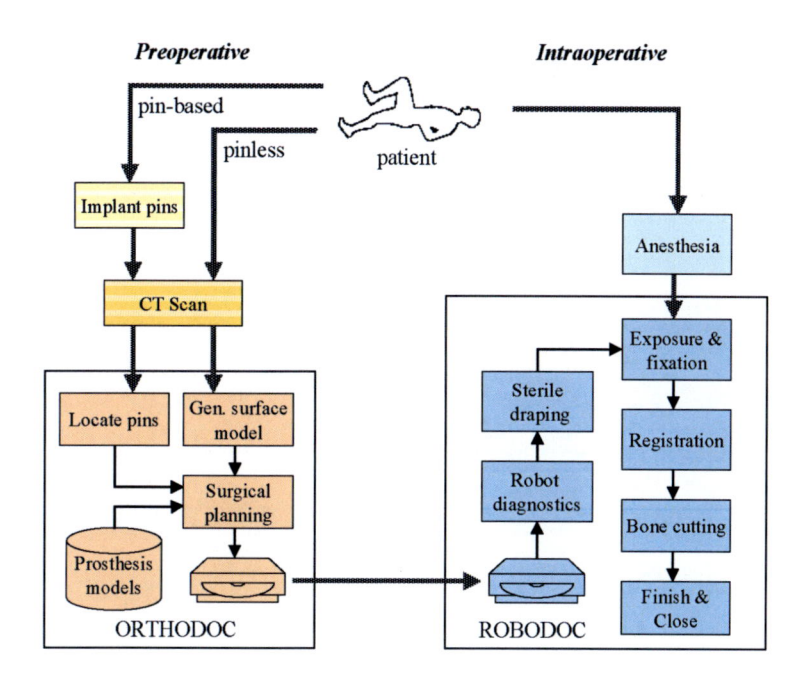

Figure 2. ROBODOC Process

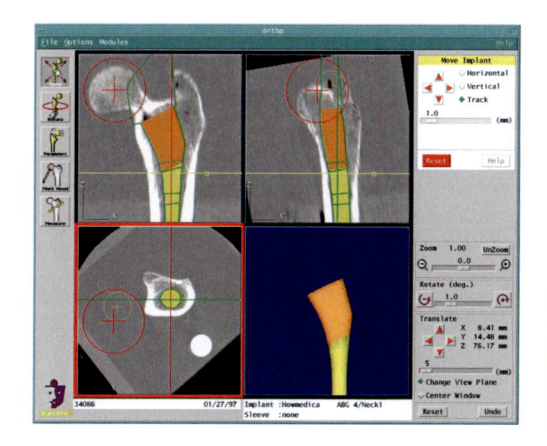

Figure 3. ORTHODOC Planning System
Notes: Green outline indicates area that will be cut by robot; bone model is not shown in 3D view.

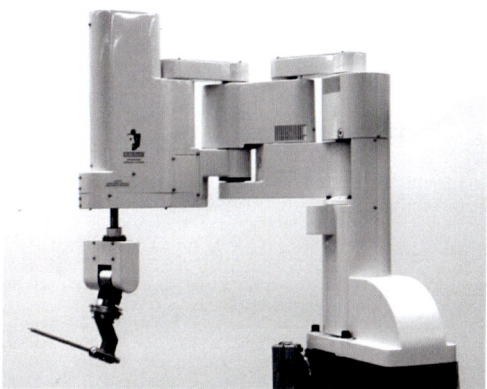

Figure 4. ROBODOC® Manipulator Arm

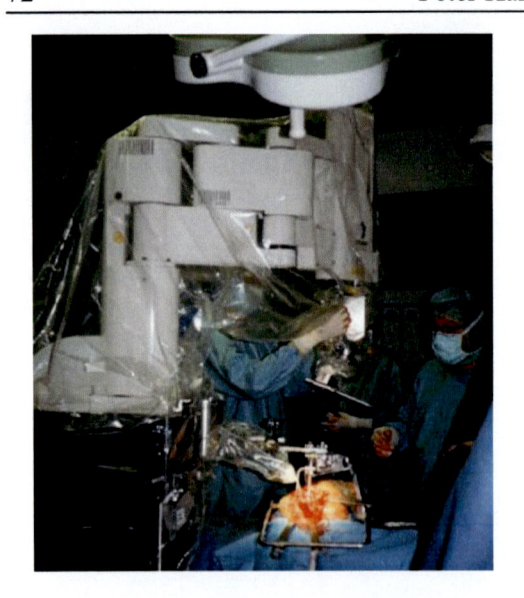

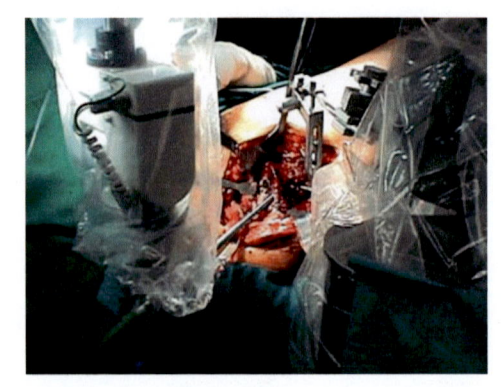

Figure 5. ROBODOC system in clinical use for THA

ROBODOC executes the preoperative plan by machining the specified prosthesis cavity in the femur (see Fig. 5). This requires the bone to be rigidly attached to the robot. A bone motion monitor (BMM) is used as a safety sensor to detect motion of the bone relative to the robot (i.e., fixation failures). In addition, accurate cavity placement requires a registration between the patient's anatomy in the preoperative plan (i.e., the bones in the CT scan) and the anatomy of the actual patient. The preoperative plan is specified in image (CT) coordinates whereas intraoperative localization of the patient can be obtained in robot coordinates, so registration implies finding the transformation between image and robot coordinates.

Initially, ROBODOC used a "pin-based" registration method, which required the implantation of titanium bone screws (pins) in the femur prior to the CT scan. Registration was accomplished by defining at least three reference points on the pins and then identifying them in both the CT and robot coordinate systems. Because the pins are titanium, the ORTHODOC software could easily locate them in the CT data using image processing techniques. The robot system identified the physical pins via a tactile search, using feedback from its wrist-mounted force sensor [38]. ROBODOC initially used three registration pins, with the centers of the pin heads serving as the three reference points, but shortly afterwards transitioned to a two-pin method, where the third reference point was obtained by creating a "virtual pin" based on the center and axis of the distal pin. In this case, a longer distal pin was required to enable accurate determination of the pin axis in the CT data.

Although pin-based registration is reliable, it involves an additional, preliminary surgery to implant the pins prior to the CT scan and was also the source of postoperative knee pain for many patients. This motivated the development of the "pinless" DigiMatch^{TM} Single Surgery System [39], which uses anatomical features instead of metal pins as fiducials. Registration is accomplished by collecting a set of points on the surface of the bone, using a passive digitizing arm registered to the robot coordinate system, and then applying optimization methods to match this "cloud of points" to a three-dimensional model of the bone created from the CT data. Once an acceptable registration is obtained, the digitizer locates a pair of "recovery markers" (i.e., pins that were intraoperatively inserted prior to registration). If registration subsequently needs to be re-established (e.g., due to bone motion), it can quickly be performed by locating the two recovery markers. The DigiMatch System was first used clinically in March 1998.

Regardless of the method of registration, ROBODOC performs a workspace check prior to beginning the machining process [40]. This ensures that the entire cavity is within the robot's workspace, which provides a more accurate shape than would otherwise be obtained if the robot or bone had to be repositioned (and therefore re-registered) during the cutting procedure. Once cutting has commenced, ROBODOC provides a visual display of its progress on the computer monitor. As the robot mills the cavity, the monitor displays the CT data overlaid with a model of the prosthesis cavity. The completed portion of the cavity is displayed in one color while the remaining portion is displayed in another. This is similar to the visualization provided by most navigation systems. During cutting, the control software continuously monitors the force sensor and adjusts the cutter feed rate based on the sensed force and on parameters specific to the prosthesis design and cutting tool [41]. This enables the robot to adapt to the patient's anatomy by slowing down in regions of hard cortical bone and speeding up in other regions.

Although initially used for THA, from the beginning the developers intended to extend the technology to TKA. This goal was realized in March 2000, when ROBODOC performed the first robot-assisted TKA surgery (shortly before the first CASPAR TKA surgery). ROBODOC has also been used for RTHA [42, 43] and some preliminary work on minimally-invasive THA has been reported [44].

4.2. Externally-mounted semi-active or passive robots

This group consists of image-guided robots that either position a mechanical guide [9, 10, 14] (passive) or provide active motion constraints [17, 18] (semi-active). Most of these systems require a preoperative plan that is based on a three-dimensional image modality such as CT. A notable exception is the system developed at the University of Washington, which uses specially constructed three-dimensional templates for intraoperative planning [9, 10].

4.2.1. Example: Acrobot

The Acrobot system [17, 18] was developed at the Imperial College in London, England, and is being commercialized by The Acrobot Company, Ltd. The name Acrobot is derived from Active Constraint Robot, which describes the manner in which this system is used. Specifically, the surgeon performs the bone cutting by pushing on the robot's handle, while relying on the robot software to keep the cutting tool within the desired cut volume. This is often referred to as a semi-active mode of operation. The Acrobot developers believe that this "hands on" (semi-active) control mode will be preferred by surgeons over the automated (active) operation of systems such as ROBODOC and CASPAR.

The system actually consists of two robots: a larger robot used as a gross positioning device and a smaller one that provides the active constraints (see Fig. 6). Technically, the Acrobot is the smaller robot, although the entire system (including the preoperative planner)

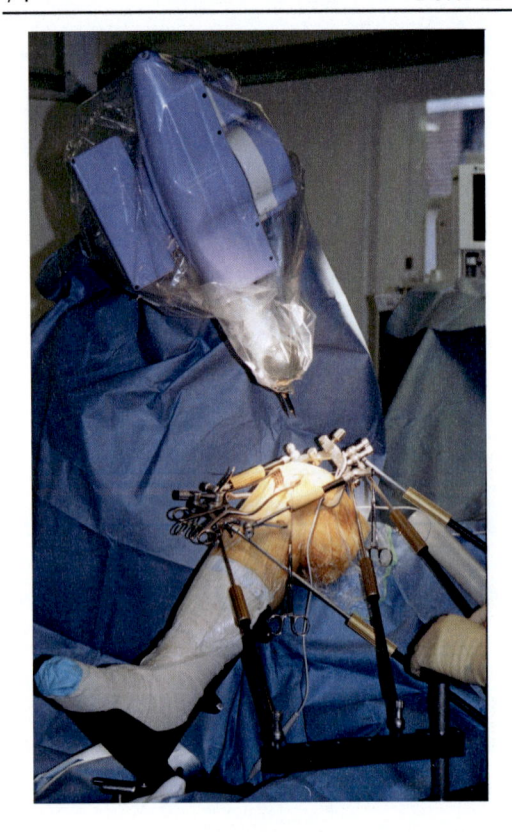

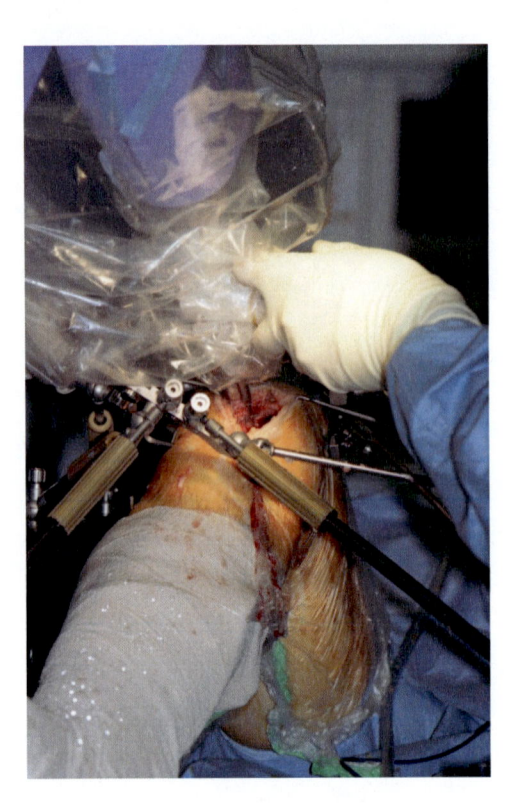

Figure 6. Acrobot system in clinical use for UKA
Credit: Courtesy of Acrobot Company Limited, UK

is referred to as the Acrobot System. The Acrobot (small robot) has a spherical kinematic design, with two rotational axes (yaw and pitch) and one prismatic axis (extension). These three axes have similar low mechanical impedances, which allow the surgeon to easily backdrive the robot while feeling the contact forces with the environment. The handle includes a force sensor to measure the force exerted by the surgeon.

The gross positioning device is used to position the small robot in the vicinity of the cut volume. Once the Acrobot is properly positioned, the gross positioning device is powered off and braked in position. This process is repeated, as required, to move the Acrobot to the appropriate positions for the resection planes corresponding to the femoral and tibial prosthesis components. A six-axis gross positioning device is described for TKA [17], whereas a three-axis device is described for UKA [18].

The Acrobot System currently uses a preoperative CT image for planning and requires intraoperative registration between the CT image and the patient. Initially, the registration was based on fiducials (pins) but, as with ROBODOC, the developers realized that a "pinless" method would be necessary for clinical use. Therefore, the current registration method requires the surgeon to use the robot to collect several points (typically 20-30) on the bone surface and then applies the iterative closest point (ICP) algorithm [45] to match this set of points to the 3D bone model created from the preoperative CT data. Once an acceptable registration is achieved, the surgeon locates several fidicual points on the clamps that are attached to the femur and tibia. If registration needs to be repeated during the procedure, it can quickly be performed by re-finding these fiducial points. This technique is analogous to the one used by the ROBODOC "pinless" registration technique, which touches recovery markers that were installed intraoperatively [39].

The active constraint control is achieved by a two-level controller. The inner loop is a joint position/velocity control loop with friction, gravity, and guiding force compensation. The outer loop adjusts the desired position and velocity, the control gains, and the guiding force compensation parameter for the inner loop based on the distance to the constraint boundary and the magnitude and direction of the force applied by the user (as measured by the force sensor). The robot's workspace is divided into 3 regions: RI (inside the safe region), RII (inside the safe region, but near the boundary), and RIII (the "no-go" region).

In region RI, the control gains are low to allow the surgeon to feel the cutting forces, and the robot's desired velocity is proportional to the measured handle force (admittance control). The guiding force compensation is 0.

In region RII, the control gains increase as the distance to the boundary decreases, thereby increasing the robot's stiffness as the tool approaches the boundary. The robot's velocity is still based on the sensed handle force, but the admittance gain for the direction towards the boundary is decreased proportional to the distance to the boundary (i.e., the gain in this direction approaches 0 as the tool approaches the boundary). Finally, the guiding force compensation is increased as the tool approaches the boundary. The net result is that the robot becomes stiffer as it is pushed towards the boundary, but forces in any direction parallel to, or away from, the boundary result in low impedance motion as in region RI.

In region RIII, the desired position is set to the nearest boundary point and the desired velocity is non-zero only when the user pushes the handle towards the safe region (RI or RII). The guiding force compensation is set to oppose any measured force component that is directed towards the "no-go" region.

Acrobot has been used clinically for TKA [17] and for minimally-invasive UKA [18], which is shown in Fig. 6.

4.3. Bone-mounted active robots

This group consists of robots that mount to the bone and are used in an active mode [23, 25]. The MARS robot [24], currently developed for spine procedures, is similar to these systems except that it operates as a passive system. All of these robot are based on a parallel kinematic design, which compared to a serial kinematic design has higher rigidity at the expense of a smaller workspace. Because the robots are already attached to the bone, they do not require a large workspace to perform their task, so this is an acceptable tradeoff. In the case of THA, the Arthrobot system relies on manually-performed distal reaming to determine the correct prosthesis placement; this circumvents the workspace problem that would otherwise have occurred if the robot attempted to machine the distal femur.

4.3.1. Example: Mini Bone-Attached Robotic System (MBARS)

MBARS [25] is a bone-mounted parallel robot developed at the Institute for Computer Assisted Orthopaedic Surgery (ICAOS) at Western Pennsylvania Hospital and the Robotics

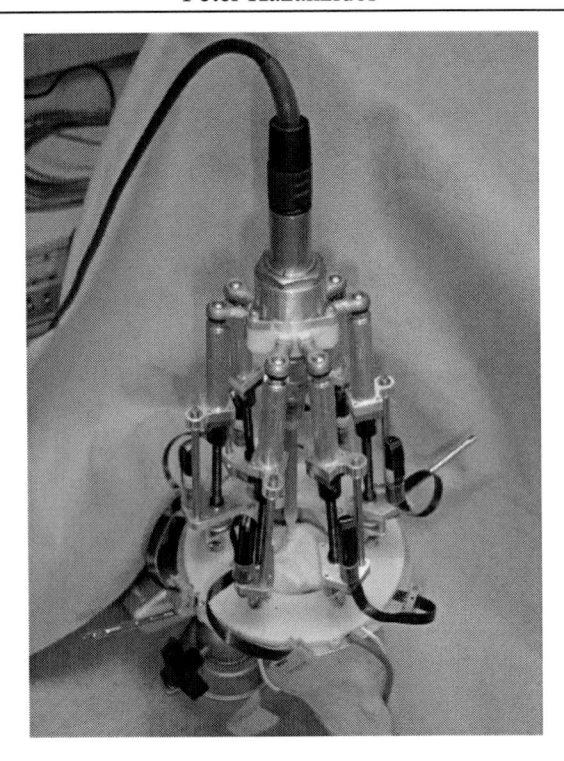

Figure 7. Mini Bone-Attached Robotic System (MBARS)
Credit: Alon Wolf, Ph.D.

Institute at Carnegie-Mellon University[2]. It was designed to assist with patello-femoral arthroplasty (PFA), a partial knee replacement procedure where artificial components are attached to the patella and the trochlear groove (distal end of the femur). The conventional technique uses a template to mark the area of the trochlea that must be cut and then relies on manual resurfacing, using osteotomes and high-speed burrs, to create the desired cavity. MBARS was created to facilitate this procedure.

The first prototype of MBARS, mounted on an artificial femur, is shown in Figure 7. It has six linear actuators connected in parallel between two rigid platforms. The lower (reference) platform is attached to the distal femur via three Steinman pins. The upper platform supports a rotary cutting tool and moves it relative to the lower platform to machine the trochlea (distal femur). The low level motor control is provided by a custom electronics board, installed in the robot housing, that contains a PIC microprocessor, PWM amplifier, and sensor interface for each of the six brushed DC motors. This design simplifies the cabling because only 6 wires (for power and the I2C control bus) are required to connect the robot to the higher-level control computer.

The prototype implementation uses a preoperative 3D image for planning. The surgeon marks the patellar tracking line on the preoperative image and the software then positions the artificial component. The cutting paths are calculated using a cell decomposition technique. The authors mention that an image-free technique is in development. The conventional technique uses only preoperative X-ray images, and so an image-free technique

---

[2]The primary author has since moved to the Technion in Israel.

would be more acceptable because it would not require additional imaging. The image-free technique would use the robot, in conjunction with a force sensor and haptic interface, to scan the bone surface. This would bring the additional benefit of not requiring a registration of the preoperative image to the robot coordinate system.

MBARS has been used experimentally with artifical femurs (sawbones). The entire process of preparing the cavity required about two minutes, which is likely to be faster than the average time required for manual preparation. Accuracy studies are currently being performed.

4.4. Bone-mounted passive robots

These systems generally have a small number of active degrees of freedom (e.g., 2) to move a saw guide between the different cut planes for the femoral component of a TKA prosthesis. The systems contain additional degrees of freedom (active or passive) to align themselves with the desired prosthesis orientation [26–28].

4.4.1. Example: Praxiteles

Praxiteles [26], named after the ancient Greek sculptor, is being developed for TKA by Praxim-Medivision (LaTronche, France) in collaboration with the Université Joseph Fourier (La Tronche, France) and the University of British Columbia (Vancouver, Canada). It attaches to the distal femur and consists of 2 motorized degrees of freedom (dof), which position a saw guide around the distal femur, and 2 passive dof which are used to align the motorized dof with the cutting planes for the femoral component of the knee prosthesis.

The first prototype required fixation on both sides (medial and lateral) of the distal femur and was therefore not suitable for minimally-invasive TKA. The second prototype (Fig. 8) was designed to overcome this limitation by attaching to just the medial side of the distal femur. In addition, the passive milling tool guide was redesigned to improve the ergonomics and kinematics (i.e., by allowing the tool to rotate and slide in the cutting plane while maintaining the fixed, minimally-invasive, entry point).

Praxiteles is being integrated with the Surgetics Station®, a navigation system produced by Praxim-Medivision that offers image-free navigation for TKA.

4.5. Hand-held semi-active robots

These systems have extremely small workspaces and operate by using their limited motion to compensate for positioning errors due to inherent human limitations and/or hand tremor. They can thus be considered as devices that augment human performance. These robots are semi-active because they do not cut bone until they are manually advanced by the surgeon. The systems in this category follow two basic approaches: i) use motorized degrees of freedom to correct for small positioning errors [29, 30], and ii) use computer control to enable the cutter when the surgeon holds the tool in the correct position [31, 32].

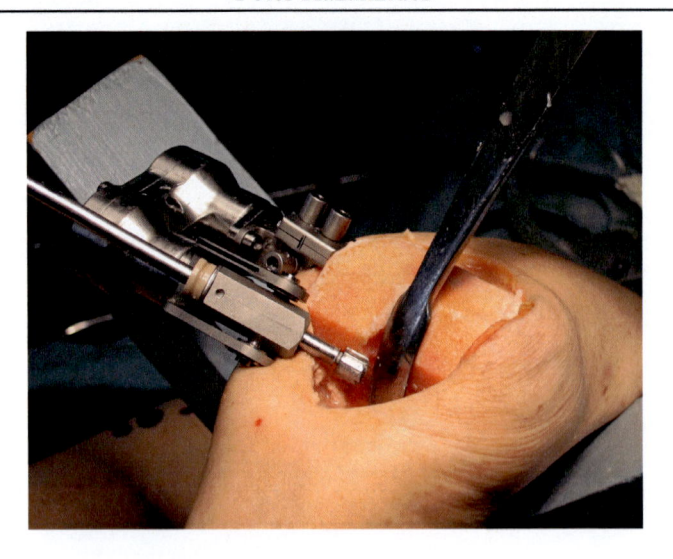

Figure 8. Praxiteles for minimally-invasive TKA
Credit: Christopher Plaskos, Praxim-Medivision

4.5.1. Example: Precision Freehand Sculptor (PFS)

The Precision Freehand Sculptor (PFS) [31, 32] is under development at the Robotics Institute at Carnegie Mellon University and the Institute for Computer Assisted Orthopaedic Surgery (ICAOS) at The Western Pennsylvania Hospital in Pittsburgh. The basic concept is that a tracking system monitors the position of the hand-held cutting tool and the computer enables the cutter only when it is held in a region where cutting should occur. The computer provides a visual display of the cutter's position relative to the desired cut region, allowing the user to also participate in the feedback loop. The accuracy that can be achieved is dependent on the tool speed, the calibration of the system (e.g., registration between tracking system and cutting tool), the tracking system accuracy, and the response time of the system and/or user.

Two prototypes were constructed to test different methods of stopping the cutter [31]. The first prototype, called the "clutch tool," uses a clutch to engage or disengage the blade from the drive shaft. Because it does not include a brake, the blade spins up quickly but takes several seconds to spin down. The second prototype, called the "shaver'," contains an actuator that extends and retracts the cutting blade behind a guard. This prototype was also tested with the blade continuously extended (always cutting) to evaluate the performance of computer-controlled blade retraction versus the user's response time. When used in this mode, the tool was called the "navigated shaver."

Accuracy testing was performed by cutting a simple faceted shape in wax and then measuring the actual shape with an accurate digitizing system. The results show higher errors for the "clutch tool" (maximum error greater than 6 mm) compared to the "shaver" and "navigated shaver," which produced similar errors (maximum errors less than 2 mm).

An improved version of the "shaver" tool (Fig. 9) was recently evaluated in six artificial femurs by cutting a 3-faceted shape to accept a unicondylar knee prosthesis [32]. Three femurs were wrapped in foam and cut through a small incision to simulate a minimally-

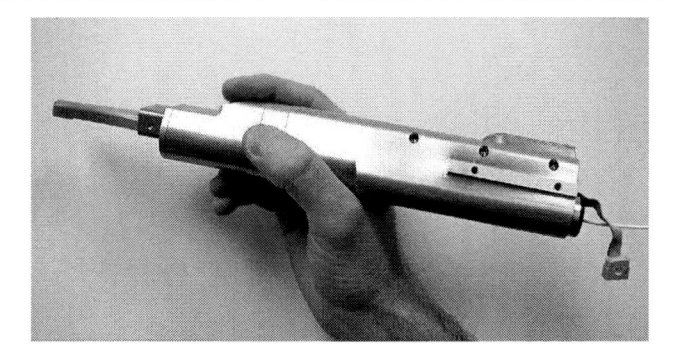

Figure 9. Precision Freehand Sculptor (PFS)
Credit: Gabriel Brisson, Carnegie Mellon University

invasive approach, whereas the other three femurs were cut with a completely open approach. The actual shape was measured by a laser scanner system. In this experiment, the actual shape was registered to the desired shape by minimizing RMS error, so the results reflect only the dimensional accuracy that can be achieved; placement error (for example, due to registration error) is not evaluated. The results show an RMS cutting error that is less than 0.2 mm for all cases (minimally-invasive or open), except for one outlier at 0.27 mm.

5. User Experiences with Orthopaedic Robots

In this section, we focus on the experiences of surgeons and researchers who used the commercially available ROBODOC and CASPAR systems and include a small clinical trial conducted with Acrobot. The largest number of clinical studies involve the implantation of the femoral component in THA since that was the first orthopaedic application addressed by both ROBODOC and CASPAR. The literature includes significantly more ROBODOC studies due to its longer history (first clinical use in 1992).

The user experiences with these robot systems can be grouped into the following general categories:

1. In-vitro experiments using cadaver bones or artificial bones to evaluate parameters that are unique to the robotic technique [46, 47] or to compare the robotic technique to the manual technique [48–54].

2. Controlled clinical studies with a small number of patients [55–59].

3. Clinical experiences resulting from use of the robot system, often with a large patient population, but generally without a control group of comparable size [60–62].

5.1. In-Vitro Experiments

Several experiments have been performed to compare the accuracy of the robotic technique to the manual technique, based on various anatomic parameters [48–50]. Another experiment measured the overall accuracy of the ROBODOC and CASPAR systems using a specially constructed phantom [63]. Other experiments investigated the primary stability achieved by the robot to that achieved by manual implantation [51–53] and the quality of the prosthesis-bone contact [54]. A few experiments were performed to investigate parameters unique to the robotic procedure, such as the possibility of nerve damage due to implantation of fiducial markers (pins) [46] and the effectiveness of irrigation to prevent thermal necrosis during bone milling [47].

In [48], 14 femurs were CT scanned and planned with ORTHODOC, the planning component of the ROBODOC System. These femurs were separated into manual implantation and robot implantation groups and a second CT scan was performed after implantation of the femoral component. The robot group showed better results for the implant-bone interface in the medial calcar region (1.6 mm for the robot group vs. 5.1 mm for the manual group) and for the anteversion angle errors (0.4 degrees for the robot group vs. 10.8 degrees for the manual group). Other parameters, such as the neck-shaft (CCD) angle and the neck length, were comparable between the two groups.

A similar study was reported in [49], with additional results in [50]. In this experiment, 10 matched pairs of femurs were split into robot and manual groups. All femurs were CT scanned and planned using ORTHODOC. They were CT scanned again after implantation and analyzed on the ORTHODOC workstation. The initial study [49] compared the original physiologic values to the values achieved after implantation – it did not account for changes that were intentionally introduced during the planning phase. Although this is useful information, it does not evaluate the ability of the robot or manual instrumentation to accurately execute the preoperative plan. These results ("planned versus postoperative parameters") are provided in a later publication [50]. The femurs prepared by the robot showed smaller average errors compared to those prepared manually for all parameters: leg length (0.3 mm vs. 6.8 mm), medial-lateral offset (-0.2 mm vs. 0.6 mm), CCD angle (-0.1 deg vs. -0.6 deg), antetorsion angle (1.3 deg vs. 4.5 deg). The earlier report [49] also mentions that a blind radiographic analysis indicated that the robot group demonstrated better-fitting hip stems.

A quantitative comparison of the prosthesis-bone interface achieved by manual preparation and robot-assisted preparation was recently reported [54]. In this study, 5 cadaver femurs were prepared using manual instrumentation and 5 were prepared using the CASPAR system. After insertion of the prosthesis, each femur was encased in resin and sectioned into 2.5 mm slices. These slices were digitized and the prosthesis-bone contact and the average gap heights were measured. The results showed a better fit for the robot-prepared femurs, with an average full contact area of 93% and average gap height less than 0.2 mm, compared to 60% contact area and an average gap height of 0.8 mm for the manual femurs.

A geometric accuracy study of the ROBODOC and CASPAR systems was performed using a specially-constructed phantom [63]. The phantom consisted of several parts that modeled the left and right femurs and surrounding soft tissue. The femur model was designed to accommodate an insert. Two different types of inserts were created: 1) a scan insert that included a guiding structure visible in the CT image, and 2) a milling insert that had mechanical properties similar to human bone. The goal of the planning phase was to align the prosthesis model provided by the planning software with the guiding structure visible in the CT image. The robot machined the cavity in the milling insert according to the plan and the position of the cavity was subsequently measured by a coordinate measuring machine. The authors measured the robot repeatability by creating two plans (one for

ROBODOC and one for CASPAR) and executing each plan four times with the respective system. The standard deviations of the measured values were approximately 0.25 mm in all three linear directions (both systems), 0.4 degrees (CASPAR) or 0.6 degrees (ROBODOC) for antetorsion, and 0.2 degrees for the other two angles (both systems). The overall system accuracy was measured by performing the complete procedure 7 times with ROBODOC and 4 times with CASPAR. The standard deviations of the measured values were approximately 0.5 mm in the two directions perpendicular to the femur shaft (both systems), 0.3 mm (CASPAR) or 1.6mm (ROBODOC) along the femur shaft, 0.6 degrees (CASPAR) or 0.9 degrees (ROBODOC) for the antetorsion angle, and 0.3 degrees for the other two angles (both systems). The authors state that the overall accuracy was similar for both systems and "the apparent differences between the systems are probably due to both the statistical uncertainty in the data collected and the motivation and experience of the various people participating in the study during the preoperative planning stage." [63]

Thomsen et al. investigated the stability of 7 [51], and later 8 [52], different femoral stems implanted following cavity preparation by a robot system (ROBODOC and/or CASPAR) and by manual instrumentation. This study used synthetic femurs designed to mimic actual bone. All measured displacements were negligible except for the rotational stem displacement, so only those results were reported. The results were mixed: some prostheses were more stable in the manual group, whereas others were more stable in the robot group. Only one prosthesis was tested with both robot systems – in this case, the femurs prepared by ROBODOC showed the best stability, whereas the femurs prepared manually and by CASPAR were equivalent.

Nogler et al. [53] studied the primary stability of one type of prosthesis in 6 pairs of cadaver bones prepared manually and by the ROBODOC System (initially 7 pairs, but 1 femur was damaged during testing). As in [51], they found larger motion (less stability) in the femurs prepared by ROBODOC, though the difference was not statistically significant.

Nogler et al. [46] also performed a cadaver study to investigate the cause of postoperative knee pain, which has been frequently reported for the pin-based ROBODOC System [58,59]. The distal registration pin used by ROBODOC was implanted in the medial condyle in 20 cadaver knees. The investigators discovered that at least one nerve was injured in 11 of the 20 knees and suggest that the lateral condyle may be a better implantation site because there are fewer neural structures. Of course, this issue is also resolved by the "pinless" (DigiMatch) registration procedure introduced for ROBODOC [39].

Finally, Nogler et al. [47] tested whether irrigation could provide adequate cooling to prevent thermal damage to the bone during total hip revision surgery, where ROBODOC machines the old cement. They found that proper irrigation reduced the temperature below the safe level of 70 °C in all places except the distal plug, where "the irrigation stream was impeded by the cutter in the narrow cavity." They recommend a new design where the irrigation stream can be provided through the cutter.

5.2. Controlled Clinical Studies

Controlled clinical studies have been performed on three continents (North America [55,64], Europe [58], and Asia [59]) to compare the clinical outcome of ROBODOC THA surgery to that obtained by the conventional (manual) method. A controlled clinical study was also performed with the CASPAR System for TKA surgery [65] and with the Acrobot System for UKA surgery [18]. It is difficult to make definitive conclusions because in orthopaedic procedures such as THA and TKA, the clinical outcome often cannot be completely evaluated until 10 or 20 years after the surgery. Most studies available now consist of shorter follow-up periods, such as 2 or 3 years. As a result, these studies primarily report on perioperative differences, such as surgical time and complication rates, and on short term evaluations such as post-operative radiographic analyses, patient-reported pain measures, and reports of early failures.

Several reports resulted from the U.S. clinical trials initiated to collect supporting data for an application for FDA clearance of ROBODOC. There were three different FDA-authorized clinical trials:

1. A 10-patient feasibility study performed at Sutter General Hospital (Sacramento, CA) from 1992-1993 to demonstrate safety of the system.

2. A multi-center controlled clinical trial, started in 1994, to compare the pin-based ROBODOC System to the manual technique [55]. This trial was abandoned shortly after the pinless ROBODOC System was introduced in 1998.

3. A multi-center controlled clinical trial, begun in 2001, to compare the pinless ROBODOC System to the manual technique [64].

Bargar et al. [55] report on the first 120 patients (136 hips) that were enrolled in the multi-center U.S. trial of the pin-based ROBODOC System. The followup period was between 3 months and 2 years. The results show a significantly longer average surgical time for the robot group (258 minutes) compared to the control group (134 minutes), although it was noted that some of this was due to the learning curve. Blood loss with the robot group was also higher (1189 cc vs. 644 cc) and seemed to correlate directly with surgical time. There were no intraoperative fractures in the robot group, compared to three fractures in the control group. There were no statistically significant differences in the pain scores. The authors note that the most positive results of the robot-assisted procedure were the radiographic analysis of prosthesis fit and alignment (positioning) and they speculate that "these improved radiographic results for patients in the ROBODOC® group represent surrogate variables that indicate probable improvement in long term clinical performance."

Early results of the second multi-center clinical trial (pinless ROBODOC) are based on 6-month followup of the first 88 patients (68 ROBODOC and 20 control) [64]. The average surgery time is still longer with the robot (120.6 minutes) compared to the manual technique (82.7 minutes), but the difference (37.9 minutes) is much less than in the original multi-center clinical trial. Average blood loss is a little higher in the robot group, but the difference is not statistically significant. There is no statistically significant difference in 6-month pain scores (Harris Hip Scores). There was one revision in the ROBODOC group due to a prosthesis failure, but there were no device-related complications.

Honl et al. [58] present the results of a controlled clinical study of the pin-based ROBODOC System for THA performed in Hamburg, Germany. This trial included 154 patients (80 robot and 74 control), who all received the S-ROM prosthesis (J&J DePuy) and were followed for 2 years postoperatively. Although this study confirmed certain advantages of the robotic technique (better prosthesis position, leg length and pain scores at 6 and

12 months), overall it presents a negative result. The most critical problems encountered with the robotic technique were a higher dislocation rate (18% vs. 4%), a higher revision rate due to causes other than infection (15% vs. 0%), a longer OR time (by 25 minutes), a higher nerve injury rate (7% vs. 1%), and a higher cost per procedure. The surgeons also experienced a rather high failure rate of the robot (13 patients, or 18%) – in these cases, the procedure was completed manually and the patients were subsequently excluded from the study. The authors indicate that the dislocation problems were due to "insufficiency of the abductor muscles." This occurred because the robot often had to remove a large portion of the greater trochanter (where the abductor muscles attach) to be able to machine the cavity in the preoperatively planned position. In [58, Fig. 5], the authors show preoperative (ORTHODOC) plans with the same patient for 3 different prostheses: the S-ROM (used for the study), the Osteolock (Stryker-Howmedica), and the "anatomic" ABG (Stryker-Howmedica). The ORTHODOC software indicates the entire volume that will be machined by the robot, including the "precut" area that must be machined by the robot to gain access to the cavity. In this figure, it is clear that the S-ROM and Osteolock plans require removal of a significant portion of the greater trochanter (lateral side of "precut" area). In contrast, the ABG plan preserves a larger portion of the greater trochanter and is therefore less likely to interfere with the attachment of the abductor muscles. The authors also note that the ROBODOC software has since been improved (i.e., the "precut" area requires less lateral machining), but they do not have results with this software.

Nakamura et al. [59] present the results of a controlled clinical study of the pin-based ROBODOC System for THA performed in Osaka, Japan. This trial included 153 hips (78 robot and 75 control), who all received the Versys Fiber Metal Taper stem (Zimmer Inc.) and were followed for 24-37 months postoperatively. As in all other studies, they report a longer average surgery time (121 minutes vs. 108 mins), but in this case the robot group had significantly less average blood loss (559 ml vs. 666 ml). The robot group had no intraoperative fractures, compared to 5 in the control group. The robot group also had fewer incidences of postoperative thigh pain, although there were 2 cases of knee pain due to the pins. There were 2 dislocations in the robot group compared to 1 dislocation in the control group. The robot group had significantly better pain scores (JOA hip scores) at 6 and 24 months postoperatively. The 2 year radiographs showed bone ingrowth in both groups, though the manual group had more proximal stress shielding.

Two controlled clinical trials were performed to evaluate specific parameters. One study [56] focused on postoperative gait analysis because the authors were concerned about the possibility of impaired hip abductor function due to the extended exposure and fixation requirements of the ROBODOC System. The study included 50 hips (25 robot and 25 manual, not randomized). Neither group (robot or manual) achieved normal gait at 6 months, but the impairment was equivalent between the two groups. The authors therefore concluded that "the robotic procedure did not impair hip abductor function more than the conventional method." Another study, with 50 ROBODOC hips and 25 manual hips, used transesophageal echocardiography and hemodynamic monitoring to investigate the incidence of intraoperative embolisms. The results indicated that ROBODOC "may reduce the risk of clinically significant pulmonary embolism during cementless THA." [57]

Siebert et al. [65] present the results of a clinical study of the (pin-based) CASPAR System for TKA that was performed in Kassel, Germany, starting in March 2000. This trial included 70 robot-prepared knees that were compared to 52 historical controls. The patients in the robot group received the LC Search Evolution® prosthesis (Aesculap Inc.) because it was the only one supported by CASPAR at the time, whereas the control group received the NexGen® prosthesis (Zimmer Inc.). The average operating time for the robot-assisted procedure was 135 minutes, which is reported to be longer than the manual procedure. A learning curve was observed in that operating times decreased from 220 minutes to about 90 minutes. There were no major adverse events related to the use of the robotic system. Postoperatively, the robot group showed a higher accuracy in achieving the planned tibio-femoral alignment, with an average error of 0.8 degrees (range 0-4.1 degrees) compared to the control group's average error of 2.6 degrees (range 0-7 degrees).

A randomized double-blind (patient and evaluator) clinical study was performed with the Acrobot robot for UKA [18]. This study included 13 patients operated by Acrobot and 15 patients operated by the conventional technique. The primary outcome measurement was the difference between the planned prosthesis position and the actual prosthesis position, which was measured via a postoperative CT scan. The results showed that the tibio-femoral alignment for all 13 patients operated by Acrobot was less than 2 degrees, whereas only 6 of the 15 patients that received the conventional operation had tibio-femoral alignments in this range. The pain scores measured at 6 months postoperative were also better for the patients operated by Acrobot. As with the other robot systems, the average surgery time was longer when the Acrobot was used (104 minutes vs. 88 minutes).

5.3. Routine Clinical Use

By far, the largest number of ROBODOC surgeries were performed at the Berufsgenossen-schaftliche Unfallklinik (BGU) in Frankfurt, Germany, which eventually had 3 ROBODOC Systems in routine clinical use [60]. BGU surgeons have reported on their experiences with the ROBODOC System (both pin-based and pinless) for THA, RTHA, and TKA. A recent publication [60] reports on the results of performing the ROBODOC THA procedure for 4000 patients. There were no intraoperative fractures, which is a significant result given the size of the group. Other complications, such as infections (0.84%), nerve lesions (1.9%), muscular deficiency (1.7%), and deep vein thrombosis (1.6%), were reported to be comparable to the manual technique. The average surgery time started at 210 minutes, but has since decreased to 90-100 minutes, which is about 20 minutes longer than the manual technique. The hips had high primary stability and there was no subsidence in spite of immediate full-weight bearing.

An earlier report [55], included the results of 900 patients, where 30 of the patients were RTHA. This report provides some details of the technical difficulties encountered with the system:

- In 7.1% of the cases, the CT scan had to be repeated due to detected motion.

- In 11% of the cases, intraoperative registration (pin finding) had to be repeated due to bone motion detected by ROBODOC.

- Registration pins were implanted in 932 femurs, but 32 femurs (3.4%) could not be completed by the ROBODOC System due to various technical difficulties.

For 42 patients, bilateral hip surgery was performed with a mean interval of 312 days between surgeries. The CT scan that was performed prior to the second surgery enabled the surgeons to evaluate the postoperative result (prosthesis placement) from the first surgery. The authors found that deviations in implant position were between 0.4 and 1 mm and deviations in anterversion angle were 1 degree or less.

Of the 30 RTHA cases, 23 were performed using the primary THA module, where the cement or fibrous tissue was removed as a consequence of machining the cavity for the new femoral stem. The other 7 were performed by using the ROBODOC revision module, which allows the surgeon to define a custom cavity that corresponds to the cement to be removed, in the preoperative CT image. Additional information about the revision module is presented in [42, 43].

Clinical experience with ROBODOC for TKA is presented in [61], which reviews the experience with the first 100 patients at BGU Frankfurt and in [66], which discusses 50 ROBODOC patients in Jeonnam, Korea. At BGU Frankfurt, the robot could not be used in 5 cases due to various technical problems and those patients were excluded from the results. The surgical time was initially 130 minutes, but was reduced to 90-100 minutes as a result of the learning curve. This is reported to be only slightly longer than the manual technique. The authors report that their preliminary results indicate that the robot technique achieves correct alignment and rotation of the prosthesis. Disadvantages include software tissue management, the need for rigid fixation, and the use of pins for registration. The Korean study concludes that "the surgical robot was helpful for obtaining balanced soft tissue tension and a more reliable normal kinematic pattern" [66].

Compared to ROBODOC, there are relatively few reports of clinical use of the CASPAR System. In one study [62], 10 of 16 CASPAR patients were postoperatively evaluated with CT. The authors reported that the measured anteversion angles differed from the plan by an average of 7.8 degrees and the medial and lateral placements differed by 1.8 mm and 1.2 mm, respectively. These results are worse than the manufacturer claims and are worse than results reported for in-vitro experiments with cadaver bones [48]. The authors speculate that this may be due to patient motion.

6. Discussion of User Experiences

Use of a surgical robot system such as ROBODOC or CASPAR for THA or TKA surgery is currently a controversial topic, due to the conflicting results (positive and negative) that have been published. It appears that both sides of the debate agree with the following three points:

1. The robot system provides a higher level of accuracy for prosthesis placement and fit. This is especially evident in the in-vitro experiments and in radiographic analysis of in-vivo (clinical) results. Whether or not this higher accuracy is clinically relevant is the subject of ongoing debate.

2. The surgery time is longer for the robotic technique. For THA, the average time is extended by about 15-30 minutes, after the initial learning curve. There is less data for TKA, but the average surgery time appears to be slightly longer.

3. It is a disadvantage to require an extra procedure to implant registration markers (pins) prior to the preoperative CT scan. Besides the obvious issues of higher cost and greater risk to the patient, there have been numerous reports of postoperative knee pain, subsequent to THA, due to the pins. This issue is resolved by newer developments, such as the DigiMatch (pinless) technique introduced for ROBODOC [39].

The most serious criticism of the robotic technique is the high revision rate, mostly due to postoperative dislocation, that was reported in [58]. This study is often referenced by others as evidence that the robot system introduces "considerable morbidity" in THA, despite the fact that this negative outcome has not been observed in any other controlled clinical study [55,59] or during routine clinical use of the system for thousands of surgeries [60]. Furthermore, the authors of this study make the following comment:

> Robotic surgery allows an exact intraoperative translation of the preoperative planning, whereas there is a certain variability with the manual approach. This is illustrated by the higher accuracy with regard to limb length and varus-valgus alignment of the prosthetic stem in the group treated with robotic implantation. [58]

So, if the robot precisely executes the preoperative plan, but the clinical outcome is unsatisfactory, is the problem due to the robot or to the preoperative plan? With regards to the study reported in [58], Bargar makes the following comment:

> A careful review of the study in question seems to show that the cause of the instability was damage to the abductor muscles. This appears to be due to improper implant selection and failure to protect the soft tissues at the time of the surgery. When planning a case on the workstation, if there is excessive overhang of the trochanter over the projected cut path of the robot, the case should be excluded. [64]

Surgeons have often mentioned the learning curve associated with using the robot system in surgery, but it appears that there is also a learning curve for the 3-dimensional preoperative planning that directs the robot. Careful planning is especially important because current robot systems do have limitations, such as the lateral clearance in the proximal femur that is necessary to machine the cavity for some prosthesis designs. The planning workstation clearly indicates the entire cut volume, as shown in [58, Fig. 5] and Fig. 3, so the surgeon must evaluate whether it is acceptable; if not, the surgeon should either change the plan or exclude the patient from the robotic procedure.

Another concern with the robotic technique is the result of in-vitro studies [51–53], with synthetic or cadaver bones, that suggest that robotic preparation may produce lower primary stability than manual implantation for some prosthesis designs. This result seems counter-intuitive, but there are two important issues to consider. First, Thomsen [52] speculates that for some anatomic prostheses, lower stability may occur because "the robot needs additional space for maneuvering the drill head around the curved shoulder thus resulting in gaps between stem and bone bed." This is a valid point. Although manual preparation is less precise, the instrumentation allows the surgeon to create cavities that cannot be duplicated by the straight shaft cutters currently used by robot systems. For example, it is possible to "cut around corners" using a flexible reamer or to insert a broach along a curved path. The second issue is that, for any given prosthesis, it is not trivial to specify the dimensions of the cavity that should be machined by the robot. Should this cavity be based on the prosthesis dimensions (taking into account the manufacturer's recommendations for press-fit, overcutting, etc.), the broach dimensions, the cavity that would actually be created by the broach, or some other data? In practice, specification of the prosthesis cavity is a collaborative effort between the robot manufacturer and the prosthesis manufacturer and often includes (unpublished) in-vitro studies similar to the published ones [51–53]. These published studies suggest that the optimal cavity specification may not yet have been achieved for all prosthesis designs. In theory, for a straight-stem implant, the robot can always achieve equivalent results to the manual technique – after all, one could digitize the manually created cavity and reproduce it with high precision using the robot.

Another criticism of the robot technique is the reliability with which it can complete the surgery. This is often called the "failure rate," though it should be made clear that "failure" in this case does not mean a clinical failure, but rather that the robot system ceased to operate. Often, this is due to a safety check in the robot software that causes it to fail to a safe state (i.e., turn off). In [58], the "failure rate" was rather high (18%), with nearly 70% of these failures due to persistent "force freezes" (i.e., forces that exceed the safety threshold) when cutting sclerotic bone. This is a known problem with ROBODOC that has been experienced at many centers and there are anecdotal reports of surgeons occasionally "helping" ROBODOC to cut the bone, for example by using their hands to stabilize the cutter or by manually removing hard pieces of bone. ISS responded by introducing hardware improvements, such as a better cutting system, and software improvements, such as adaptively changing the cutting feed rate based on the sensed force [41], but much of this was not available prior to the cited study. It should be noted that other centers have reported significantly lower "failure rates," such as 3.4% for the first 932 patients at BGU Frankfurt [55].

A major advantage of the robotic technique is the accuracy with which it can execute the preoperative plan. The in-vitro studies reported average positional errors less than 1 millimeter and average angular errors less than 1.5 degrees [48, 50]. Clinically, somewhat lower accuracy can be expected due to factors such as uncompensated patient motion during CT scanning or during surgery. There is one study of 10 CASPAR patients that reported unusually large clinical errors in position and orientation [62] but larger studies, such as the 42 bilateral hip patients at BGU Frankfurt [55], measured errors that were more consistent with the in-vitro results. Whether or not this increased accuracy is clinically significant is the subject of further study.

Another benefit of the robot system is that there appear to be fewer intraoperative fractures. Also, there is one study [57] suggesting that fewer pulmonary embolisms may occur during the robot-assisted procedure.

There is disagreement in the literature on how other parameters, such as the incidence of nerve damage, amount of blood loss, and postoperative pain scores, compare between the robotic and manual techniques.

7. Conclusion

Orthopaedic procedures are a natural target for robotic technology because they often require bones to be machined or cut. Computer numerical control (CNC) machines have replaced most manual tools in the fabrication of parts in the industrial world, and it was hypothesized that computer-controlled machines could have the same impact in orthopaedic surgery. It has been noted that most prostheses are manufactured using CNC technology, so it would be logical to use that technology intraoperatively to create the matching cavity in the bone. Of course, it is impractical to use a conventional CNC for surgery because the part (bone) would have to be brought to the CNC,[3] but a robot can bring CNC-like capabilities to the bone in the operating theatre. Of course, robotic assistance is not limited to bone machining. For example, current procedures can be made less invasive through the use of small, dextrous robots and/or by the robot's ability to use registered preoperative or intraoperative images to "see" hidden anatomy.

Many research systems have been created and two commercial systems, ROBODOC and CASPAR, were installed in at least 100 hospitals, mostly in Europe, and performed surgery on more than 10,000 patients. Use of these systems became controversial, especially in Germany, with surgeons and patients reporting both positive and negative results. Two points that all sides seem to agree on are:

- The robot procedure requires a longer surgery time and has higher surgical costs, compared to the conventional technique.

- The robot can execute a preoperative plan more accurately than the conventional technique.

Clearly, a new technology cannot be successful unless it reduces costs and/or provides a clinical benefit. In their current form, it appears that ROBODOC and CASPAR do not reduce surgical costs. Robot proponents have argued that some costs are saved because the unused manual instrumentation does not need to be cleaned and sterilized. Also, if clinical results are better, there could be an overall cost savings to society (e.g., shorter recovery times, lower revision rates), but this has yet to be proven. At this time, it is not proven whether the superior accuracy provided by the robot system is clinically relevant.

Furthermore, the experiences with ROBODOC and CASPAR have shown that introduction of this new technology creates a significant learning curve. This has been well documented for the robotic phase, often by showing a reduction in average surgery time as the operating room staff gains experience with the technology. The clinical results seem to indicate that there is also a learning curve for the planning phase. In particular, the poor outcomes reported in [58] (high dislocation rates leading to high revision rates) appear to be due to sub-optimal surgical plans, rather than intraoperative problems with the robot.

Fortunately, the mixed results for ROBODOC and CASPAR have not deterred continued research in this field. A recent trend has been the development of small robots designed to mount directly to the target bone or to be held by the surgeon. In the latter case, the robot actuators are used to compensate for human errors. The developers of these systems

---

[3]Though an engineer once asked why the femur couldn't be excised from the patient, machined on a CNC, and then reinserted into the body.

have undoubtedly been influenced by the feedback that large floor-mounted robots, such as ROBODOC and CASPAR, are too bulky and occupy too much space in the operating theatre. Perhaps an even more important argument is that these small systems are likely to be less costly than their large predecessors. One potential issue with bone-mounted robots is whether they can be firmly attached to the bone without causing damage (e.g., fractures) or requiring more invasive exposure in actual clinical settings. Of course, the key question is whether any of these new systems can reduce costs, improve clinical outcomes, or preferably both. Otherwise, they may realize their technical goals but fail to achieve clinical and commercial success.

Acknowledgments

I thank Russell H. Taylor for introducing me to the field of medical robotics in 1989 at the IBM T.J. Watson Research Center (Yorktown Heights, New York), and then for giving me the opportunity in 2002 to broaden my experience by joining him at the Engineering Research Center for Computer-Integrated Surgical Systems and Technology (CISST ERC) at Johns Hopkins University (Baltimore, Maryland). I acknowledge my many colleagues and friends from my twelve years at Integrated Surgical Systems, Inc. (Sacramento and Davis, California), who bravely traveled down the often rocky road of clinical development and commercialization of the ROBODOC System. I received photographs and information from Brian Davies (Acrobot), Alon Wolf (MBARS), Christopher Plaskos (Praxiteles), and Gabriel Brisson (PFS). I thank Suzanne Byerley for her careful review of this chapter.

References

[1] Pott PP, Scharf HP, Schwarz MLR. Today's state of the art in surgical robotics. *Computer Aided Surgery*. 2005 Mar;10(2):101–132.

[2] Taylor RH, Lavallée S, Burdea GC, Mösges R, editors. *Computer Integrated Surgery: Technology and Clinical Applications*. MIT Press; 1995.

[3] Nolte LP, Ganz R, editors. *Computer Assisted Orthopedic Surgery (CAOS)*. Hogrefe and Huber; 1999. Composed of papers from '95 and '96 CAOS Symposia.

[4] DiGioia AM, Jaramaz B, Picard F, Nolte LP. *Computer and Robotic Assisted Knee and Hip Surgery*. Oxford University Press; 2004.

[5] Stiehl JB, Konermann WH, Haaker RG, editors. *Navigation and Robotics in Total Joint and Spine Surgery*. Springer-Verlag; 2004.

[6] Taylor RH, Stoianovici D. Medical Robotics in Computer-Integrated Surgery. *IEEE Trans on Robotics and Automation*. 2003 Oct;19(5):765–781.

[7] Paul HA, Bargar WL, Mittelstadt B, Musits B, Taylor RH, Kazanzides P, et al. Development of a Surgical Robot for Cementless Total Hip Arthroplasty. *Clinical Orthopaedics and Related Research*. 1992 Dec;285:57–66.

[8] Buechel FF, Stiehl JB. Total Knee Arthroplasty. In: Stiehl JB, Konermann WH, Haaker RG, editors. *Navigation and Robotics in Total Joint and Spine Surgery*. Springer-Verlag; 2004. p. 175–179.

[9] Garbini JL, Kaiura RG, Sidles JA, Larson RV, Matsen FA. Robotic Instrumentation in Total Knee Arthroplasty. In: *Orthopaedic Research Society (ORS)*. San Francisco, CA; 1987. p. 413.

[10] Matsen FA, Garbini JL, Sidles JA, Pratt B, Baumgarten D, Kaiura R. Robotic Assistance in Orthopaedic Surgery: A Proof of Principle Using Distal Femoral Arthroplasty. *Clinical Orthopaedics and Related Research*. 1993 Nov;296:178–186.

[11] Taylor RH, Mittelstadt BD, Paul HA, Hanson W, Kazanzides P, Zuhars JF, et al. An Image-Directed Robotic System for Precise Orthopaedic Surgery. *IEEE Trans on Robotics and Automation*. 1994 Jun;10(3):261–275.

[12] Mittelstadt B, Kazanzides P, Zuhars J, Williamson B, Cain P, Smith F, et al. The Evolution of a Surgical Robot from Prototype to Human Clinical Use. In: Taylor RH, Lavallée S, Burdea GC, Mösges R, editors. *Computer Integrated Surgery: Technology and Clinical Applications*. MIT Press; 1995. p. 397–407.

[13] Kazanzides P. Robot Assisted Surgery: The ROBODOC Experience. In: *Intl. Symp. on Robotics (ISR)*. vol. 30. Tokyo, Japan; 1999. p. 281–286.

[14] Kienzle III TC, Stulberg SD, Peshkin M, Quaid A, Lea J, Goswami A, et al. Total Knee Replacement: Computer-assisted surgical system uses a calibrated robot. *IEEE Engineering in Medicine and Biology*. 1995 May/Jun;14(3):301–306. Special Issue on Robots in Surgery.

[15] Marcacci M, Dario P, Fadda M, Marcenaro G, Martelli S. Computer-Assisted Knee Arthroplasty. In: Taylor RH, Lavallée S, Burdea GC, Mösges R, editors. *Computer Integrated Surgery: Technology and Clinical Applications*. MIT Press; 1995. p. 417–423.

[16] Malvisi A, Marcacci M, Martelli S, Campion G, Fiorini P. A Robotic System for Total Knee Replacement. In: *IEEE/ASME Intl. Conf. on Advanced Intelligent Mechatronics*. Como, Italy; 2001. p. 1047–1052.

[17] Jakopec M, y Baena FR, Harris SJ, Gomes P, Cobb J, Davies BL. The Hands-On Orthopaedic Robot "Acrobot": Early Clinical Trials of Total Knee Replacement Surgery. *IEEE Trans on Robotics and Automation*. 2003 Oct;19(5):902–911.

[18] Rodriguez F, Harris S, Jakopec M, Barret A, Gomes P, Henckel J, et al. Robotic clinical trials of uni-condylar arthroplasty. *Int J of Medical Robotics and Computer Assisted Surgery*. 2005 Dec;1(4):20–28.

[19] Meister D, Pokrandt P, Both A. Milling Accuracy in Robot Assisted Orthopaedic Surgery. In: *IEEE Conf. of Industrial Electronics Soc*. (IECON). Aachen, Germany; 1998. p. 2502–2505.

[20] Petermann J, Azar AP, Gotzen L. Ligament reconstruction in the knee: the use of the CASPAR system. In: Stiehl JB, Konermann WH, Haaker RG, editors. *Navigation and Robotics in Total Joint and Spine Surgery*. Springer-Verlag; 2004. p. 257–272.

[21] Kerschbaumer F, Kuenzler S, Wahrburg J. Minimally Invasive Total Hip Replacement – Application of Intraoperative Navigation and Robotics. In: Stiehl JB, Konermann WH, Haaker RG, editors. *Navigation and Robotics in Total Joint and Spine Surgery*. Springer-Verlag; 2004. p. 145–150.

[22] Brandt G, Zimolong A, Carrat L, Merloz P, Staudte HW, Lavallée S, et al. CRIGOS: a compact robot for image-guided orthopedic surgery. *IEEE Trans on Information Technology in Biomedicine*. 1999 Dec;3(4):252–260.

[23] Chung JH, Ko SY, Kwon DS, Lee JJ, Yoon YS, Won CH. Robot-Assisted Femoral Stem Implantation Using an Intramedulla Gauge. *IEEE Trans on Robotics and Automation*. 2003 Oct;19(5):885–892.

[24] Shoham M, Burman M, Zehavi E, Joskowicz L, Batkilin E, Kunicher Y. Bone-Mounted Miniature Robot for Surgical Procedures: Concept and Clinical Applications. *IEEE Trans on Robotics and Automation*. 2003 Oct;19(5):893–901.

[25] Wolf A, Jaramaz B, Lisien B, DiGioia AM. MBARS: mini bone-attached robotic system for joint arthroplasty. *Int J of Medical Robotics and Computer Assisted Surgery*. 2005 Jan;1(2):101–121.

[26] Plaskos C, Cinquin P, Lavallée S, Hodgson AJ. Praxiteles: a miniature bone-mounted robot for minimal access total knee arthroplasty. *Int J of Medical Robotics and Computer Assisted Surgery*. 2005 Dec;1(4):67–79.

[27] Ritschl P, Machacek F, Fuiko R, Zettl R, Kotten B. The Galileo System for Implantation of Total Knee Arthroplasty. In: Stiehl JB, Konermann WH, Haaker RG, editors. *Navigation and Robotics in Total Joint and Spine Surgery*. Springer-Verlag; 2004. p. 281–286.

[28] Bernardoni M, Orlandini L. A computer aided cutting guide positioner to improve bone-cutting precision in total knee arthroplasty. In: *Computer Assisted Orthopaedic Surgery (CAOS)*. Marbella, Spain; 2003.

[29] Pott P, Schwarz M, Köpfle A, Schill M, Wagner A, Badreddin E, et al. ITD - a hand-held manipulator for medical applications: concept and design. In: *Computer Assisted Orthopaedic Surgery (CAOS)*. Marbella, Spain; 2003.

[30] Devos T, Martin P, Picard FJM, Borchers M, Cabanial N, Dassier A. A hand-held computer-controlled tool for total knee replacement. In: *Computer Assisted Orthopaedic Surgery (CAOS)*. Helsinki, Finland; 2005. p. 88–89.

[31] Brisson G, Kanade T, Di Gioia AM III, Jaramaz B. Precision Freehand Sculpting of Bone. In: *MICCAI*. vol. 3217. St. Malo, France; 2004. p. 105–112.

[32] Brisson G, Jaramaz B, Di Gioia A III, Kanade T. A Handheld Robotic Tool for Less Invasive Bone Shaping. In: *Computer Assisted Orthopaedic Surgery (CAOS)*. Montreal, Canada; 2006. p. 72–75.

[33] Sugita N, Warisawa S, Mitsuishi M, Suzuki M, Moriya H, Kuramoto K. Development of a Novel Robot-Assisted Orthopaedic System Designed for Total Knee Arthroplasty. In: *MICCAI*. vol. 3217. Saint-Malo, France; 2004. p. 153–160.

[34] Maillet P, Nahum B, Blondel L, Poignet P, Dombre E. BRIGIT, a Robotized Tool Guide for Orthopedic Surgery. In: *IEEE Intl. Conf. on Robotics and Automation*. Barcelona, Spain; 2005. p. 211–216.

[35] Mantwill F, Schulz AP, Faber A, Hollstein D, Kammal M, Fay A, et al. Robotic systems in total hip arthroplasty – is the time ripe for a new approach? *Int J of Medical Robotics and Computer Assisted Surgery*. 2005 Dec;1(4):8–19.

[36] de la Fuente M, Ohnsorge JAK, Schkommodau E, Jetzki S, Wirtz DC, Radermacher K. Fluoroscopy-based 3-D reconstruction of femoral bone cement: a new approach for revision total hip replacement. *IEEE Trans on Biomedical Engin*. 2005 Apr;52(4):664–675.

[37] Picard F, Moody JE, DiGioia III AM. Clinical classification of CAOS systems. In: *Computer and Robotic Assisted Knee and Hip Surgery*. Oxford University Press; 2004. p. 43–48.

[38] Kazanzides P, Zuhars J, Mittelstadt B, Taylor RH. Force Sensing and Control for a Surgical Robot. In: *IEEE Intl. Conf. on Robotics and Automation*. Nice, France; 1992. p. 612–617.

[39] Cohan S. ROBODOC achieves pinless registration. *Industrial Robot: An Intl Journal*. 2001 Sep;28(5):381–386.

[40] Stocco L. Path Verification for Unstructured Environments and Medical Applications. In: *ASME Design Automation Conf., Symp. on Mechanisms and Devices for Medical Applications*. Pittsburgh, PA; 2001. p. 1103–1108.

[41] Zuhars J, Hsia TC. Nonhomogeneous material milling using a robot manipulator with force controlled velocity. In: *IEEE Intl. Conf. on Robotics and Automation*. vol. 2. Nagoya, Japan; 1995. p. 1461–1467.

[42] Taylor RH, Joskowicz L, Williamson B, Guéziec A, Kalvin A, Kazanzides P, et al. Computer-Integrated Revision Total Hip Replacement Surgery: Concept and Preliminary Results. *Medical Image Analysis*. 1999 Sep;3(3):301–319.

[43] Nogler M, Krismer M. Cement removal with the ROBODOC System in Total Hip Arthroplasty Stem - Revision. In: Stiehl JB, Konermann WH, Haaker RG, editors. *Navigation and Robotics in Total Joint and Spine Surgery*. Springer-Verlag; 2004. p. 151–154.

[44] Sahay A, Witherspoon LW, Bargar WL. Computer Model-Based Study for Minimally Invasive THR Femoral Cavity Preparation using the ROBODOC System. In: *Computer Assisted Orthopaedic Surgery (CAOS)*. Chicago, IL; 2004. p. 314–316.

[45] Besl PJ, McKay ND. A Method for Registration of 3-D Shapes. *IEEE Trans on Pattern Anal and Machine Intell.* 1992 Feb;14(2):239–256.

[46] Nogler M, Maurer H, Wimmer C, Gegenhuber C, Bach C, Krismer M. Knee pain caused by a fiducial marker in the medial femoral condyle: A clinical and anatomic study of 20 cases. *Acta Orthop Scand.* 2001 Oct;72(5):477–480.

[47] Nogler M, Krismer M, Haid C, Ogon M, Bach C, Wimmer C. Excessive heat generation during cutting of cement in the Robodoc hip-revision procedure. *Acta Orthop Scand.* 2001 Dec;72(6):595–599.

[48] Jerosch J, Peuker E, von Hasselbach C, Lahmer A, Filler T, Witzel U. Computer assisted implantation of the femoral stem in THA – an experimental study. *International Orthopaedics (SICOT)*. 1999 Nov;23(4):224–226.

[49] Gossé F, Wenger KH, Knabe K, Wirth CJ. Efficacy of Robot-Assisted Hip Stem Implantation. A Radiographic Comparison of Matched-Pair Femurs Prepared Manually and with the Robodoc® System Using an Anatomic Prosthesis. In: *MICCAI*. vol. 1935. Pittsburgh, PA; 2000. p. 1180–1184.

[50] Knabe K, Hurschler C, Stukenborg-Colsman C, Gossé F. An Anatomically Shaped Prosthesis Stem – In Vitro Comparison Between Robot-Assisted and Manual Implantation. In: Stiehl JB, Konermann WH, Haaker RG, editors. *Navigation and Robotics in Total Joint and Spine Surgery*. Springer-Verlag; 2004. p. 132–139.

[51] Thomsen MN, Breusch SJ, Aldinger PR, Birke A, Nägerl H. Robotically-milled bone cavities: A comparison with hand-broaching in different types of cementless hip stems. *Acta Orthop Scand.* 2002 Aug;73(4):379–385.

[52] Thomsen M. Robotically Milled Bone Cavities in Comparison with Hand-Broaching in Total Hip Replacement. In: Stiehl JB, Konermann WH, Haaker RG, editors. *Navigation and Robotics in Total Joint and Spine Surgery*. Springer-Verlag; 2004. p. 123–131.

[53] Nogler M, Polikeit A, Wimmer C, Brückner A, Ferguson SJ, Krismer M. Primary stability of a ROBODOC® implanted anatomical stem versus manual implantation. *Clinical Biomechanics.* 2004 Feb;19(2):123–129.

[54] Prymka M, Wu L, Hahne HJ, Koebke J, Hassenpflug J. The dimensional accuracy for preparation of the femoral cavity in HIP arthroplasty: A comparison between manual- and robot-assisted implantation of hip endoprosthesis stems in cadaver femurs. *Archives of Orthopaedic and Trauma Surgery*. 2006 Jan;126(1):36–44.

[55] Bargar WL, Bauer A, Börner M. Primary and Revision Total Hip Replacement using the Robodoc® System. *Clinical Orthopaedics and Related Research.* 1998 Sep;354:82–91.

[56] Bach CM, Winter P, Nogler M, Göbel G, Wimmer C, Ogon M. No functional impairment after Robodoc total hip arthroplasty: Gait analysis in 25 patients. *Acta Orthop Scand.* 2002 Aug;73(4):386–391.

[57] Hagio K, Sugano N, Takashina M, Nishii T, Yoshikawa H, Ochi T. Effectiveness of the ROBODOC system in preventing intraoperative pulmonary embolism. *Acta Orthop Scand.* 2003 Jun;74(3):264–269.

[58] Honl M, Dierk O, Gauck C, Carrero V, Lampe F, Dries S, et al. Comparison of Robotic-Assisted and Manual Implantation of a Primary Total Hip Replacement, A Prospective Study. *J of Bone and Joint Surgery.* 2003 Aug;85-A(8):1470–1478.

[59] Nakamura N, Sugano N, Nishii T, Miki H, Kakimoto A, Yamamura M. Comparison between robotic-assisted system and manual implantation of primary cementless total hip arthroplasty; A short-term result. In: *Computer Assisted Orthopaedic Surgery (CAOS).* Helsinki, Finland; 2005. p. 346–347.

[60] Börner M, Wiesel U. Clinical Experiences with ROBODOC in Total Hip Arthroplasty. In: Stiehl JB, Konermann WH, Haaker RG, editors. *Navigation and Robotics in Total Joint and Spine Surgery.* Springer-Verlag; 2004. p. 140–144.

[61] Börner M, Wiesel U, Ditzen W. Clinical Experiences with ROBODOC and the Duracon Total Knee. In: Stiehl JB, Konermann WH, Haaker RG, editors. *Navigation and Robotics in Total Joint and Spine Surgery.* Springer-Verlag; 2004. p. 362–366.

[62] Mazoochian F, Pellengahr C, Huber A, Kircher J, Refior HJ, Jansson V. Low accuracy of stem implantation in THR using the CASPAR-system. *Acta Orthop Scand.* 2004 Jun;75(3):261–264.

[63] Schneider J, Kalender W. Geometric Accuracy in Robot-Assisted Total Hip Replacement Surgery. *Computer Aided Surgery.* 2003;8(3):135–145.

[64] Bargar WL. Update on the second ROBODOC multicenter trial. In: *Computer Assisted Orthopaedic Surgery (CAOS).* Chicago, IL; 2004. p. 347–348.

[65] Siebert W, Mai S, Kober R, Heeckt PF. Technique and first clinical results of robot-assisted total knee replacement. *The Knee* 2002 Sep;9(3):173–180.

[66] Seon JK, Song EK, Yoon TR, Lee JY, Lee YS. Gap balancing in robot assisted total knee arthroplasty. In: *Computer Assisted Orthopaedic Surgery (CAOS).* Helsinki, Finland; 2005. p. 419–420.

Chapter 6

ROBOTICS IN GENERAL SURGERY

Jacques Marescaux, Ali Alzahrani and Francesco Rubino
University Louis Pasteur,
Strasbourg, France

INTRODUCTION

The motivation to develop surgical robots is rooted in the desire to overcome the limitations of current laparoscopic technologies and to expand the benefits of minimally invasive surgery. Robotic-assisted surgery in fact has been envisioned to extend the capabilities of human surgeons beyond the limits of conventional laparoscopy. With the introduction of robotic and computer technologies surgical movements and images could, for the first time, be digitized and transmitted. These information can be modified to filter and exclude non-finalized movements (i.e. physiologic tremor of the surgeon)[1] resulting in greater dexterity and higher precision[2-3]. Robotic devices that cancel physiological tremor have been used for vitreoretinal microsurgery[4]. Others have reported efficient performance of sutured coronary artery bypass anastomoses in a plastic model using robotic enhancement technology[5]. Although there are, admittedly, few cases in which such a higher degree of precision is needed in general surgery; robotic assistance has been successfully used for a large variety of procedures.

Surgical robotics however should be defined as a computer interface between the surgeon and the patient, which is often referred to as "computer-assisted surgery" (CAS).

Intrinsic properties of current surgical robots include three-dimensional view, reliability and precision and enhanced dexterity. However, current robotic systems, at least those used in general surgery are not autonomous robot but simply "master-slave" telemanipulators, where the manipulation of the masters is transmitted to a computer that filters, scales, and relays the surgeon's movements to the robotic arms. Transmission of surgical gestures through dedicated telecommunication lines can also enable performance of remote surgery where an experienced surgeon can operate on patients in a remote location and assist novice surgeons by telementoring.

In this chapter, we will review the evolution of robotic technology and its clinical applications in general surgical procedures including our personal experience at the European Institute of Telesurgery (EITS).

TELEROBOTIC SYSTEMS IN GENERAL SURGERY

The concept of telemanipulators is based on a computer console that is positioned away from the patient and robotic arms placed at operating table. The distance between the two subsystems could range between a few meters in the same room to remote distances. By 1998, two commercially available surgical robot systems emerged meeting varying levels of U.S. Food and Drug Administration (FDA) approval for human use. The two systems are "Zeus" system, developed by Computer Motion in, California, and the daVinci system, developed by Intuitive Surgical in Sunnyvale, California. Both systems cost approximately $1 million. On June 30, 2003, the two previously competing companies announced their merger. A third system called Laprotek is being developed in Boston, Massachusetts, by endoVia. This system still requires regulatory clearance by FDA .

A team from Germany, has been working on a new telerobotic system called Advanced Robotic Telemanipulator for Minimally Invasive Surgery (ARTEMIS) and demonstrated its feasibility in an experimental endoscopic surgery, but for clinical application still it requires further technical development[6].

Althgough, both Zeus and da Vinci systems were designed specifically to accomplish completely endoscopic coronary artery bypass grafting 7, they also have been used in a variety of general surgical procedures, urology, gynecology, thoracic surgery and vascular surgery.

APPLICATIONS OF ROBOTIC TECHNOLOGY IN GENERAL SURGERY

Although the technology was developed initially for use in cardiac surgery, its applications into many different surgical disciplines has expanded over the last 5 years. There are several clinical studies that have clearly demonstrated the feasibility and safety of using the surgical robots for human surgery. Our group performed robotic-assisted laparoscopic cholecystectomy in 25 patients with no robot-related morbidity and with operative time and patient recovery similar to those of conventional laparoscopy[8]. Although our results, consistent with other's reports, did not demonstrate obvious advantages to the patient over conventional laparoscopy, we were able to predict that the potential advantages of computer assisted surgery lie into the inherent ability to convert a surgical gesture into digitized data. This digitized format can then interface with other forms of digitized data, such as pre or intraoperative imaging studies, or be transmitted over a distance.

Cadiere and coworkers reported robot-assisted laparoscopic antireflux procedures, gastroplasties, inguinal hernias, prostatectomies[9]. Falcone et al.[10] reported successful robotic assistance for reversal of tubal ligation using 8-0 sutures. In these published experiences, there was no morbidity related to the use of the robotic system, however, there is a common feeling that robotic assistance is most beneficial when microsuturing within the abdomen or in very confined spaces. Other areas of general surgery in which robotic technology has been applied include mainly Nissen fundoplication, obesity surgery, colorectal surgery, pancreatic surgery, esophageal surgery and adrenalectomy. Complex procedures such as esophagectomy, rectal resections, pancreatico-duodenectomy and gastric cancer surgery have been performed using the DaVinci robotic system, in different centers. Giulianotti, et al.[11], reported 13 robotic assisted laparoscopic pancreatic procedures for benign and malignant pathology. Pancreaticoduodenectomy was performed in 8 patients and distal panceatectomy in 5. The mean operative time in the robotic cases was 490 minutes (range, 360-660 minutes) for pancreatoduodenectomy and 270 minutes (range, 210-360 minutes) for distal pancreatectomy, compared to an average of 250 minutes and 170 minutes respectively, in their open experience for the same type of procedures. Morbidity and mortality of robotic-assisted pancreaticoduodenectomy were 37.5% and 12.5%, respectively (32.1% and 5.6% in open surgery), and 20% and 0% in robotic-assisted distal pancreatectomy (28.5% and 0% in open surgery). The mean postoperative hospital stay was similar in both the robotic and open pancreatic surgery. The use of robotics might have also potential benefits in rectal surgery (nerve sparing total mesorectal excision) when dealing with a deep and narrow pelvis, or when intracorporeal anastomoses are required.

BENEFITS AND LIMITATIONS OF ROBOTIC-ASSISTED SURGERY

The potential advantages of robotic systems are numerous because they overcome many of the inherent problems of laparoscopic surgery and still offer the patient all the benefits of minimally invasive surgery. They enhance dexterity and improve the surgeon's precision by computerizing the movement of the surgical instruments and creating a software program that controls the relationship between instrument's handle (master), at the surgeon's console and the tip inside the patient .This program incorporates algorithms like filtering the tremors and scaling the motion to increase precision and dexterity. Instruments with more degrees of freedom can greatly enhance the surgeon's ability to manipulate the tissues through these instruments and further improve the dexterity. Another important advantage is improved ergonomics. The surgeon sits comfortable at a remote console, without the need to twist and turn in awkward positions to move the instruments and visualize the monitor as in laparoscopic surgery. The 3-dimensional view with depth perception may be another improvement over the conventional laparoscopic 2-D camera views.

With currently available robotic systems there are, however, several disadvantages. Virtually in any kind of application in general surgery, so far, robotic assistance typically requires longer operative time compared to conventional laparoscopy, although this drawback might possibly be corrected, at least in part, with experience of the surgical team.

Furthermore, at this early stage of technology, the robotic systems are very expensive. Indeed, the cost of this technology makes it difficult to propose robotic assistance for standard laparoscopic procedures. It is possible that with improvements in technology the cost will fall. Table 1 summarizes current benefits and limitations of robotic technology in general surgery.

Table 1. Benefits and limits of current robotic systems

Benefits	Limits
o Ergonomy	o Lack of reliable force feedback
o Voice-controlled camera holder (ZEUS)	o No automatic-tool changer
o 3D visualisation	o Fewer energy-directed instruments than in conventional laparoscopy
o Dexterity (ambidextrous)	
o Precision (tremor-filtring scaling)	o Cost
o Range of motion (6° of freedom)	o Ethical issues
	o Lack of evidence-based clinical data

REMOTE TELESURGERY

A unique aspect of robotic-assisted surgery is the ability of the surgeon to operate while separated from the operative field. Through telecommunication lines, digitized information can be transmitted to distant locations, enabling surgeons to operate on patients located remotely. Telesurgery or telepresence surgery combines the advances of telecommunications with robotic technology. Surgery could be carried out in remote locations where there are a lack of surgical expertise (from battlefields to developing nations) or to assist or teach new surgical procedures.

Challenges to this concept are many, but the most important limitations have been the reliability (or quality of service) of the telecommunication lines and the issue of latency (the delay time from when the hand motion is initiated by the surgeon until the remote manipulator actually moves and the image is shown on the surgeon's monitor). Our preliminary studies estimated in about 300 milliseconds (ms), the maximum time delay compatible with safe performance of surgical manipulations and we measured a mean time delay of 155 ms over transoceanic distances[12,13] when using dedicated terrestrial optical fibers. On September 7th 2001, our group performed the world's first human long-distance operation using then Zeus surgical system (Computer Motion Inc, Santa Barbara, CA), between New York, NY (USA) and Strasbourg, (France), demonstrating the feasibility and safety of performing a complete surgical procedure from a remote location. The two sites were connected through a high-speed terrestrial optical fibre network (FranceTelecom/Equant) that transports data through dedicated connections using "Asynchronous Transfer Mode" (ATM) technology. A bandwidth of 10Mb/s was reserved through network interconnecting applications at both sites using a Network Termination Unit (NTU), which provides a "multiservice" path to different applications. Round trip delay by ATM transport ranged between 78 and 80 ms. Adding 70 ms for video coding and decoding, plus a few milliseconds for rate adaptation and Ethernet to ATM packet conversion, motions done by the surgeon in NY were perceived within 155ms on his video screen in NY.

More recently, Anvari and colleagues reported the establishment of a remote telerobotic surgical service between a teaching hospital (St. Joseph's Hospital in Hamilton, Canada) and a community hospital (North Bay General Hospital) more than 400 km away[14]. Nissen fundoplications, sigmoid resections, right hemicolectomies, anterior resection, and inguinal hernia repairs have been carried out with this technology. The telesurgical robotic system used was the Zeus TS microjoint system. The telecommunication link was provided by a commercially available IP/VPN (Internet Protocol-Virtual Private Network) network with QOS (Quality of Service) used to link the 2 hospitals at a bandwidth of 15 Mbps. This service includes an active line and a fully redundant (active backup) line enabling the telerobotic surgeon to use the second line immediately if there is a failure of the first line. There were no major intraoperative complications or problems related to the telecommunication lines, except for a temporary disturbance in signal transmission during the first case. The disruption was so short in duration that there was no impact on the course of surgery, as the telerobotic surgeon was able to use the second telecommunication line. The results from this study corroborate our findings with the Lindberg operation and encouraged these authors to plan a Surgical Support Network for provision of telementoring, and telerobotic surgery between 8 teaching hospitals and 32 rural communities in Canada over the next 3 years.

There are still several limitations for routine performance of remote telesurgery.

Today, the cost of remote teleoperations is one of the main issues. The robotic machines cost approximately $1 million. For our research development other significant costs were involved such as the use of telecommunication lines and human resources, including several professionals, such as surgeons, computer scientists, and engineers. Of course, the costs of remote surgery when performed on a routine basis would have to cover solely the cost of the robotic machine and the teletransmission. It is difficult at present to give an exact estimate of the cost of the telecommunication component, because this varies depending on the distance and location of the sites connected (i.e., transoceanic connections would reasonably be more expensive than connections within the same continent or country).

It seems reasonable however, that if remote surgery achieves the goals of increasing access to healthcare and improving training and efficiency with enhanced outcomes, it may prove less costly to healthcare systems. The cost of technologies is also expected to decrease with time.

The lack of face-to-face contact between the patient and the surgeon is an important aspect of telesurgery that might be an issue in malpractice actions. Because telesurgery may involve more than one state or country, conflicts of jurisdictions may also arise. Other legal issues also need to be addressed, such as whether the surgeon should or not be liable for errors related to delays in transmission or equipment failure or whether a special consent should be obtained, and who is the person responsible for it.

The possibility to have active intervention from remote locations opens new avenues for surgical education. Telesurgery can in fact significantly improve outcomes through teaching and mentoring in order to reduce the learning curve of surgeons for new procedures, thus possibly help better standardizing surgical care throughout the world. Telesurgery could also be an opportunity for cost-savings. For instance, it has been estimated that between 44,000 and 98,000 deaths annually occur due to errors in hospital care and that as much as 54% of surgical errors could be prevented [15]. Through the ability to provide active intervention of remote experts, robotics may well reduce the learning curve effect on errors and reduce morbidity and its related costs. Many surgical procedures indeed still depend on the operator's skills and experience and that the learning curve significantly influences outcomes.

One example for all is rectal cancer surgery, where it has been demonstrated that surgeon's skills and experience represent the most important prognostic factor[16].

THE IMPACT OF VIRTUAL REALITY TECHNOLOGIES IN ROBOTIC ASSISTED SURGERY

Implementation of virtual reality (VR) and simulation in robotic surgery may create additional and significant opportunities to improve surgical care.

Virtual reality indeed provides a safe training environment where errors can be made without consequences to a patient and the learning process is based upon learning the cause of failure. VR can be used to improve the teaching of surgical anatomy, in particular when dealing with an inner anatomic structure of a complex and non-transparent organ such as the liver. These systems are capable to continuously track the hand motions as well as the trainee's actions allowing for real-time monitoring and displaying of the student's skills. Skills as well as precision and appropriateness of the student's actions can therefore be analysed to monitor individual's improvement. VR can be used to reach and teach trainees in distant locations. Silverstein et al.[17] used a teleimmersive virtual reality environment for simultaneously teaching liver segments and portal vein anatomy to senior surgical residents at two different locations. Authors reported effective acquisition of the new knowledge with no difference between those residents who were with the instructor and those at the remote location as shown by a 24-questions examination test administered prior and after the anatomy workshop.

A further application of VR is the preoperative simulation and planning of robotic assisted procedures. Combining virtual laparoscopy with a virtual ZEUS robotic system we are currently experimenting the possibility to simulate the surgical gestures required for a specific procedure in a given patient with the system able to process these informations and anticipate possible conflict between robotic arms and therefore helping planning the ideal robotic arm positioning for a smoother operation.

Augmented reality (AR) is a technology that allows superimposing computer-generated images on the real vision of the world in a real-time. Thus, the 3-D reconstruction can be superimposed on the real patient for providing additional help and make inner structures visible on the surface, for instance, of the liver through a virtual transparency. At the EITS we have developed our own real-time augmented reality system for hepatic surgery. Two cameras provide a 3D video view of the physical model; by superimposing the virtual model we obtain a virtual transparency of the physical model. Images are then displayed on a head-mounted displayer that combines the virtual and real images. We have preliminary used AR in experimental simulation of radiofrequency ablation in both plastic and animal models with promising results. This research prompted us to perform the first augmented reality-assisted operation in general surgery. Indeed, we recently reported the first image-guided interactive laparoscopic adrenalectomy in humans, using AR technology[18]. The AR was generated from pre-operative CT-derived 3D images of intra-abdominal organs, manipulated by an independent operator in real-time from a distant site through a fibre-optic network. Seven different visible anatomical landmarks were used for registration of the virtual and the real image. Visible landmarks were chosen on the skin (ribs margin, and three trocar sites) and inside the abdomen (inferior vena cava and two laparoscopic tools). Thus, virtual images of the adrenal gland, tumour and blood vessels were superimposed onto the conventional laparoscopic view in real-time. AR accurately predicted the exact site of the adrenal vein and led to its safe isolation through a virtual transparency of the fatty tissue in which it was embedded.

Potential advantages of the intraoperative use of AR include the adaptation of dissection planes or resection margins and the avoidance of injury to invisible structures. AR could aid the novice surgeon to identify and dissect critical anatomic landmarks as well as be used for a more interactive form of telementoring by a distant expert. Applied to robotic assisted surgery, AR might improve efficacy of robotic procedures and help perfect preoperative planning and simulation with the final goal to rehearse the procedure, digitize gestures and replicate the "best performance" automatically by using a robotic system. This process may lead to the automation of surgical procedures, especially simple, yet invasive procedures such as percutaneous techniques (i.e. radiofrequency liver tumors ablation).

THE FUTURE OF ROBOTIC TECHNOLOGY IN GENERAL SURGERY

Robotic surgery is evidently still in its infancy and not at all cost effective, at least in general surgery and with currently available robotic systems. However, robotic surgery has a very promising future if the technology will allow to go beyond some of the current issues and allow to implement all the conceptual advantages of robotics. Indeed, developments that facilitate remote surgery and that can make this technology widely available are likely going to boost this type of practice with potential benefits for standardization of surgical care and surgical education. There is no doubt, that significant changes and improvement are needed to fully exploit the advantages of robotic surgery, that is, in general to improve human capabilities. The solution lies in the development of the concept of computer-assisted surgery and implementation of novel imaging technologies such as virtual and augmented reality with robotic mechanics. With further development of these concepts and of technology, the use of automation and miniaturization features, robotic surgery may indeed prove more efficient than conventional approaches in general surgery.

REFERENCES

1. Garcia-Ruiz A, Gagner M, Miller JH, Steiner CP, Hahn JF. Manual vs robotically assisted laparoscopic surgery in the performance of basic manipulation and suturing tasks. *Archives of Surgery* 1998 Sep; 133(9): 957-61.

2. Damiano RJ Jr, Ehrman WJ, Ducko CT, Tabaie HA, Stephenson ER Jr, Kingsley CP, Chambers CE. Initial United States clinical trial of robotically assisted endoscopic coronary artery bypass grafting. *Journal of Thoracic and Cardiovasular Surgery* 2000 Jan; 119(1): 77-82.

3. Reichenspurner H, Boehm D, Reichart B. Minimally invasive mitral valve surgery using three-dimensional video and robotic assistance. *Seminars in Thoracic and Cardiovascular Surgery* 1999 Jul; 11(3): 235-40.

4. Gomez-Blanco M, Riviere CN, Khosla PK. Intraoperative tremor monitoring for vitreoretinal microsurgery. *Studies in Health Technology and Informatics* 2000; 70: 99-101.

5. Garcia-Ruiz A, Smedira NG, Loop FD, Hahn JF, Miller JH, Steiner CP, Gagner M. Robotic surgical instruments for dexterity enhancement in thoracoscopic coronary artery bypass graft. *Journal of Laparoendoscopic Advanced Surgical Techniques* 1997; 7(5): 277-8.

6. Schurr MO, Buess G, Neisius B, Voges U. Robotics and telemanipulation technologies for endoscopic surgery. A review of the ARTEMIS project. Advanced Robotic Telemanipulator for Minimally Invasive Surgery. *Surgical Endoscopy* 2000 Apr ; 14(4): 375-81.

7. Falk V, Diegler A, Walther T, Autschbach R, Mohr FW. Developments in robotic cardiac surgery . *Current Opinion in Cardiology* 2000; 15(6): 378-387.

8. Marescaux J, Smith MK, Folscher D, Jamali F, Malassagne B, Leroy J. Telerobotic laparoscopic cholecystectomy: initial clinical experience with 25 patients. *Annals of Surgery* 2001; 234(1): 1-7.

9. Cadiere GB, Himpens J, Germay O, Izizaw R, Degueldre M, Vandromme J, Capelluto E, Bruyns J. Feasibility of robotic laparoscopic surgery: 146 cases. *World Journal of Surgery* 2001; 25(11): 1467-77.

10. Falcone T, Goldberg JM, Margossian H, Stevens L. Robotic-assisted laparoscopic microsurgical tubal anastomosis: a human pilot study. *Fertility and Sterility* 2000; 73(5): 1040-2.

11. Pier Cristforo Giulianotti, et al. Robotics in General Surgery Personal Experience in a Large Community Hospital. *Archives of Surgery* 2003; 138(7): 777-784.

12. Marescaux J, Leroy J, Gagner M, Rubino F, Mutter D, Vix M, Butner SE, Smith MK. Transatlantic robot-assisted telesurgery. *Nature* 2001; 413(6854): 379-80.

13. Marescaux J, Leroy J, Rubino F, Smith M, Vix M, Simone M, Mutter D. Transcontinental robot-assisted remote telesurgery: feasibility and potential applications. *Annals of Surgery* 2002; 235(4): 487-92.

14. Anvari, M, McKinley C, Stein H. Establishment of the World's First Telerobotic Remote Surgical Service: For Provision of Advanced Laparoscopic Surgery in a Rural Community. *Annals of surgery* 2005 Mar; 241(3): 460 – 464.

15. Kohn LT, Corrigan JM, Donaldson MS. To err is human: building a safer health system. Washington, DC: *National Academy Press*, 1999.

16. McArdle CS, Hole D. Impact of variability among surgeons on postoperative morbidity and mortality and ultimate survival. *British Medical Journal* 1991 Jun; 302(6791):1501-5.

17. Silverstein JC, Dech F, Edison M, Jurek P, Helton WS, Espat NJ. Virtual reality: immersive hepatic surgery educational environment. *Surgery* 2002; 132(2):274-7.

18. Marescaux J, Rubino F, et al. Augmented-reality-assisted laparoscopic adrenalectomy. *JAMA*. 2004 Nov 10; 292(18): 2214-5.

In: Robotics in Surgery: History, Current and Future Applications ISBN 1-60021-386-3
Editor: Russell A. Faust, pp. 105-135 © 2007 Nova Science Publishers, Inc.

Chapter 7

THE ROLE OF ROBOTICS IN UROLOGIC SURGERY

Sanjeev Kaul[1], Gabriel P Haas[2] and Mani Menon[3]
[1] Vattikuti Urology Institute, Henry Ford Hospital
2700 West Grand Boulevard, K-9, Detroit, MI USA
[2] State University of New York Upstate Medical University
Department of Urology, 750 East Adams Street, Syracuse, NY USA
[3] Vattikuti Urology Institute, Henry Ford Hospital, Detroit, MI, USA
[3] Case Western Reserve University, Cleveland, Ohio, USA

INTRODUCTION

Minimally invasive urologic surgery using the da Vinci surgical system is being increasing embraced by the surgeon and patient alike. Robot assisted operations offer the surgeon outstanding visualization of anatomy with magnification and depth perception. The increased degrees of freedom of movement provide improved access to difficult locations and greater precision in tissue handling. The surgeon benefits from decreased fatigue while the patient is the recipient of all the advantages of minimally invasive surgery such as less post operative pain, less analgesic requirement, earlier discharge, quicker recovery and early return to work. These advantages have resulted in rapid acceptance of the da Vinci surgical system. There has been an exponential proliferation of the number of robots installed as well as the number of procedures performed in the United States and abroad. This chapter will summarize the state of the art in urologic robotic surgery describing the procedures and expected outcomes.

THE ROBOT

A robot is broadly defined as a mechanical device that is controlled using a computer system. There are two broad classifications of surgical robots; offline and online. The offline robots, which include the "Probot"[1], "Neuromate"[2] and "Robodoc"[3] were preprogrammed to perform repetitive automatic movements under computer control, without human intervention. These systems are mostly used in Neurosurgery and Orthopedics to perform specific limited tasks. Online robots are mechanical devices that are controlled primarily by the surgeon through a computer interface. These robots, which include the Zeus Telepresence system and the da Vinci surgical system[4,5], are different in that they are two component systems; a control console that is under human control and a mechanical effector device that reproduces the control movements within the body.

Computer Motion, the company that designed and marketed the Zeus system merged with Intuitive Surgicals, makers of the da Vinci, in 2003. Subsequently, further manufacture of the Zeus system has been discontinued; however existing systems are still in use in some institutions.

The da Vinci System uses a kinematic structure, permitting the surgeon to use open surgical "intuitive" movements while maintaining the benefits of minimally invasive access. The instruments are capable of 7 degrees of freedom; (yaw, pitch, insertion, rotation), and an additional 3 degrees of freedom are delivered by the EndoWrist Instruments. The da Vinci System incorporates a natural stereoscopic vision which uses two independent cameras to provide independent right and left eye images which are superimposed to give a 3D image.

PROSTATE CANCER

Prostate cancer remains the most common non- skin cancer in men in 2005 and the second leading cause of cancer mortality[6]. It is estimated that 232,090 new cases of prostate cancer will be diagnosed in the United states in 2005; 83% present with clinically localized stage, for whom 5 year survival approaches 100%[6]. Patients with localized disease are commonly treated with surgery, radiation therapy or cryotherapy. The patients usually determine their own treatment choice based on physician advice and patient preference. Although the overall survival may be similar for each approach, the morbidity of therapy and the effect on the patients quality of life may vary significantly depending on the chosen treatment strategy. As a result, patients' select their treatment based on their desire for minimally invasive treatment, cancer control and preservation of continence and erectile function. Historically, radical prostatectomy has been associated with significant blood loss, prolonged recovery, loss of potency and poor urinary continence. Walsh's description of the anatomy of the dorsal vein complex and cavernous nerves and subsequent elucidation of the anatomical nerve sparing radical prostatectomy has revolutionized surgical treatment of organ confined prostate cancer, decreasing post operative morbidity and improving both oncologic results and post operative potency[7]. However recovery following open surgery was prolonged and there was a need for development of minimally invasive alternatives. By the 1990's, laparoscopic operations in general, gained acceptance for their minimally invasive alternative to open surgery. In 2000, Guillonneau and Vallencian[8] reported on the feasibility of Laparoscopic radical prostatectomy. Despite the outpouring of enthusiasm, the operation remained difficult to perform, lengthy, physically demanding, and associated with a steep learning curve[9]. While a few surgeons with extensive experience have been able to master the technique with relative ease, others continued to struggle, keeping this surgery beyond the scope of the average urologist. The introduction of the da Vinci brought laparoscopic surgery within the repertoire of the non laparoscopic surgeon. Abbou[10], Pasticier[11] and Binder[12] independently performed successful robot assisted radical prostatectomy and reported their anecdotal experience in 2000. Dr Menon from the Vattikuti Urology Institute developed and popularized the technique of robotic radical prostatectomy (Vattikuti Institute prostatectomy).[13-15] Over 1800 procedures have been performed to date at the Vattikuti Urology Institute.

TECHNICAL CONSIDERATIONS (ROBOTIC RADICAL PROSTATECTOMY)

There are two approaches to robotic radical prostatectomy; transperitoneal and extraperitoneal.

1. Transperitoneal technique (Vattikuti Institute Prostatectomy)[16]

The transperitoneal approach to Robotic radical prostatectomy was developed and popularized by Menon et al. at the Vattikuti Urology Institute. It differs from the original Montsouris technique in that the dissection proceeds in an antegrade manner and the first step is transection of the bladder neck. This permits all subsequent dissection to proceed in the direction of telescope vision in an antegrade fashion.

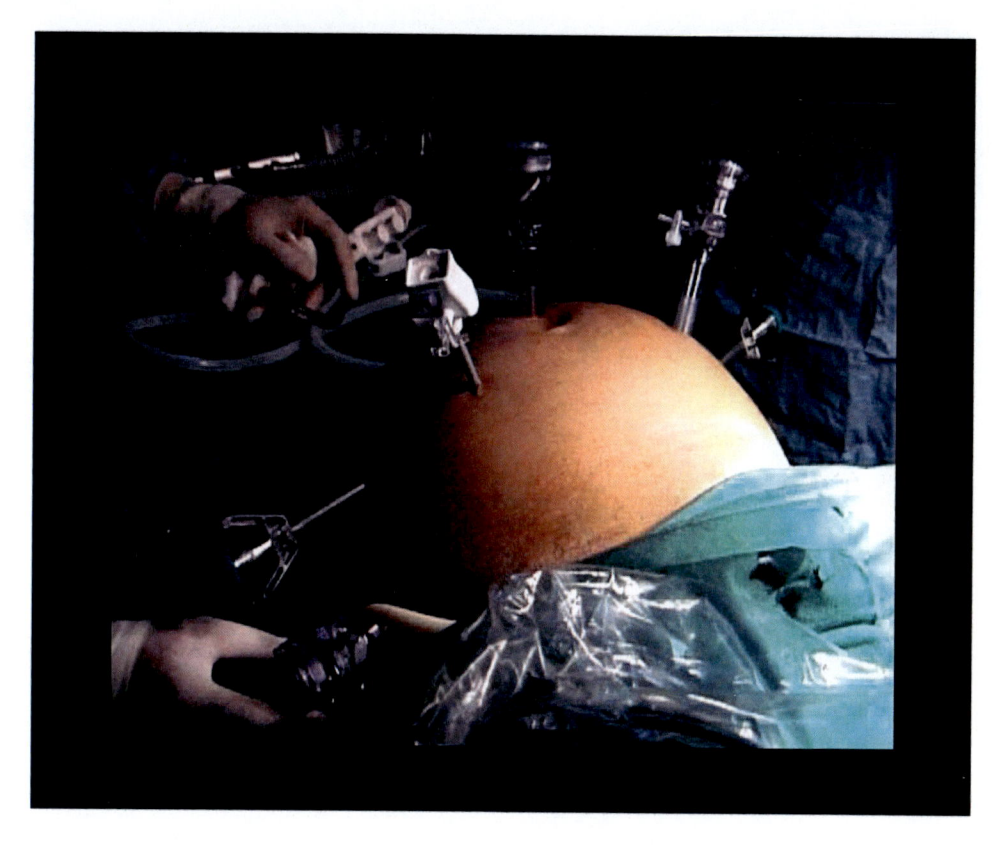

The patient is placed supine, strapped to the table and placed in steep (45 degrees) Trendelenberg position. A total of 6 ports are used in an inverted V shaped configuration. The veress needle is used to establish the pneumoperitoneum and a 12mm port is placed to the left of the umbilicus (camera port). A 30 degree up lens is then used to place the remaining ports under direct vision; two 8mm ports placed as mirror images of each other, 10 to 12 cm from the camera port and two finger breadths below it. Two ports are placed in the right lower quadrant, a lateral 12mm port just superior to the right anterior superior iliac spine for retraction and passage of sutures and a medial 5mm port for suction and irrigation midway between and slightly inferior to the umbilicus and right robotic port. Finally a 5mm left lateral port is placed as a mirror image of its right sided counterpart **(Fig 1)**. The robot is then docked and the robotic instrument ports and the camera port are fixed to the arms of the robot. This procedure takes approximately 15 minutes.

A. Visualization of the Operative field: A celioscopy is performed to identify and lyse adhesions and mobilize the sigmoid colon.

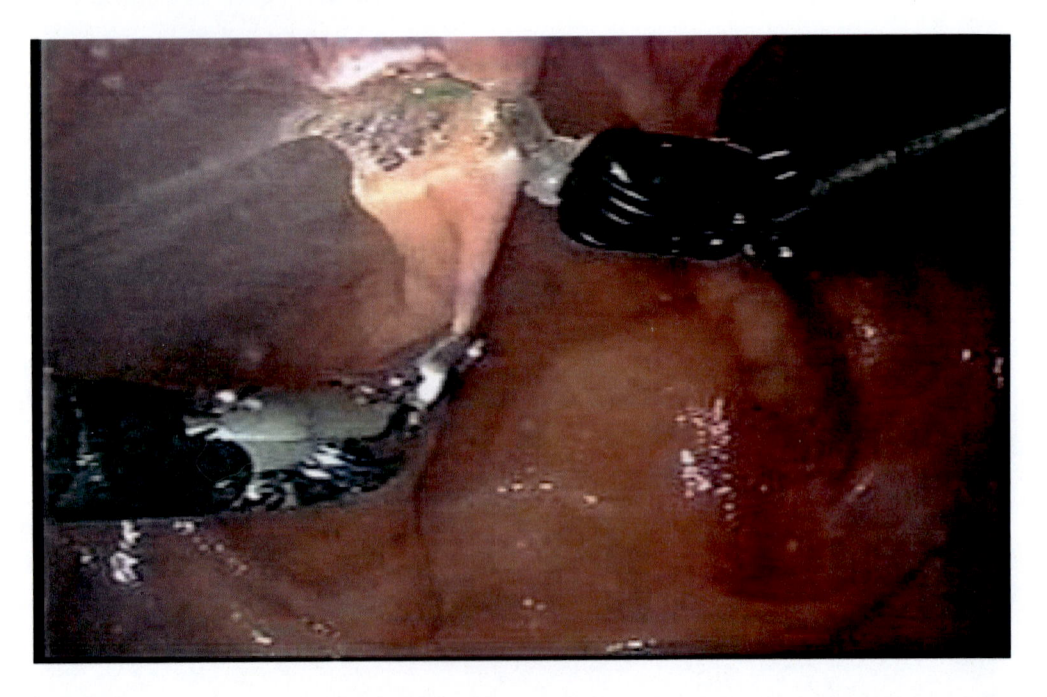

B. Mobilization of the Bladder: (Fig 2) This step is performed using a 30-degree upward-looking lens. A transverse peritoneal incision is made extending from the left to the right medial umbilical ligament and extended in an inverted U shaped manner to the level of the vasa on either side. The space of Retzius is developed after transecting the medial and median umbilical ligaments. This dissection allows the bladder, prostate and bowel to drop and the remainder of the operation to be performed in the extraperitoneal space.

C. Lymph node dissection: (Fig 3) A 0-degree lens is used for optimum visualization and 1:3 scaling is used for added precision. Lymphadenectomy is performed as indicated. A round tip scissors and a bipolar Maryland forceps are used for the dissection. The assistant holds the nodal package with an atraumatic laparoscopic grasper and the tissue overlying the external iliac vein is incised and lymph nodal package pushed medially. The limits of the dissection are the external iliac vein superiorly, the femoral canal distally, the obturator nerve inferiorly and the bifurcation of the common iliac vein proximally. The dissection starts at the lymph node of Cloquet at the femoral canal and continues toward the bifurcation of iliac vessels. The obturator nerve lies on the floor of this dissection and is carefully preserved. The magnification allows us to identify the vascular and lymphatic branches, including occasional accessory obturator vessels, which are carefully controlled by bipolar forceps or small clips. The lymph node package is removed through the 12 mm port and sent for permanent section; The nodal package is sent for frozen section only if the nodes appear enlarged.

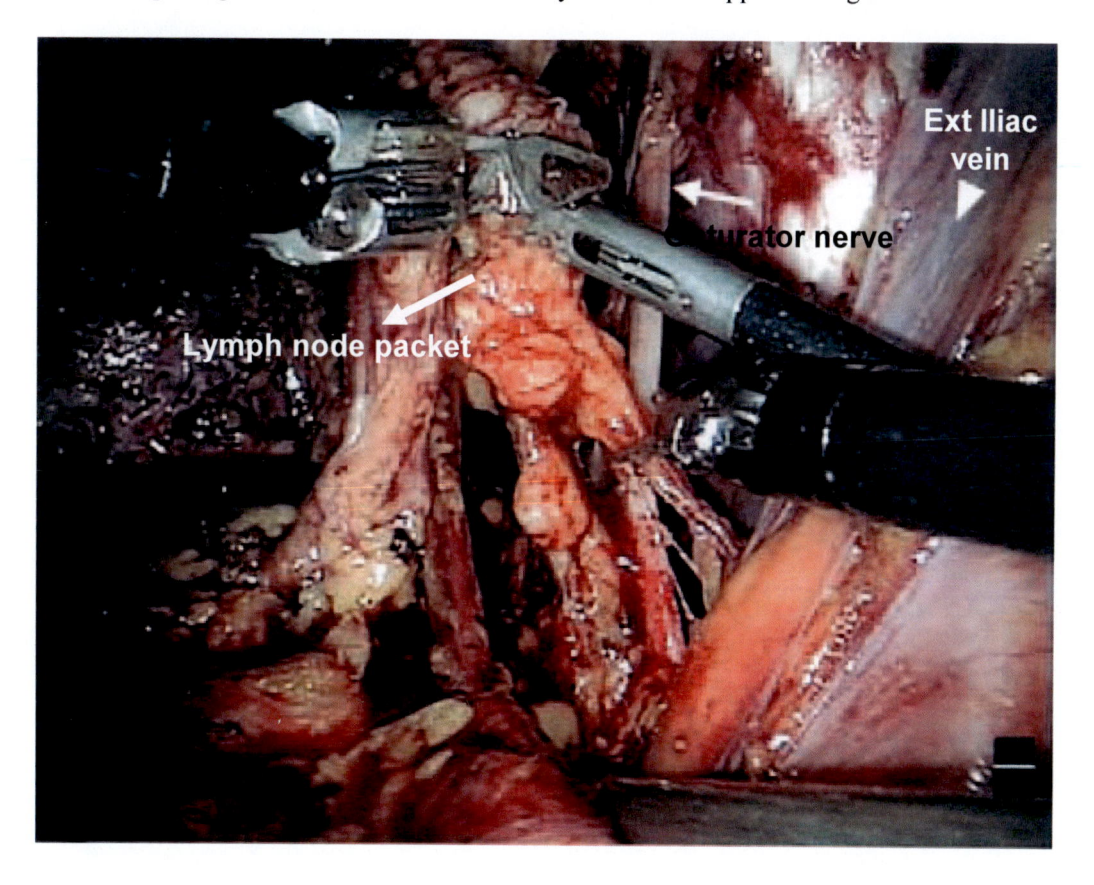

D. Exposure of prostatic apex and endopelvic fascia: The 0-degree lens with 1:2 scaling is used for this part of the dissection. This fascia is incised using the da Vinci™ hook. Once incised, no additional electrocautery is utilized. The forceps is used to provide medial countertraction on the prostate and the hook is used to bluntly dissect the levator fascia off the prostatic surface. The posterior limit of dissection is the perirectal fat with the neurovascular bundles, seen running longitudinally to the apex. Dissection is carried distally until the urethra with the surrounding puboperinealis muscle is exposed and proximally until the prostatovesical junction is identified by a prominent lip of adipose tissue; the perivesical fat.

E. Control of the Dorsal vein complex: (Fig 4) The 1:2 scale setting is used for this step. A figure-of-8 stitch is placed around the dorsal venous complex using a 6-inch long1-0 polyglactin suture on a CT-1 36 mm. taper needle. Alternatively the dorsal vein may be oversewn with a 2-0 vicryl suture on a RB-1 needle after dissection of the prostatic apex and division of the urethra. Perineal pressure provided by the assistant is helpful while placing the sutures around the dorsal vein complex.

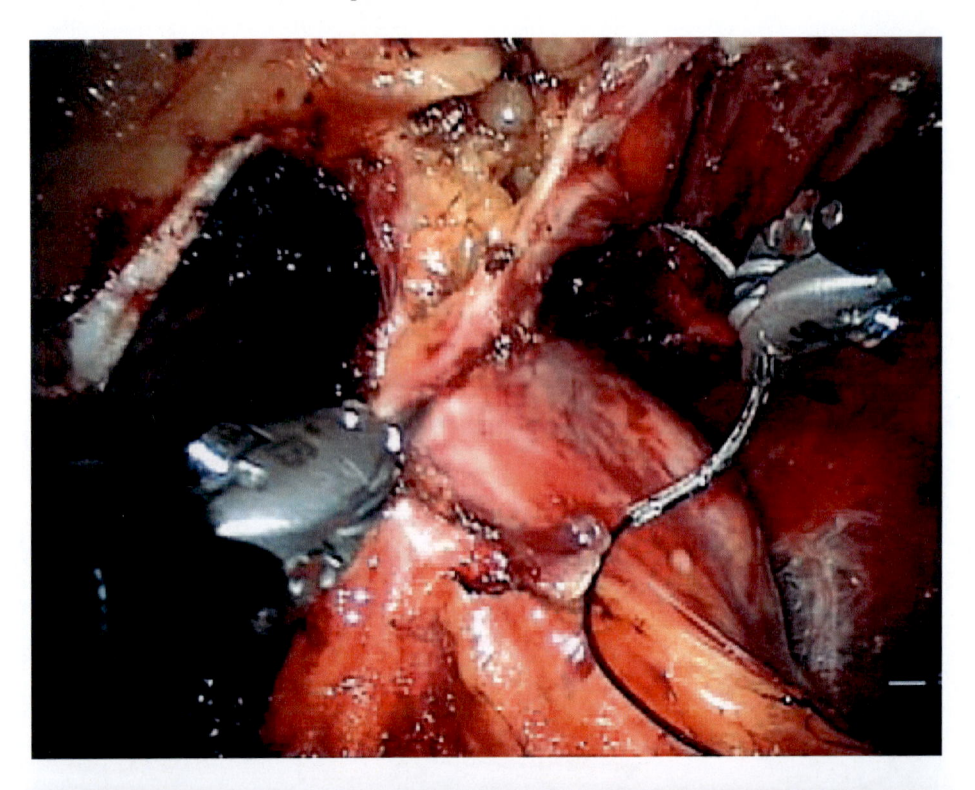

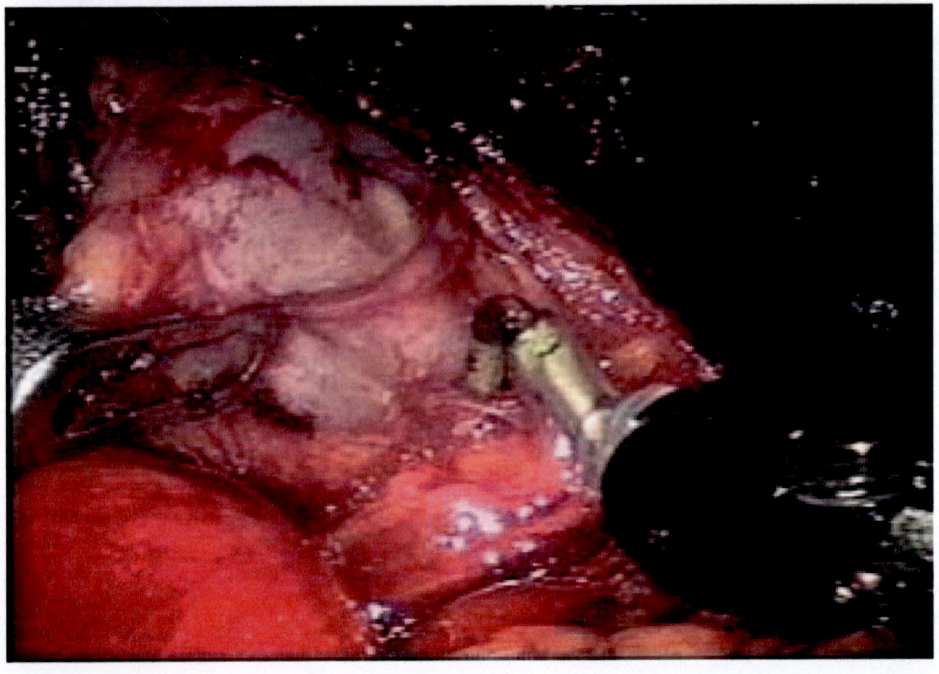

F. Bladder neck transection: (Fig 5) The assistant provides vertical traction on the anterior wall of the bladder. The balloon of the Foley's catheter is deflated to highlight the junction of the prostate and the bladder. The monopolar hook is used to incise the bladder at the prostatovesical junction till the foley's catheter is seen. The open bladder is surveyed to rule out the presence of a median lobe and determine the position of the ureteral orifices. The assistant then retracts the catheter to provide counter traction as the posterior bladder wall is cut taking care to stay well clear of the ureteral orifices. The bladder neck is not preserved and the bladder neck incision is made elliptical so that the posterior lip is slightly longer than the anterior lip. This maneuver helps in better visualization of the posterior suture line during anastomosis. Others with less experience may find it useful to place a urethral sound or traction on the catheter to identify the bladder neck junction. Using the da Vinci® Maryland forceps the surgeon grasps the cut end of the posterior bladder neck in the midline and gradually dissects it away from the prostate. The anterior layer of Denonvilliers' fascia is now exposed. It is incised, exposing the vasa and seminal vesicles. At this point the left assistant retracts the posterior lip of the prostate anteriorly whereas the right assistant depresses the bladder posteriorly. This provides a clear operative field for dissection of the vas and seminal vesicles. The vasa are transected and the seminal vesicles are skeletonized, avoiding damage to the neurovascular bundles. It is important to keep the plane of dissection as close to the surface of the seminal vesicles as possible to prevent damage to the pelvic plexus which is closely applied to the seminal vesicles laterally. Several arterioles to the seminal vesicles are encountered and require coagulation and division.

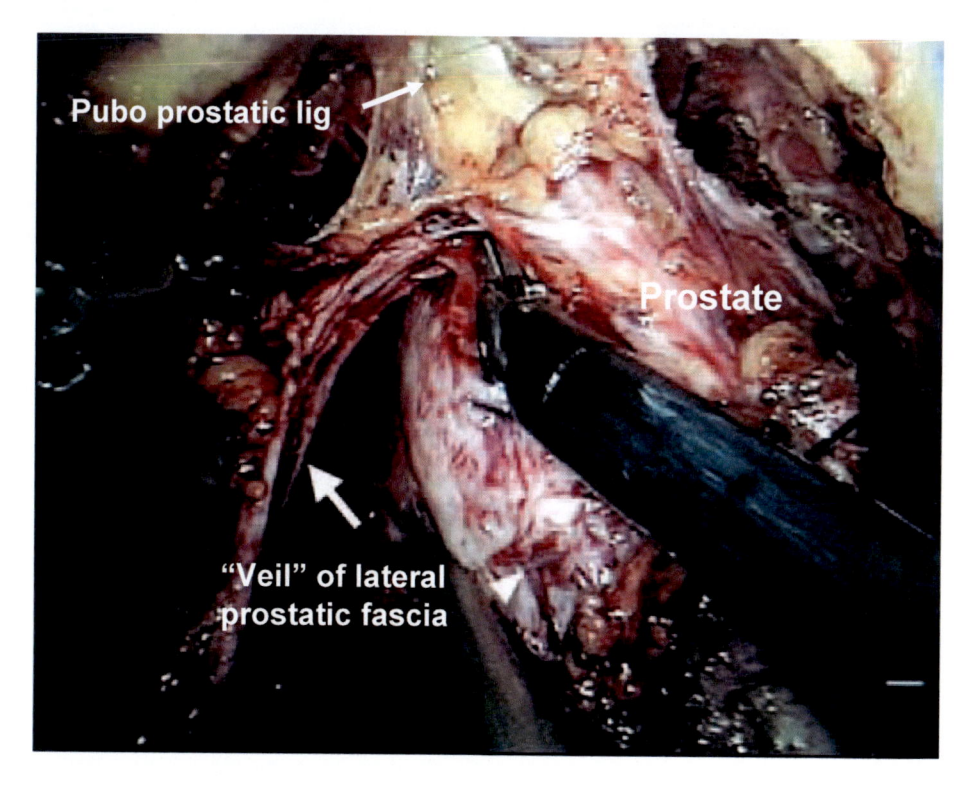

G. Posterior dissection: Once the seminal vesicles are freed the left assistant retracts the seminal vesicles anteriorly. At this point the posterior layer of Denonvilliers' fascia can be seen between the two lateral prostatic pedicles. This fascia is incised close to the prostate and a plane is developed between the prostate anteriorly and the rectum posteriorly. The plane of dissection leaves the most posterior layer(s) of Denonvilliers' fascia on the rectum and the perirectal fat well visualized. This dissection is carried down to the apex of the prostate.

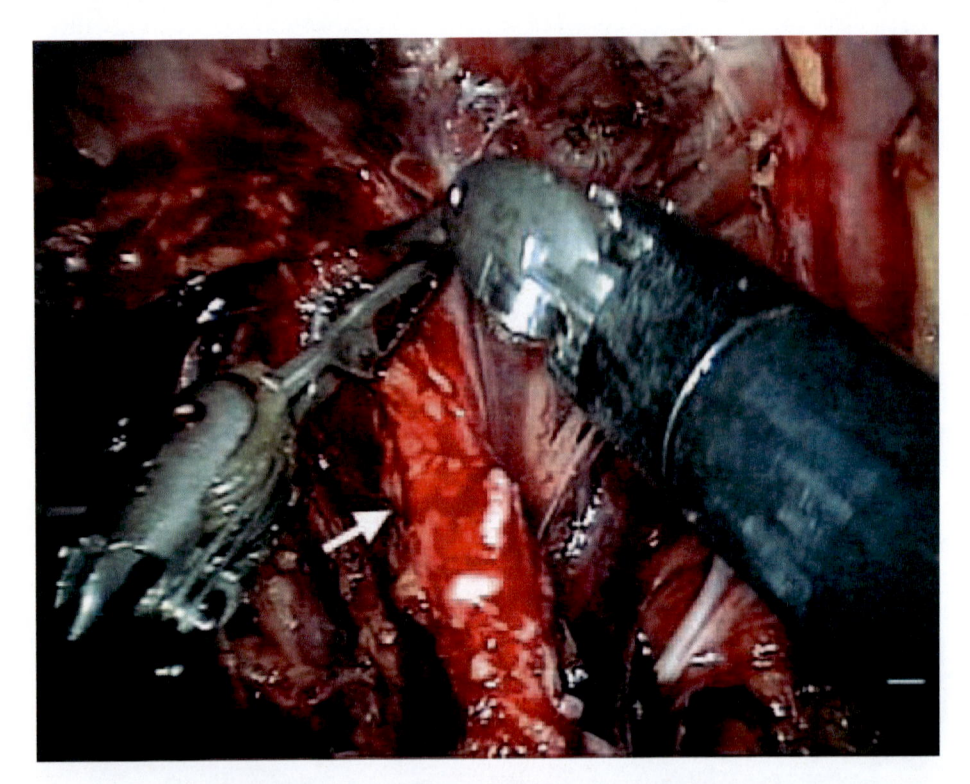

H. Preservation of Neurovascular bundles: (Fig 6 & 7) The lateral pedicles at the prostate vesical junction are controlled using Hem-o-lock™ clips and bipolar coagulation. The clips are applied close to the prostate and the pedicle is divided between them. Once the dissection enters the plane between the prostatic fascia medially and the levator fascia laterally electrocautery is avoided and the anterior nerve sparing dissection proceeds using sharp cutting with scissors and bipolar coagulation as necessary. Small arterioles entering the substance of the prostate are coagulated with bipolar forceps and divided with scissors. This dissection proceeds to the apex of the prostate distally.

I. Incision of the dorsal venous complex and urethra: (Fig 8) This is the final step of the dissection. Using a 0-degree lens with 1:2 scaling, the ligated dorsal venous complex is incised tangential to the prostate to avoid capsular incision. A plane between urethra and dorsal venous complex is gently developed to expose the anterior urethral wall. The anterior wall of the urethra is sharply transected with scissors a few millimeters distal to the apex of the prostate. The posterior wall of the urethra and rectourethralis muscle are cut under direct vision. The freed specimen should be examined for adequacy of resection margins and placed in a specimen retrieval bag.

J. Role of Frozen Sections: Periurethral tissue that is suspicious for prostatic tissue is biopsied for frozen section analysis. Presence of glands or malignancy requires resection of additional tissue to achieve negative margins.

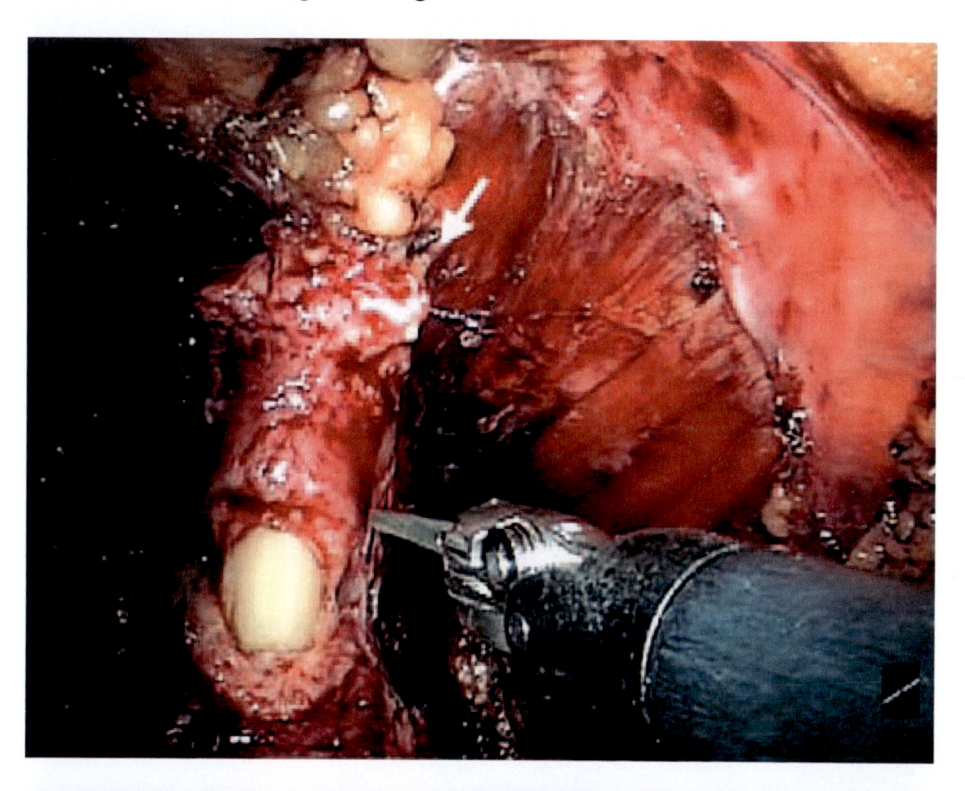

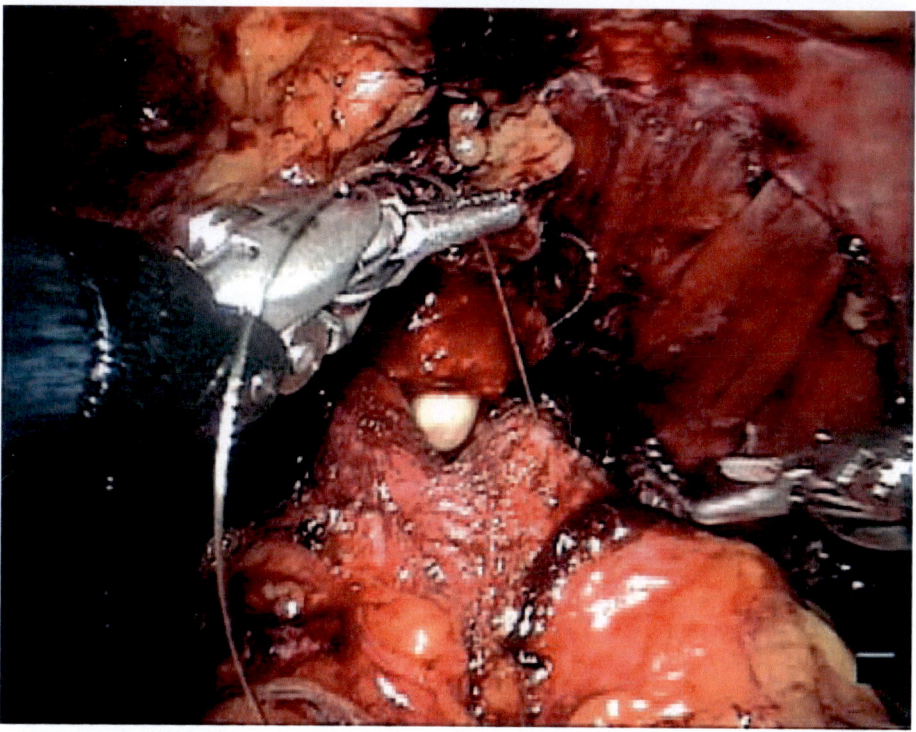

K. Urethrovesical anastomosis: (Fig 9) The urethrovesical anastomosis is performed using a running suture (two 3-0 monocryl sutures on RB-1 needles one dyed and the other undyed, each 6 inches in length and tied to each other thereby forming a double ended suture with a knot in the middle). The initial throw is placed outside in the bladder at 5 o clock and the dyed suture is pulled through so that the knot lies securely on the outside wall of the bladder posteriorly. The dyed suture is then used as a running stitch to suture the posterior bladder wall to the urethra. The dominant hand is used for the urethral pass and the nondominant hand is used for the vesical pass. About 5 or 6 throws are made posterior with the assistant on the right side placing slight tension on the suture. At the corner the surgeon reverses the suture within the bladder lumen and passes the suture outside-in on the urethra. The post suture ends at 11 o clock and is held on traction by the left assistant to prevent loosening of the stitch. The undyed suture is then used to perform the anterior part of the urethrovesial anastomosis extending from 5 o clock to 12 o clock. The two sutures are now tied to each other to complete the anastomosis. The bladder is irrigated with 200 cc saline and reinforcing sutures are placed if a leak if seen. A 20 Fr indwelling foley's catheter is placed and the balloon filled with 20 cc.

L. Retrieval of the specimen and closure of ports: A 15 Fr Jackson Pratt drain is placed in the pelvis near the anastomosis through the 5 mm left port. The bagged specimen is retrieved through the 12 mm umbilical port which is extended to remove the specimen. The fascia of the umbilical port is closed with figure of 8 sutures using No 1 Ethibond on a CT-1 needle. The skin incisions are closed with subcuticular sutures.

2. Robotic Extraperitoneal approach[17]

The extraperitoneal approach has several theoretical advantages compared to the transperitoneal approach, such as avoidance of peritoneal adhesions and the need to retract bowel and prevention of bowel injury. The patient is placed supine with a 15 degree trendelenberg tilt. A 3 cm horizontal incision is made one fingerbreadth below the umbilicus and the preperitoneal space is entered. A Bluntport Hassons canula is placed and the preperitoneum insufflated to 18 mm Hg. The space of retzius is developed by blunt dissection using a conventional laparoscope till the pubic symphsis is reached. A 5mm port is then placed in the midline 2 fingerbreadths above the symphysis to further develop the retropubic space. The right and left extraperitoneal robotic instrument ports are placed 4cm below the camera port at the pararectal line. Two additional assistant ports are placed on the right side ; one at the level of the umbilicus above the right robotic instrument port and the second to the right and in line with the right robotic instrument port. The procedure essentially follows the same steps of the Vattikuti Institute Prostatectomy but the dissection is entirely extraperitoneal. Drawbacks include less space for manipulation, greater clashes between instruments, absence of anatomical landmarks and potential for greater CO_2 absorption.

OUTCOMES

Perioperative outcomes:

The first robotic radical prostatectomy was performed in 2001. Several centers have reported on their early results, however long term results, especially for cancer control are lacking. The largest series comes from the Vattikuti Urology Institute where over 1800 cases have been performed to date and Menon et al. have reported on results of 530 patients[18].

Table 1. Peri operative outcomes of contemporary robotic prostatectomy series

Series	year	Access	Pts	Op time (min)	Blood Loss (ml)	Gle >6	Hosp Stay	Cath	Comp
Binder[12]	2001	TP	10	450	NA	NA	NA	16.7	NA
Pasticier[11]	2001	TP	5	222	800	40%	6.5	6.5	20%
Ahlering[21]	2002	TP	45	228	134	52%	1.6	7	14%
Samadi[22]	2002	TP	11	300	900	NA	NA	2 to 5	0%
Menon[19]	2002	TP	100	140	100	NA	1.2	7	NA
Bentas[23]	2003	TP	40	500	570	NA	NA	16.7	32.5%
Tewari[20]	2003	TP	200	160	153	51%	1.2	7	3.5%
Ahlering[24]	2003	TP	60	231	103	38%	1.1	7	6%
Wolfram[25]	2003	EP+TP	81	250	300	NA	NA	14	NA
Gettman[26]	2003	EP	4	274	1013	75%	5.3	4.7	0%
Cathlineau[27]	2004	EP+TP	105	180	500	NA	5.5	7	NA

Binder[15] and Pasticier[14] presented their early experience and averaged operative times of over 4 hours and blood loss in excess of 800 ml. Their catherization and hospitalization times were high primarily reflecting the practices in Europe. Menon et al.[19] in 2002, reported on results of their first 100 patients; their mean operative times were 140 min and average blood loss was 100 ml. Mean catheterization time was 7 days and mean duration of hospitalization was 1.2 days. Ahlering et al.[21] reported on results of 40 patients in 2002; mean operative time of 228 minutes and average hospital stay of 1.6 days. Since then, both Menon and Ahlering have updated their results; these and other contemporary series are detailed in Table 1.

There have been two prospective non randomized trials to date, comparing open retropubic and robotic radical prostatectomy. Tewari et al.[20] compared 100 open with 200 robotic radical prostatectomies and concluded that the operative duration was not different (163 v/s 160 min). However intraoperative blood loss was 910 ml and 150 ml for open and robotic arms respectively, and transfusion rate was greater in the open approach. There were more complications after open prostatectomy (20% v/s 5%), and the hospital stay was also longer (3.5 days v/s 1.2 days). Ninety-three percent of the robotic group and none of the open patients were discharged within 24 hours. Post operative pain and analgesic use was significantly higher in the open arm (mean pain score 3 v/s 7). They concluded that the robotic approach had significant advantages. However Ahlering et al.[24], in their prospective study of a single surgeon's open and robotic prostatectomy patients showed statistically significant differences in intra operative blood loss and duration of hospitalization. However they found no differences in post operative complications.

Sexual Function:

Few series report on sexual function outcomes following nerve sparing robotic radical prostatectomy. These are detailed in Figure 2. Bentas et al.[23] reported on 37 potent patients, of which eight recovered erections with assistance. Ahlering et al.[24] reported on potency in 9 patients; three had recovered erections adequate for intercourse. Menon and Tewari[20] reported on 200 patients of whom 82% had "return of sexual activity" and 64% had sexual intercourse. Kiyoshima et al.[28], and Tewari et al.[29] demonstrated nerves within the prostatic fascia, and Zvara et al.[30] and Sato et al.[31] showed that these nerves play a role in erectile function. Menon and Kaul et al.[32] described a technique of nerve sparing wherein the prostatic fascia with the contained nerves were preserved during robotic radical prostatectomy. They call this procedure the "Veil of Aphrodite". They performed a prospective non randomized comparison of the "Veil of Aphrodite" with standard nerve sparing and demonstrated a significantly improved intercourse rates compared to conventional nerve sparing in their hands[34]. (Table 2)

Table 2. Sexual function outcomes in contemporary robotic prostatectomy series.

Series	No pts	Age	FU	NS	Assess	Defn	Potency (%)
Bentas[23]	28	61	15	BNS	questionnaire	Inter	22%
Ahlering[24]	9	57	9	BNS	questionnaire	Inter	33%
Tewari[20]	NA	<60	6	BNS	IIEF	Inter	64%
		>60	6	BNS	IIEF	Inter	38%
Chien[33]	16	59	NA	BNS	NA	NA	31%
Menon[34]	35	60	12	VEIL	SHIM	Inter	97%
	23	57	12	BNS	SHIM	Inter	74%

Urinary Function:

One of the striking results of robotic radical prostatectomy is the rapid return of urinary continence. Menon et al. reported that 96% of their patients were pad free (or wearing one liner for security) at 6 months follow up[18]. The median time to return of continence was 42 days for robotic radical prostatectomy and 160 days for open radical prostatectomy[20]. Bentas et al. reported a 68% continence rate at 15 months and Ahlering et al. that 33% of their patients were pad free at 1 week and 81% were pad free at 3 months. It is postulated that the magnification of the robot and the improved accuracy of movements are responsible for these excellent results.

Table 3. Urinary function outcomes in robotic prostatectomy series.

Series	No pts	FU	Continence rates
Bentas[23]	40	15	68%
Ahlering[21]	45	3	81%
Ahlering[24]	60	3	76%
Menon[20]	200	6	96%
Menon[18]	530	6	96%

Oncological Results:

If robotic radical prostatectomy is to supplant the open approach, equivalent or better oncological outcomes must be demonstrated. Long term oncologic outcomes are not available since the procedure is only 3 years old; however surgical margins and PSA recurrence data are available from several centers. An often mentioned criticism of the robotic procedure is the lack of haptics and some feel that this may reflect in high positive margins; since extraprostatic cancer extension cannot be "palpated". Results available so far seem to refute this assumption. Published reports of surgical margins from contemporary series with more than 40 patients are depicted in Figure 4.

Table 4. Cancer control and margin rates following robotic radical prostatectomy.

Series	No pts	pT2 (%)	Positive margins (%)	PSA < 0.2 ng/ml
Wolfram[25]	81	68	12.7	NA
Bentas[23]	40	63	30	NA
Ahlering[24]	60	75	17	NA
Menon[19]	100	85	7	NA
Menon[20]	200	87	6	92%
Cathlineau[27]	105	71	12	98%
Tewari[18]	530	87	5	92%

BLADDER CANCER

Radical Cystoprostatectomy is the standard for the treatment of muscle invasive bladder cancer. The operation consists of two parts; removal of the bladder with the draining lymph nodes and construction of the urinary diversion, either a bowel conduit or continent reservoir. Open cystoprostatectomy is the gold standard; however the procedure has been performed laparoscopically; either totally intracorporeal or with the reservoir performed through a mini laparotomy incision. The major advantages of the laparoscopic approach versus the open approach are excellent visualization of anatomy, selective control of bleeding and strikingly diminished blood loss. These same advantages may be realized with robotic assistance. Menon et al.[35] reported the largest series of robotic radical cystoprostatectomy to date, of 24 patients. The mean operative time was 2.3 hours and mean blood loss 190 ml. Key features of the procedure are complete dissection of bilateral regional lymph nodes **(Fig 10 & 11)**; skeletonization of the external iliac vessels **(Fig 12)** and visualization of the superior and inferior vesical arteries as well as the collateral blood supply. This technique also facilitates identification and preservation of the neurovascular bundles and in females, the uterus and vagina[36]. In case of orthotopic urinary reconstruction, the authors recommend creation of the pouch through a mini laparotomy incision **(Fig 13)**. However, the urethro neovesical anastomosis is completed robotically **(Fig 14)**. Others (Becken)[37] reported a small series in which they performed the entire operation intracorporeally with the da Vinci robot. Similar experiences have been reported by others[38,39]. These early results suggest that after substantial experience is acquired in the area of robotic radical prostatectomy, the horizon may be expanded to include surgery of the bladder.

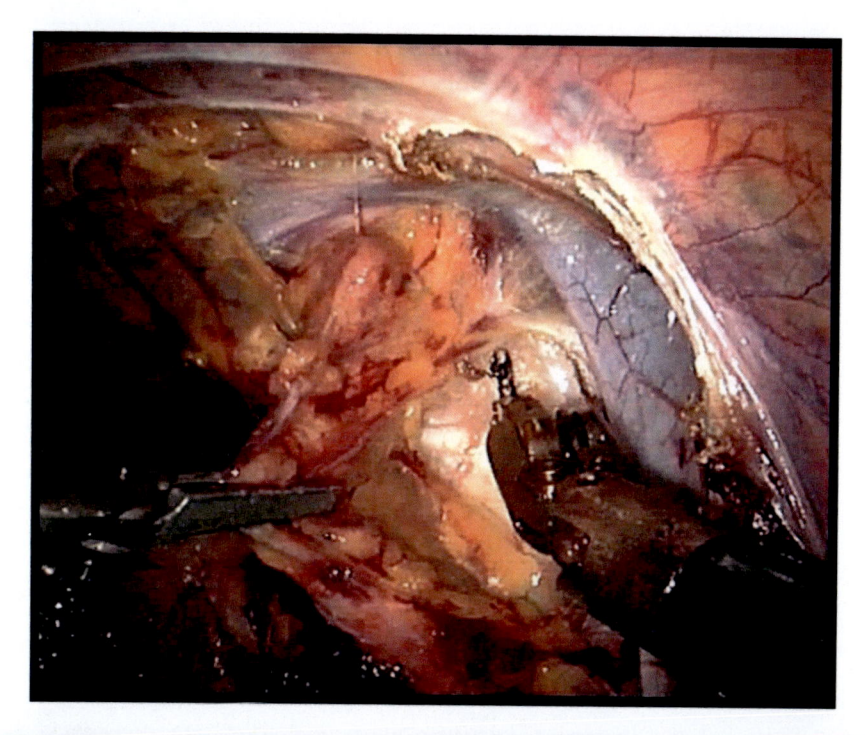

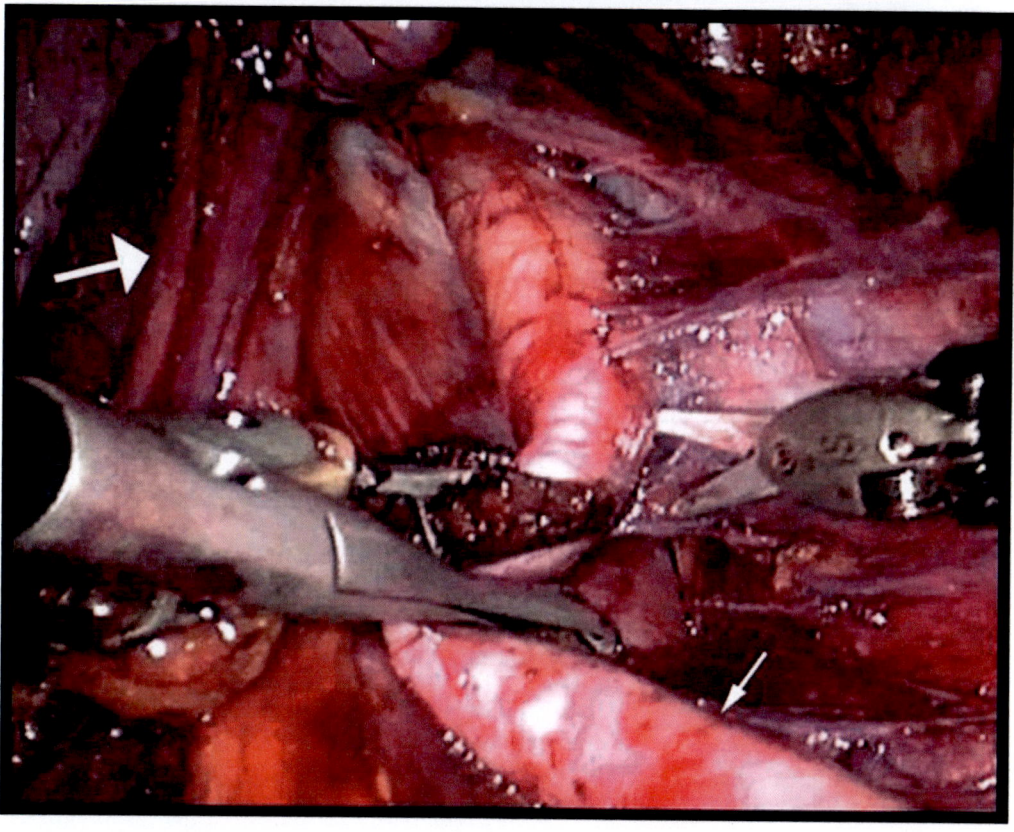

Table 5. Robotic Cystoprostatectomy series at Vattikuti Urology Institute

No of patients	17
Form of Reconstruction Ileal conduit W Pouch Serosal tunnel Double chimney T pouch & serosal tunnel	2 10 2 2
Operative time (min) Cystectomy Ileal conduit Orthotopic neobladder	 140 120 168
Mean Blood loss (ml)	<150
Positive margins	0

NEPHRECTOMY AND PARTIAL NEPHRECTOMY

Laparoscopic and hand assisted laparoscopic nephrectomy are considered the gold standard for surgical treatment of kidney diseases[40]. Laparoscopic nephrectomy technically is a straight forward operation and current opinion suggests that performing it with the da Vinci robot may be overkill and not cost effective, since the robot offers no advantages to the laparoscopic approach. However, a few reports of robotic nephrectomy do exist in literature, and these have been equivocal on the role of the da Vinci robot for nephrectomy. Marcella et al.[41] compared hand assisted and robot assisted laparoscopic nephrectomy and concluded that the robot offered no advantage. Surgeons at the Hospital Brabois in France[42] reported on their experience of 38 robotic nephrectomies and concluded that the robot permitted more accurate dissection of the hilum.

In contrast to simple and radical nephrectomy, partial nephrectomy is associated with a steep learning curve when performed laparoscopically. It requires intracorporeal suturing of the collecting system, delicate atraumatic dissection of the renal vessels and the need to keep warm ischemia time as low as possible makes partial nephrectomy ideally suited for robotic assistance **(Fig 15 to 18)**. Few centers have reported their experience with da Vinci assisted partial nephrectomy. Taneja et al.[43] reported 10 cases with a mean tumor size of 2.5 cm. Peschel et al.[44] and Gettman et al.[45] performed robotic partial nephrectomy on 13 tumors of mean size 3.5 cm. Eight patients underwent core cooling of the kidney with intra arterial catheters. Mean operating time was 215 minutes, and warm and cold ischemia times were 22 and 33 minutes respectively. Surgeons at the Vattikuti Urology Institute have performed robotic partial nephrectomy in 8 males and 2 females (unpublished data). Mean tumor size was 2 cm; range (1 to 3 cm). Mean operative time was 158 minutes and mean warm ischemia time was 21 minutes. Mean hospital stay was 1.4 days. Pathology revealed renal cell carcinoma in eight and benign adenoma (1) and lipoma (1). All resection margins were negative.

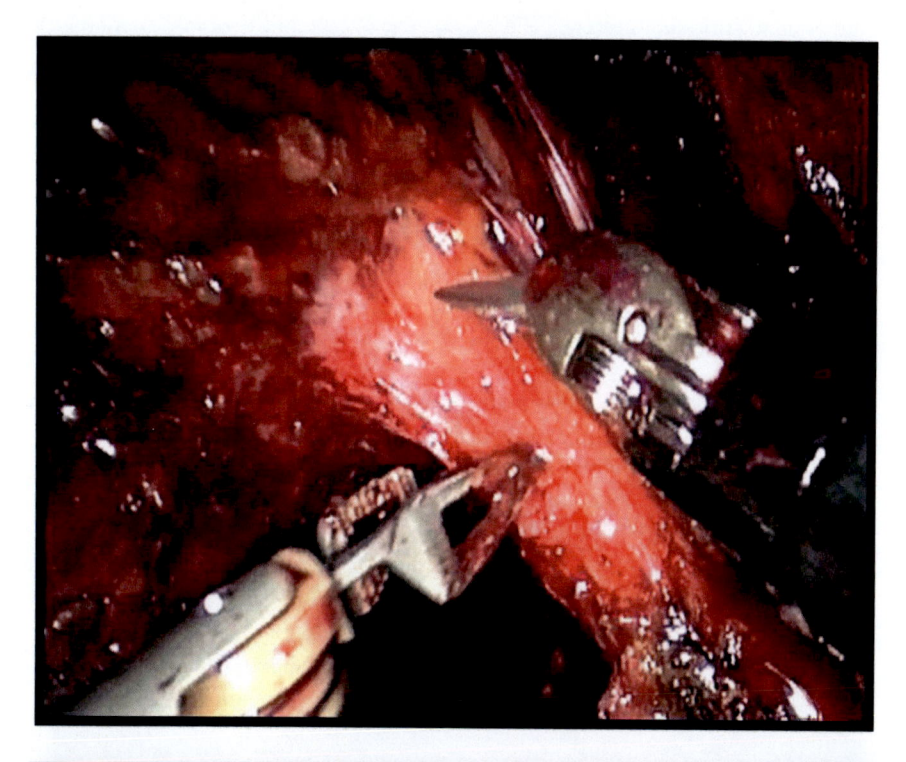

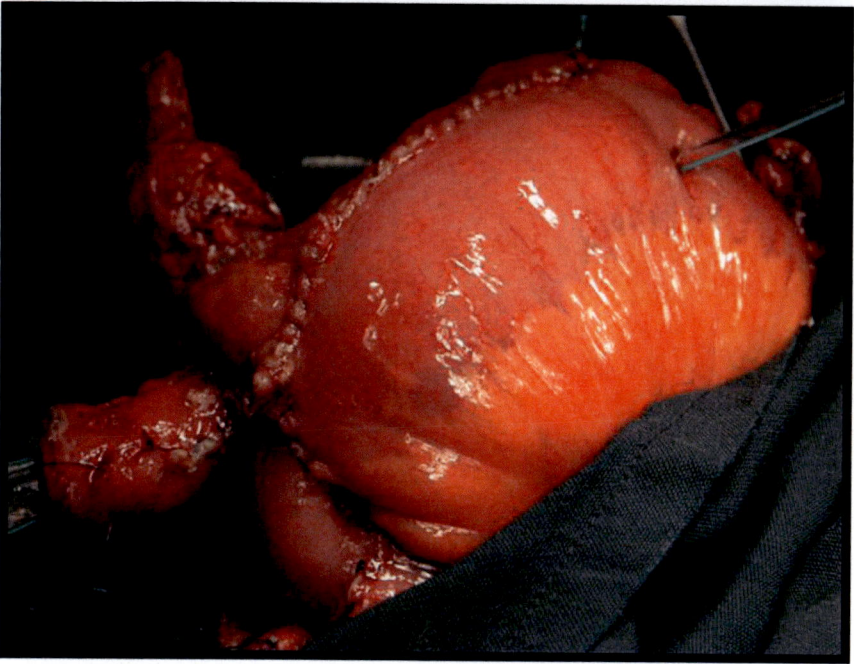

RENAL TRANSPLANTATION

The da Vinci surgical system has been used for both donor nephrectomy and transplantation of the harvested graft in the recipient.

Horgan et al.[46] reported on their experience of 12 robotic donor nephrectomies; however they used a Lap Disc hand port (Ethicon, a Johnson & Johnson Company, Piscataway, NJ) in all patients. They surmised that although the results were similar to standard laparoscopic donor nephrectomy, the robot made dissection of the renal vessels technically easier. They noted that the quality of the allograft improved because the dexterity of the robot permitted a longer length of renal vessels to be dissected and preserved with the specimen. The mean operative time was 166 minutes and a third of the patients had more than one artery. All transplanted kidneys functioned normally. The mean warm ischemia time was 79 seconds.

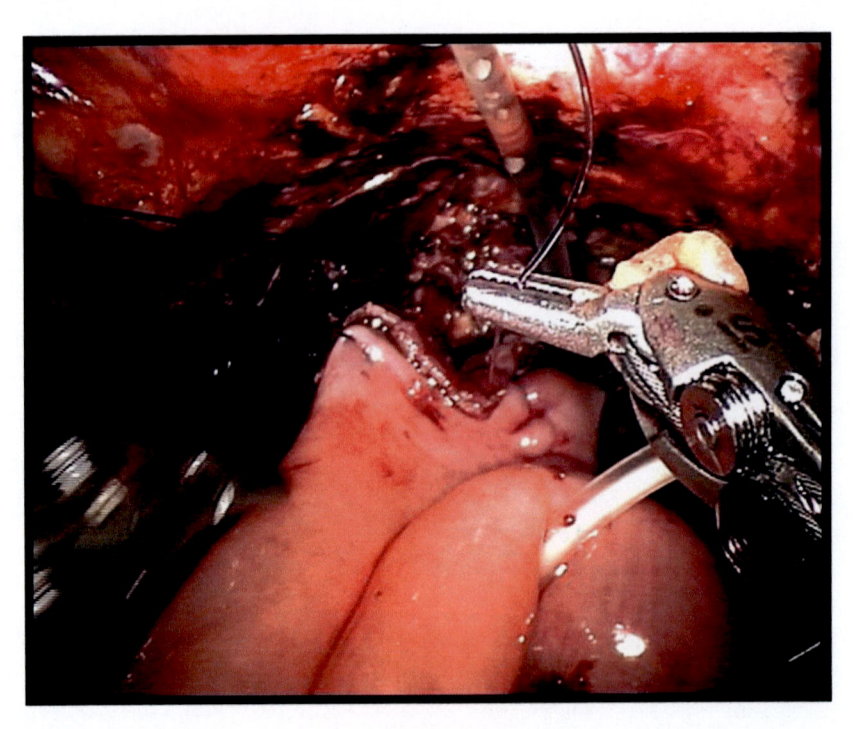

Arenas and colleagues from Henry Ford Hospital in Detroit have performed 38 pure robotic donor nephrectomies (Unpublished data, 2004). With their technique, Robotic Donor nephrectomy is a 4 port procedure; the kidney, hilum and ureter is dissected completely with the robot, which is then de docked and an Endocatch II bag introduced through the 15mm infra umbilical assistant port and placed near the kidney. A 7 cm infra umbilical incision is deepened up to but not through the linea alba in order to preserve the pneumoperitoneum. The renal artery and vein are then secured with Weck clips and an EndoGIA (USSC-Tyco, Norwalk, CT) stapler respectively and the kidney is bagged. The incision is then deepened into the peritoneum and the bagged kidney delivered to be perfused. Mean warm ischemia time was less than 3 minutes and all grafts functioned normally.

Abbou et al.[47] described a cadaveric renal transplantation with the da Vinci robot. The dissection of the Iliac vessels and preparation of the renal bed was performed with robotic assistance, as was the vascular and the ureterovesical anastomosis.

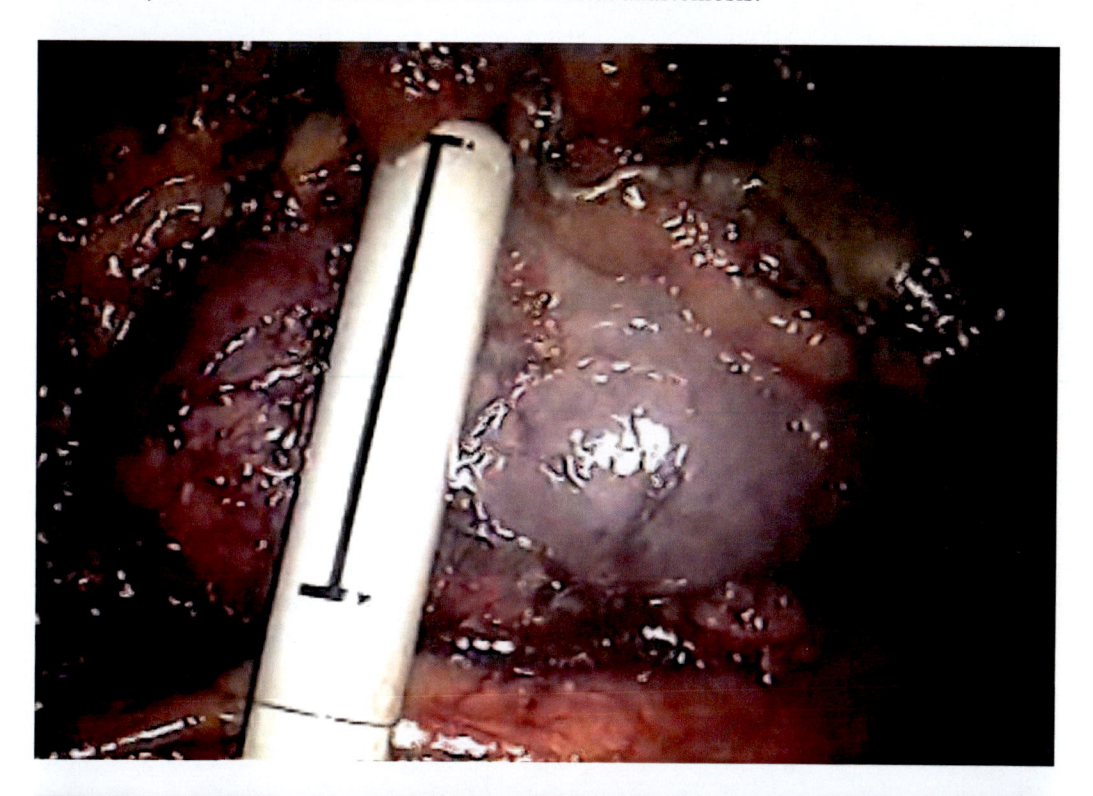

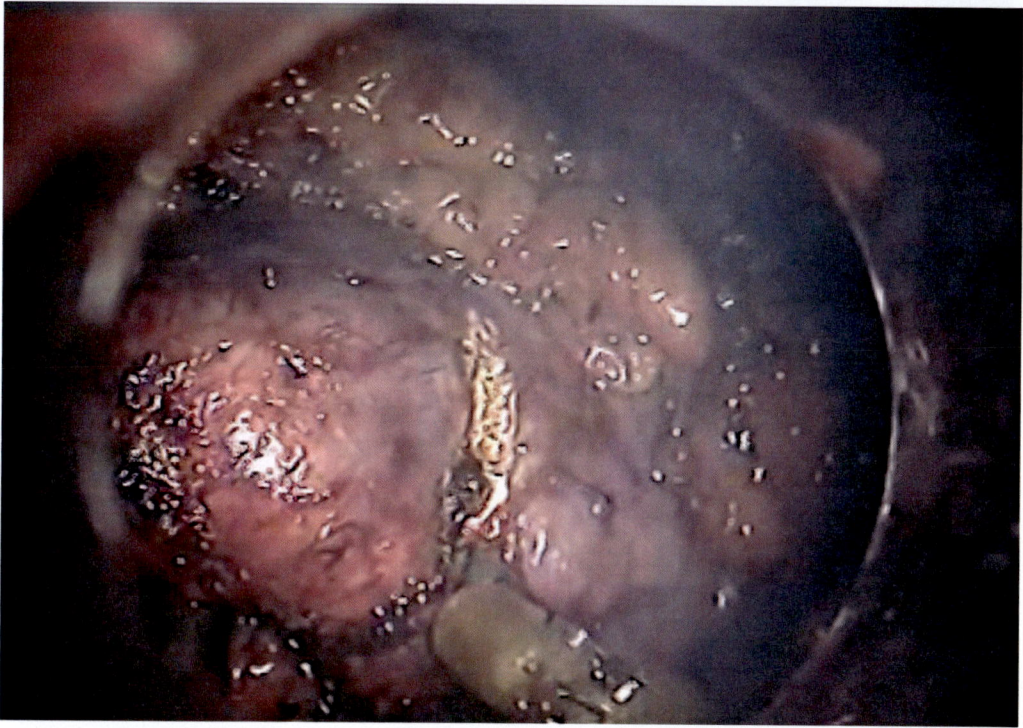

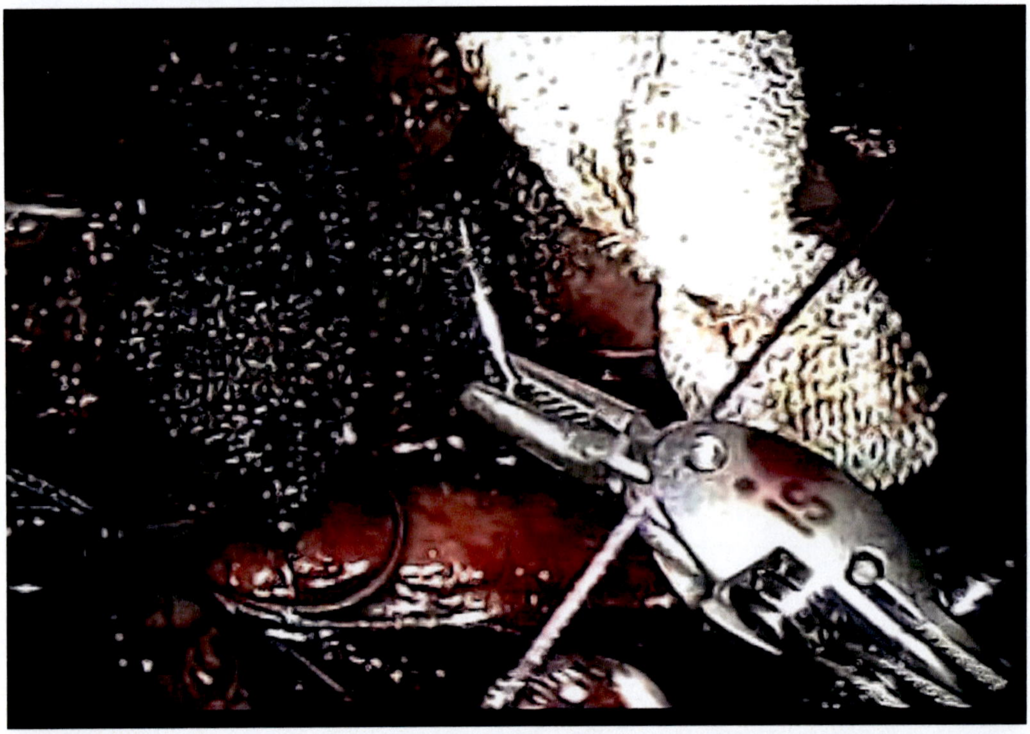

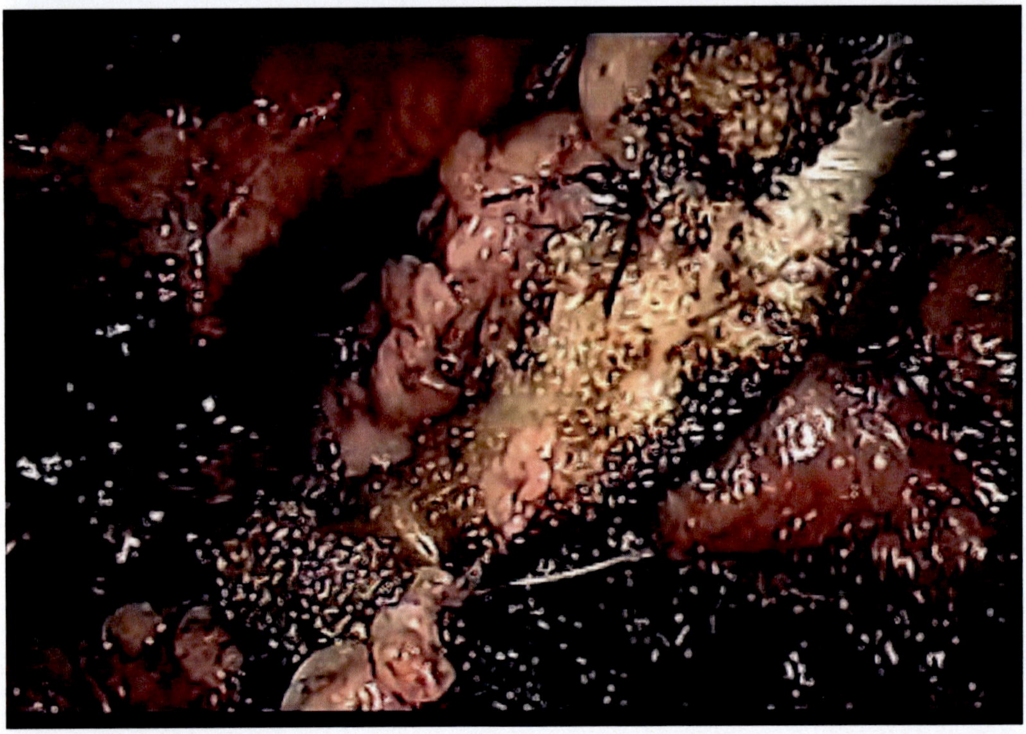

PYELOPLASTY

Several minimally invasive treatments for UPJ obstruction are currently available including endopyelotomy; both retrograde and antegrade, endopyeloplasty, laparoscopic pyeloplasty and robotic pyeloplasty. The endourologic approaches have not replicated the long term success rates of open surgery and are contraindicated in the presence of crossing vessels. Pure laparoscopy is technically demanding as it requires intracorporeal suturing which is technically demanding[48]. Pyeloplasty is ideally suited to using a robotic interface since the endowristed instruments and seven degrees of freedom of the instruments makes intracorporeal suturing less demanding and more accurate.

Technical Considerations:

There are two approaches to gain access to the UPJ; transmesocolic and retrocolic. Four ports are generally used for the procedure; three robotic ports and a 12mm assistant port.

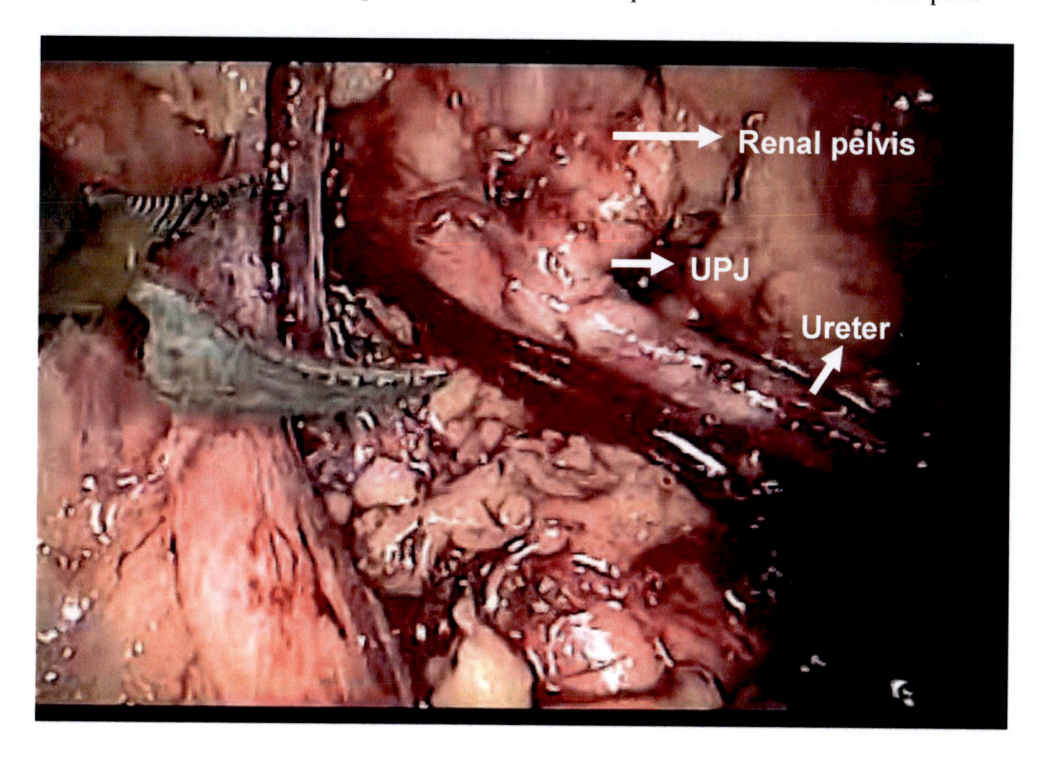

The transmesocolic approach is preferred in children; a small incision is made within an avascular area of the mesocolon to approach the UPJ. Advantages include lack of mobilization of the colon and reduced risk of injury to the renal vasculature or spleen on the left. The retrocolic approach is the traditional approach in which an incision is made along the line of Toldt to mobilize the colon. Subsequently the Gerota's fascia is incised and the renal pelvis dissected clear of the renal artery and vein **(Fig 19)**.

A careful search is made for crossing renal arteries at the UPJ and these are carefully preserved. Principles of open surgery such as excision of redundant pelvis, creation of dependent UPJ and tension-free anastomosis are respected **(Fig 20)**.

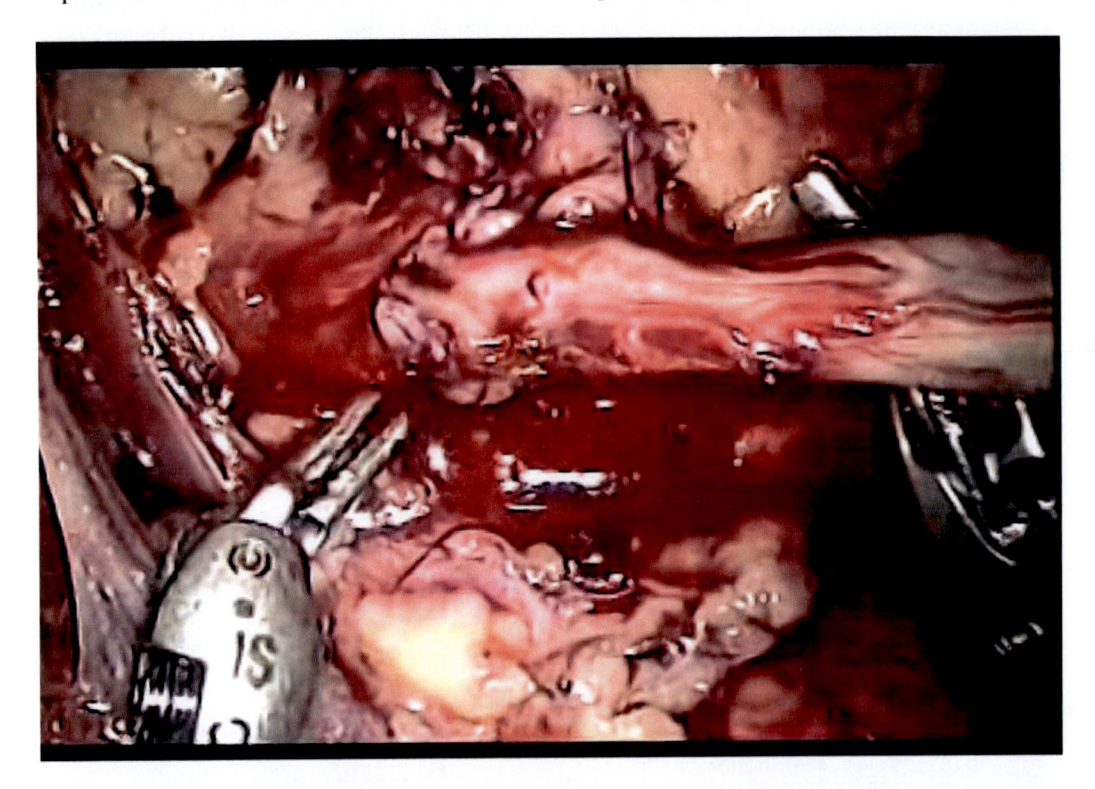

Sung and colleagues[49] used the Zeus and da Vinci systems to perform pyeloplasty on pigs and concluded that the da Vinci system was faster and more accurate than the Zeus system. Gettman et al.[50] first described da Vinci assisted Anderson Hynes pyeloplasty in 9 patients in 2002. They used 4 ports; three robotic and a 12 mm assistant port. They reported operative times of 139 minutes and suturing time of 62 minutes. Eleven percent patients underwent re exploration to repair a pelvic defect. All patients had non obstructive renal system on follow up. In a study comparing da Vinci and Conventional laparoscopic pyeloplasty (Anderson Hynes and Fengerplasty) they concluded that in both techniques the da Vinci robot was significantly faster in terms of both operative times and suturing times[50]. Subsequently several centers have published their results of robotic pyeloplasty[51-53], some of which are detailed in Table 2. The follow up in these series is relatively short and the definition of successful surgery is variable (Renogram documented $t^{1/2} < 20$ min, IVP documented non obstruction and absence of pain).

Table 2 Outcomes of robotic pyeloplasty series

Series	No pts	Mean Op time (min)	Mean Blood loss (ml)	Hospital stay (d)	Complications (%)	Success rate (%)
Gettman et al.[50]	9	140	<50	4.7	11	100
UCI[54]	13	350	71	2	7.6	100
Peschel et al.[55]	49	124	< 50	NA	2	100
Munver et al.[56]	15	190	37	3.1	0	100
Patel et al.[57]	10	210	58	0.76	0	100
Peters et al.[58] (pediatric)	14	144	NA	NA	4	94

ADRENALECTOMY

Laparoscopic adrenalectomy is considered as the gold standard for management of benign adrenal diseases. As with many laparoscopic procedures, robotic assistance has been evaluated for management of benign adrenal tumors. Gill and colleagues[59] first compared laparoscopic and robotic adrenalectomy using the Zeus system. Although the operative times were longer for the robotic group, they could repair an IVC injury without open conversion using robot assisted intra corporeal suturing. Horgan et al.[60] reported the first case of da Vinci assisted robotic adrenalectomy in 2001 and since, several small series of da Vinci assisted adrenalectomy have been published[61-64]. The procedure involves 5 ports on the right and four on the left; the fifth port serving as a liver retractor. The steps of surgery essentially duplicate the steps of conventional laparoscopic adrenalectomy. Benica et al.[61] compared robotic and conventional laparoscopic adrenalectomy and concluded that the outcomes were similar in both groups, however the robotic procedure was considerably more expensive. Mean operative time was 133 minutes for the robotic group and hospital stay was 5.7 days. This seems excessive given that laparoscopic adrenalectomy is a daycare procedure, with patients discharged with 24 hours. Lack of progression and excessive bleeding in 4 of the 9 robotic patients necessitated conversion to open surgery. Brunaud and colleagues[62] have published the largest series to date, of 14 patients. They reported operative times of 97 minutes. These results represent the learning curve of these institutions and are certain to improve as the experience improves.

PEDIATRIC UROLOGY

The initial concern that the bulk of the da Vinci Robot would preclude its use in children has been found to be unfounded. Several da Vinci procedures have been performed in children and infants with excellent results.

The recommended 7 cm distance between each of the three robotic ports may be difficult to achieve in small infants. However recent introduction of 5 mm robotic instruments has spurred interest in robotic pediatric urology applications. Pedraza et al.[65] described a single case of robotic assisted appendicovesicostomy in a 7 seven year old boy with posterior urethral valves. The entire procedure, using 4 ports was performed with the da Vinci system in 6 hours. Craig Peters from Boston Childrens Hospital has performed both extravesical Lich Gregoir and transvesical Cohen's reimplantation in children[57]. Twenty one children underwent a unilateral ureteral reimplant and 3 children, a bilateral reimplant. Operative times ranged from 2 hours for the unilateral to 3 hours for the bilateral procedure. At a follow up of just under 9 months 21 of the 27 patients have a satisfactory outcome. The early experience of robotic pediatric urological surgery appears promising and this field is certain to expand in the years to come. The expected miniaturization of the robotic system, telescope and instruments is expected to further encourage expansion of pediatric urological applications.

FEMALE UROLOGY

Two robotic assisted female urologic procedures have been described in literature. Di Marco et al. described 5 cases of robot assisted sacrocolpopexy for uterine prolapse[66]. The initial dissection was completed using standard laparoscopy and the robot was utilized for suturing of the graft. The authors concluded that the superior optics and dexterity of the robot permitted more accurate suture placement while avoiding the sacral and vaginal veins. Urologists at the University of California at Irvine have used the da Vinci to repair a vesico vaginal fistula[67]. The initial dissection was performed using conventional laparoscopy and the robot was used for suturing the vaginal and bladder wall. The authors felt that the robot permitted improved accuracy of suturing. The patient was voiding normally at 6 weeks follow up.

RETROPERITONEAL LYMPH NODE DISSECTION (RPLND)

Laparoscopic retroperitoneal lymph node dissection was first performed by Rutalis et al. in 1992. Laparoscopic RPLND is considered to be the most technically demanding laparoscopic procedure in all of urology, and its practice is restricted to a select few centers[69-71]. Current literature suggests that Lap RPLND is feasible for both Stage I and II NSGCT and that its efficacy parallels open surgery.

Currently, no reports on robotic RPLND exist in the medical literature, although conceptually it is ideally suited to robotic assistance given the fine dissection required, especially for nerve sparing RPLND. As the experience with the da Vinci robot expands, RPLND is sure to come within the purview of the robot.

CONCLUSION

Robot assisted minimally invasive surgery is here to stay. The ability to perform precise tissue manipulation under outstanding visualization enables the surgeon to carry out complex tasks with excellent results. The Vattikuti Urology Institute; which has the largest single institution experience of robotic radical prostatectomy in the world, has demonstrated that robotic radical prostatectomy is a safe and effective operation with markedly improved recovery of potency and urinary continence, compared to alternative approaches. It is predicted that robotic radical prostatectomy will become the gold standard for the treatment of localized prostate cancer for both urologists and patients alike. Robotic assistance will be adopted for many other urological operations as well, especially in areas where current experience indicates that robotic operations have comparable outcomes to laparoscopic approach. The anticipated advantages of robotic technology will likely lead to superior results in the future.

REFERENCES

1. Harris SJ, Arambula-Cosio F, Mei Q, Hibberd RD, Davies BL, Wickham JE, Nathan MS, Kundu B. The Probot--an active robot for prostate resection. *Proceedings of the I MECH E Part H Journal of Engineering in Medicine* 1997; 211(4):317-25(9).

2. Glauser D, Fankhauser H, Epitaux M, Hefti JL, Jaccottet A. Neurosurgical robot Minerva: first results and current developments. *Journal of Image Guided Surgery* 1995; 1(5): 266-72.

3. Spencer EH. The ROBODOC clinical trial: a robotic assistant for total hip arthroplasty. *Orthopedic Nursing* 1996; Jan-Feb; 15(1):9-14.

4. Sackier J, Wang Y. Robotically assisted laparoscopic surgery. From concept to development. *Surgical Endoscopy* 1994; 8(1):63-6.

5. Sung GT, Gill IS. Robotic laparoscopic surgery: a comparison of the Da Vinci and Zeus systems. *Urology* 2001 Dec; 58(6):893-8.

6. Jemal A, Murray T, Ward E, Samuels A, Tiwari RC, Ghafoor A, Feuer EJ, Thun MJ.. Cancer statistics, 2005. *CA: Cancer Journal for Clinicians* 2005 Jan-Feb; 55(1):10-30.

7. Walsh PC, Donker PJ. Impotence following radical prostatectomy: insight into etiology and prevention. *Journal of Urology* 1982; 128(3): 492-7.

8. Guillonneau B, Vallancien G. Laparoscopic radical prostatectomy: the Montsouris technique. *Journal of Urology* 2000 Jun;163(6):1643-9.

9. Guillonneau B, Cathelineau X, Doublet JD, Vallancien G. Laparoscopic radical prostatectomy: the lessons learned. *Journal of Endourology* 2001; 15(4):441-5.

10. Abbou CC, Hoznek A, Salomon L, Olsson LE, Lobontiu A, Saint F, Cicco A, Antiphon P, Chopin D. Laparoscopic radical prostatectomy with a remote controlled robot. *Journal of Urology* 2001; 165(6pt1):1964-6.

11. Pasticier G, Rietbergen JB, Guillonneau B, Fromont G, Menon M, Vallancien G. Robotically assisted laparoscopic radical prostatectomy: feasibility study in men. *European Urology* 2001 Jul; 40(1):70-4.

12. Binder J, Kramer W. Robotically-assisted laparoscopic radical prostatectomy. *BJU International* 2001; 87(4): 408-10.

13. Menon M, Tewari A, Peabody J. The VIP Team. Vattikuti Institute prostatectomy: technique. *Journal of Urology* 2003 Jun; 169(6): 2289-92.

14. Tewari A, Srivasatava A, Menon M; Members of the VIP Team. A prospective comparison of radical retropubic and robot-assisted prostatectomy: experience in one institution. *BJU International* 2003 Aug ; 92(3): 205-10.

15. Menon M. Robotic radical retropubic prostatectomy. *BJU International* 2003 Feb; 91(3):175-6.

16. Menon M, Tewari A, Peabody JO, Shrivastava A, Kaul S, Bhandari A, Hemal AK. Vattikuti Institute prostatectomy, a technique of robotic radical prostatectomy for management of localized carcinoma of the prostate: experience of over 1100 cases. *Urology Clinics of North America* 2004 Nov; 31(4): 701-17.

17. Gettman MT, Hoznek A, Salomon L, Katz R, Borkowski T, Antiphon P, Lobontiu A, Abbou CC. Laparoscopic radical prostatectomy: description of the extraperitoneal approach using the da Vinci robotic system. *Journal of Urology* 2003 Aug; 170(2 Pt 1): 416-9.

18. Tewari A, Kaul S, Menon M. Robotic radical prostatectomy: a minimally invasive therapy for prostate cancer. *Current Urology Reports* 2005 Feb; 6(1):45-8.

19. Menon M, Shrivastava A, Sarle R, Hemal A, Tewari A. Vattikuti Institute Prostatectomy: a single-team experience of 100 cases. *Journal of Endourology* 2003 Nov; 17(9): 785-90.

20. Tewari A, Shrivastava A, Menon M, Members of the VIP Team. A prospective comparison of radical retropubic and robot assisted prostatectomy: experience in one institution. *BJU International* 2003 Aug; 92(3): 205-210.

21. Ahlering TE, Skarecky D, Lee D, Clayman, RV. Successful transfer of open surgical skills to a laparoscopic environment using a robotic interface: initial experience with laparoscopic radical prostatectomy. *Journal of Urology* 2003 Nov; 170(5):1738-41.

22. Samadi DB, Nadu A, Olsson E, Hoznek A, Salomon L, Saint F, Abbou CC, Creteil. Robot assisted laparoscopic radical prostatectomy- Initial experience in eleven patients. *Journal of Urology* 2002;167(4 suppl; Abstract 1554):390.

23. Bentas W, Wolfram M, Jones J, Brautigam R, Kramer W, Binder J. Robotic technology and the translation of open radical prostatectomy to laparoscopy: the early Frankfurt experience with robotic radical prostatectomy and one year follow-up. *European Urology* 2003 Aug; 44(2): 175-81.

24. Ahlering TE, Woo D, Eichel L, Lee DI, Edwards R, Skarecky DW. Robot-assisted versus open radical prostatectomy: a comparison of one surgeon's outcomes. *Urology* 2004 May; 63(5): 819-22.

25. Wolfram M, Brautigam R, Engl T, Bentas W, Heitkamp S, Ostwald M, Kramer W, Binder J, Blaheta R, Jonas D, Beecken WD. Robotic-assisted laparoscopic radical prostatectomy: the Frankfurt technique. *World Journal of Urology* 2003 Aug; 21(3):128-32. Epub 2003 July 8.

26. Gettman MT, Hoznek A, Salomon L, Katz R, Borkowski T, Antiphon P, Lobonitiu A, Abbou CC. Laparoscopic radical prostatectomy: description of the extraperitoneal approach using the da Vinci robotic system. *Journal of Urology* 2003 Aug; 170(2pt1):416-19.

27. Cathelineau X, Rozet F, Vallancien G. Robotic radical prostatectomy: the European experience. *Urologic Clinics of North America* 2004 Nov; 31(4):693-9.

28. Kiyoshima K, Yokomizo A, Yoshida T, Tomita K, Yonemasu H, Nakamura M, Oda Y, Naito S, Hasegawa Y. Anatomical Features Of Periprostatic Tissue And Its Surroundings: A Histological Analysis Of 79 Radical Retropubic Prostatectomy Specimens. *Japanese Journal of Clinical Oncology* 2004; 34(8): 463-8.

29. Tewari A, Peabody JO, Fischer M, Sarle R, Vallancien G, Delmas V, Hassan M, Bansal A, Hemal AK, Guillonneau B, Menon M. An operative and anatomic study to

help in nerve sparing during laparoscopic and robotic radical prostatectomy. *European Urology* 2003; 43(5): 444-54.

30. Zvara P, Spiess PE, Merlin SL, Begin LR, Brock GB. Neurogenic Erectile dysfunction: The course of nicotinamide adenine dinucleotide phosphate diaphorase - positive nerve fibers on the surface of the prostate. *Urology* 1996; 47(1):146-151.

31. Sato Y, Rehman J, Santizo C, Melman A, Christ GJ. Significant physiological roles of ancillary penile nerves on increase in intracavernous pressure in rats: experiments using electrical stimulation of the medial preoptic area. *International Journal of Impotence Research* 2001 Apr; 13(2):82-8.

32. Kaul S, Bhandari A, Hemal A, Savera A, Shrivastava A, Menon M: Robotic radical prostatectomy with preservation of the prostatic fascia: A feasibility study. *Urology* 2005; 66(6):1261-5.

33. Chien GW, Orvieto MA, Galocy RM, Zagaja GP, Sokoloff MH, Shalvav AL. Antegrade nerve preservation during robotic laparoscopic prostatectomy: the video. *Journal of Urology* 2004; 171(4 suppl; Abstract V1977): 522.

34. Menon M, Kaul S, Bhandari A, Shrivastava A, Tewari A, Hemal A. Potency following robotic radical prostatectomy: a questionnaire–based analysis of outcomes after conventional nerve sparing and prostatic fascia sparing techniques. *Journal of Urology* 2005 Dec; 174(6):2291-6.

35. Menon M, Hemal AK, Tewari A, Shrivastava A, Shoma AM, Et-Tabey NA, Shaaban A, Abol-Enein H, Ghoneim MA. Nerve-sparing robot-assisted radical cystoprostatectomy and urinary diversion. *BJU International* 2003 Aug; 92(3): 232-6.

36. Menon M, Hemal AK, Tewari A, Shrivastava A, Shoma AM, Abol-Enein H, Ghoneim MA. Robot-assisted radical cystectomy and urinary diversion in female patients: technique with preservation of the uterus and vagina. *Journal of the American College of Surgeons* 2004 Mar;198(3):386-93.

37. Beecken WD, Wolfram M, Engl T, Bentas W, Probst M, Blaheta R, Oertl A, Jonas D, Binder J. Robotic-assisted laparoscopic radical cystectomy and intra-abdominal formation of an orthotopic ileal neobladder. *European Urology* 2003 Sep; 44(3):337-9.

38. Yohannes P, Puri V, Yi B, Khan AK, Sudan R. Laparoscopy-assisted robotic radical cystoprostatectomy with ileal conduit urinary diversion for muscle-invasive bladder cancer: initial two cases. *Journal of Endourology* 2003 Nov; 17(9):729-32.

39. Balaji KC, Yohannes P, McBride CL, Oleynikov D, Hemstreet GP 3rd. Feasibility of robot-assisted totally intracorporeal laparoscopic ileal conduit urinary diversion: initial results of a single institutional pilot study. *Urology* 2004 Jan; 63(1):51-5.

40. Johnston WK 3rd, Wolf JS Jr. Laparoscopic partial nephrectomy: technique, oncologic efficacy and safety. *Current Urology Reports* 2005 Feb; 6(1):19-28.

41. Marella VK, Wise GJ, Silver DA. Adjunctive technologies in laparoscopic nephrectomy – comparison of hand-assisted and robot-assisted techniques. *Journal of Urology* 2004; 171(4 Suppl; Abstract 1284):338.

42. Hoznek A, Hubert J, Antiphon P, Gettman MT, Hemal AK, Abbou CC. Robotic renal surgery. *Urology Clinics of North America* 2004 Nov; 31(4):731-6.

43. Taneja SS, Caruso RP, Phillips CK, Stifelman MD. Robotic partial nephrectomy: Initial experience. *Journal of Urology* 2004;171(4 Suppl; Abstract 1289):339.

44. Peschel R, Neururer R, Blute ML, DiMarco DS, Bartsch G, Gettman MT. Robotic - assisted laparoscopic partial nephrectomy. *Journal of Urology* 2004; 171 (4 Suppl; Abstract 1782):471.

45. Gettman MT, Blute ML, Chow GK, Neururer R, Bartsch G, Peschel R. Robotic-assisted laparoscopic partial nephrectomy: technique and initial clinical experience with DaVinci robotic system. *Urology* 2004 Nov; 64(5):914-8.

46. Horgan S, Vanuno D, Sileri P, Cicalese L, Benedetti E. Robotic assisted laparoscopic donor nephrectomy for kidney transplantation. *Transplantation* 2002; 73(9):1474-9.

47. Hoznek A, Zaki SK, Samadi DB, Salomon L, Lobontiu A, Lang P, Abbou CC. Robotic assisted kidney transplantation: initial experience. *Journal of Urology* 2002 Apr; 167(4):1604-6.

48. Guillonneau B, Rietbergen JB, Fromont G, Vallancien G. Robotically assisted laparoscopic dismembered pyeloplasty: a chronic porcine study. *Urology* 2003 May; 61(5):1063-6.

49. Gill IS, Sung GT, Hsu TH, Merany AM. Robotic remote laparoscopic nephrectomy and adrenalectomy: an initial experience. *Journal of Urology* 2000; 164(6): 2082-5.

50. Gettman MT, Peschel R, Neururer R, Bartsch G. A comparison of laparoscopic pyeloplasty performed with the daVinci robotic system versus standard laparoscopic techniques: initial clinical results. *European Urology* 2002 Nov; 42(5): 453-7; discussion 457-8.

51. Yohannes P, Burjonrappa SC. Rapid communication: laparoscopic Anderson-Hynes dismembered pyeloplasty using the da Vinci robot: technical considerations. *Journal of Endourology* 2003 Mar; 17(2):79-83.

52. Hubert J, Feuillu B, Mourey E, Ferchaud J, Prevot L, Mangin P. Laparoscopic transperitoneal pyeloplasty using a remote controlled robotic surgical system (Da Vinci®). 37 cases. *European Urology Supplements* 2004 Feb; 3(2):86.

53. Bentas W, Wolfram M, Brautigam R, Probst M, Beecken WD, Jonas D, Binder J. Da Vinci robot assisted Anderson-Hynes dismembered pyeloplasty: technique and 1 year follow-up. *World Journal of Urology* 2003 Aug;21(3):133-8. Epub Jul 9.

54. Eichel L, Ahlering T, Clayman R. Role of Robotics in laparoscopic urologic surgery. *Urologic Clinics of North America* 2004 Nov; 31(4):781-92.

55. Peschel R, Neururer R, Bartsch G, Gettman MT. Robotic pyeloplasty: technique and results. *Urologic Clinics of North America* 2004 Nov;31(4):737-41.

56. Munver R, Del Pizzo JJ, Sosa RE, Poppas DP. Minimally invasive surgical management of ureteropelvic junction obstruction: laparoscopic and robot-assisted laparoscopic pyeloplasty. *Journal of Long-Term Effects of Medical Implants*. 2003; 13(5):367-84.Review.

57. Patel V. Robotic ureteral reconstruction. *Journal of Endourology* 2003; 17 (Suppl 1):A220.

58. Peters CA. Laparoscopic and robotic approach to genitourinary anomalies in children. *Urologic Clinics of North America* 2004 Aug; 31(3):595-605.

59. Desai MM, Gill IS, Kaouk JH, Martin SF, Sung GT, Bravo EL. Robotic assisted laparoscopic adrenalectomy. *Urology* 2002; 60(6):1104-7.

60. Horgan S, Vannuno D. Robots in laparoscopic surgery. *Journal of Laparo-endoscopic & Advanced Surgery Techniques Part A* 2001 Dec; 11(6):415-19.

61. Beninca G, Garrone C, Rebecchi F, Giaccone C, Morino M. Robot-assisted laparoscopic surgery. Preliminary results at our Center. *Chirurgia Italiana* 2003 May-Jun; 55(3):321-31.

62. Brunaud L, Bresler L, Ayav A, Tretou S, Cormier L, Klein M, Boissel P. Advantages of using robotic Da Vinci system for unilateral adrenalectomy: early results. *Annals de Chirurgie* 2003 Oct; 128(8):530-5.

63. Bentas W, Wolfram M, Brautigam R, Binder J. Laparoscopic transperitoneal adrenalectomy using a remote-controlled robotic surgical system. *Journal of Endourology* 2002 Aug;16(6):373-6.

64. D'Annibale A, Fiscon V, Trevisan P, Pozzobon M, Gianfreda V, Sovernigo G, Morpurgo E, Orsini C, Del Monte D. The da Vinci robot in right adrenalectomy:

considerations on technique. *Surgical Laparoscopic Endoscopy & Percutaneous Techniques* 2004 Feb; 14(1):38-41.

65. Pedraza R, Weiser A, Franco I. Laparoscopic appendovesicostomy (mitrofanoff procedure) in a child using the da Vinci robotic system. *Journal of Urology* 2004 Apr; 171(4):1652-3.

66. Di Marco DS, Chow GK, Gettman MT, Elliot DS. Robotic assisted laparoscopic sacrocolpopexy for treatment of vaginal vault prolapse. *Urology* 2004 Feb; 63(2):373-6.

67. Melamud O, Eichel L, Turbow B, Shanberg A. Laparoscopic vesicovaginal fistula repair with robotic reconstruction. *Urology* 2005 Jan; 65(1):163-6.

68. Rukstalis DB, Chodak GW. Laparoscopic retroperitoneal lymph node dissection in a patient with stage 1 testicular carcinoma. *Journal of Urology* 1992 Dec; 148(6):1907-09.

69. Steiner H, Peschel R, Janetschek G, Holtl L, Berger AP, Bartsch G, Hobisch A. Long term results of laparoscopic retroperitoneal lymph node dissection: single center 10 year experience. *Urology* 2004 Mar; 63(3):550-5.

70. Bhayani S, Ong A, Oh WK, Kantoff PW, Kavoussi LR. Laparoscopic retroperitoneal lymph node dissection for clinical stage 1 nonseminomatous germ cell testicular cancer: a long term update. *Urology* 2003 Aug; 62(2):324-7.

71. Rassweiler JJ, Frede T, Lenz E, Seemann O, Alken P. Long term experience with Laparoscopic retroperitoneal lymph node dissection in the management of low stage testis cancer. *European Urology* 2000 Mar; 37(3):251-60.

In: Robotics in Surgery: History, Current and Future Applications   ISBN 1-60021-386-3
Editor: Russell A. Faust, pp. 137-146   © 2007 Nova Science Publishers, Inc.

Chapter 8

FEMALE UROLOGIC ROBOTIC SURGERY: GYNECOLOGIC INDICATION FOR ROBOTIC-ASSISTED LAPAROSCOPY SACROCOLPOPEXY FOR THE TREATMENT OF HIGH GRADE VAGINAL VAULT PROLAPSE

Daniel S. Elliott[1], David S. DiMarco[2] and George K. Chow[1]

[1]Mayo Clinic, Department of Urology Rochester, Minnesota, USA
[2]Urology Healthcare, Springfield, Oregon, USA

Abstract

Transabdominal sacrocolpopexy offers an excellent definitive treatment option for patients with high grade vaginal vault prolapse with long-term success rates ranging from 93-99%. However, because it is a transabdominal procedure it is associated with increased morbidity compared with vaginal repairs. We describe a novel minimally invasive technique of vaginal vault prolapse repair and present out initial experience.

The surgical technique involves placement of four laparoscopic ports: three for the Da Vinci ® robot and one for the assistant. A polypropylene mesh is then attached to the sacral promontory and to the vaginal apex using Gortex sutures. At the end of the case, the mesh material is the covered by the peritoneum. We also present our initial experience with this technique in 18 consecutive patients. The analysis focused on complications, urinary continence, patient satisfaction, and morbidity. Follow-up was conducted by provider-patient interview.

Twenty-five patients underwent a robotic-assisted laparoscopic sacrocolpopexy at our institution in the past 24 months for severe symptomatic vaginal vault prolapse. 10/25 (40%) underwent a concomitant anti-incontinence procedure. Mean follow-up was 5.1(1-12) months and mean age was 66 (47-82) years. Mean total operative time was 3.2 (2.25-4.75) hours. One patient had to be converted to an open procedure secondary to unfavorable anatomy. All but one patient were discharged from the hospital after an overnight stay; one patient left on postoperative day #2. Complications were limited to mild port site infections in two patients, which resolved with oral antibiotic therapy. One patient developed recurrent grade 3 rectocele, but had no evidence of cystocele or enterocele. Significant incontinence (>1pad/day) was present in 2 patients. All 18 patients reported being satisfied with the outcome of their surgery and all 10 would recommend it to a friend.

We present a novel technique for vaginal vault prolapse repair that combines the advantages of open sacrocolpopexy with the decreased morbidity and improved cosmesis of laparoscopic surgery. It is associated with decreased hospital stay, low complication and conversion rates, and high patient satisfaction. While our early experience is encouraging, long-term data is needed to confirm these findings and establish longevity of the repair.

Keywords: Robotics, Laparoscopy, Sacrocolpopexy, Vaginal Vault Prolapse

INTRODUCTION

Currently, there has been limited reporting and research in the obstetric and gynecological literature concerning the use of robotics. To date, robotics have been utilized only for the treatment of two benign gynecologic conditions; benign hysterectomy,[1] and, sacrocolpopexy which a treatment for posthysterectomy vaginal vault prolapse.[2,3] However, laparoscopy has been utilized extensively in gynecologic surgeries and has demonstrated itself to be a invaluable with procedures such as total and supracervical hysterectomies and for the evaluation and treatment of endometriosis.[4] More recently, laparoscopy has been reported for staging purposes of gynecologic malignancies, for the treatment of early stage endometrial cancer, and the treatment of ectopic pregnancies.[5,6,7]

To demonstrate robotics potential benefit to other areas of gynecology, this chapter will focus on the emerging benefit discovered for the treatment of vaginal vault prolapse.

It has been estimated that one in nine women will undergo a hysterectomy in their lifetime, and up to 10% of these women will need surgical repair for treatment of a major, symptomatic vaginal prolapse.[8] The search for the type of repair that offers the best combination of the most effective, safest, and is most durable for the treatment of vaginal vault prolapse is an ongoing process as evidenced by the multiple surgical approaches to this problem. Clearly, no one surgical approach is ideal for every patient. However, as the known risk factors for prolapse, such as age, obesity and hysterectomy, continue to increase in the United States, so does the need for continuing the search for better means to repair vaginal vault prolapse.[9,10,11]

Currently, the transabdominal sacrocolpopexy has been shown, on multiple studies, to have one of the highest long-term success rates for durable repair of severe vault prolapse (93-100%).[12-20] In addition to a high success rate and durable results, other advantages of the sacrocolpopexy approach with the use of synthetic material to repair vault prolapse can be summarized as follows:

1. Support of the vaginal vault to the anterior surface of the sacrum preserves (or restores) the normal axis of the vagina.

2. Maximal vaginal depth can be preserved which is especially important in patients who desire continued sexual activity and in patients with an already foreshortened vagina from previous surgery.

3. Use of synthetic suspensory material can provide a source of strength in patients where the native tissue with prolapse is weak.[12]

Potential candidates for the open procedure tend to be younger patient and those who are more active and are more likely to be leading an active life-style. Other important indications are concurrent medical conditions such as chronic cough, COPD and asthma. These conditions place chronic and repeated increased intra-abdominal pressure on the repair. Unfortunately, due to the morbidity of the open transabdominal procedure, many patients are unable to tolerate the surgery. Therefore, many of these patients are treated via a transvaginal approach.

Goals of every surgical repair of vaginal vault prolapse include restoration of proper anatomy, maintenance of sexual function, and durability. Surgical approaches to correct the prolapse include either a vaginal or an abdominal approach or a combination of both. The main advantage to vaginal approach has historically been decreased morbidity, including shorter hospitalization and convalescence.[21,22] Unfortunately, long term success rates with transvaginal repairs are consistently lower compared to the abdominal approach such as sacrocolpopexy.[23]

In an effort to balance the benefit of the open sacrocolpopexy (durable repair) with the advantage of a vaginal repair (reduced morbidity), many attempts have been made with treating the vault prolapse via laparoscopic sacrocolpopexy.[24,25] Unfortunately, technical difficulties in actually accomplishing the procedure and the potentially significant increase in operative time has greatly limited its widespread use. To address theses specific limitation of laparoscopic repairs, we feel that recent advances in robotic surgery may be an answer.

Telerobotics provides technical features such as three-dimensional vision, increased robotic instrument maneuverability, and physiologic tremor filtering. These factors provide an ergonomic environment for the surgeon that simplifies performance of complex laparoscopic tasks. We describe the technique of robotic-assisted laparoscopic sacrocolpopexy using a silicone graft. Our ultimate goal of the robotic-assisted laparoscopic sacrocolpopexy was threefold:

1. Provide the most durable repair for vaginal vault prolapse.
2. Minimize the morbidity associated with transabdominal procedures.
3. Provide a procedure that can be accomplished within a reasonable operative time.

Surgical technique

The daVinci robot is an integrated computer-based system consisting of two interactive robotic arms, a camera arm, and a remote control with three-dimensional vision capability. The daVinci robot uses instruments with 6 degrees of freedom that provide the same flexibility of the human wrist. The working robotic arms are attached to reusable 8-mm trocars, while the camera is placed through a standard 12-mm laparoscopic port. For optimal robot function and to minimize risk of collisions, the angle created by the camera port and each working robotic port should be obtuse and the distance between the ports at least one hand-breadth. With robotic surgery, the motions of the surgeon at the remote control unit are replicated by the robotic arms placed within the patient. Tactile feedback is not available with daVinci, therefore an increased reliance on visual inputs is required. During robotic surgery, an assistant surgeon is scrubbed at the operating table. The assistant performs a variety of important robot-related tasks including alignment and exchange of instruments on the robotic arms. Furthermore, the assistant performs operative maneuvers with conventional instruments including tissue countertraction, hemostasis, hemoclip application, suction, and assistance during suturing. Most importantly, the scrubbed assistant is available in the event that an emergent conversion would be required.

For the procedure, the patient is placed in the dorsal lithotomy position on the operating table. After general anesthesia is established, a nasogastric tube is placed and both arms are tucked beside the torso. The patient is prepped from the nipples to proximal thigh including the vagina.

After abdominal insufflation using a Varus needle, we place a periumbilical Visiport under direct vision to avoid visceral or vascular injury. Two standard laparoscopic ports are next introduced under direct vision. One 10mm port right subcostal lateral to the rectus and one 5 mm port one hands breadth inferior-laterally **(figure 1)**. These ports are used for retraction during the procedure. Next, two 8mm robotic ports are placed lateral to the rectus 2 fingerbreadths superior to the ileac crest.

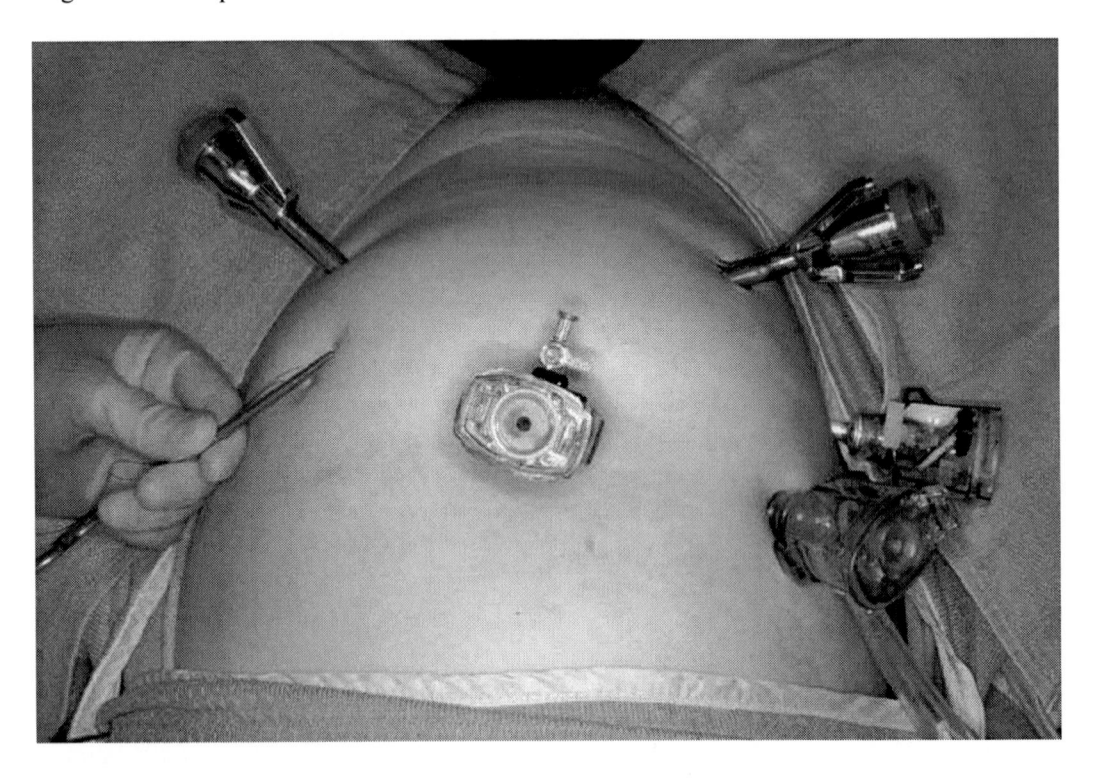

At this point, using standard laparoscopy, a retracting suture is placed through the sigmoid tenia to eventually help in exposing the sacral promontory. The next step is dissection of the bladder from the anterior vaginal wall using forceps and scissors with cautery. A customized hand-held vaginal retractor manufactured at the Mayo Clinic **(figure 2)** is used to facilitate the dissection, which should be a relatively bloodless plane. Posteriorly, the peritoneal reflection is then incised to mobilize the vagina. Both of these dissections should be carried out as distal (toward the introitus) as possible to maximize the support given by the Y-graft. After adequate vaginal mobilization the sacral dissection with careful attention to avoid sacral venous complexes is accomplished. Once the shiny periosteum is exposed, the polypropylene Y-graft (IntePro™ American Medical Systems, Minnetonka, Minnesota) **(figure 3)** is brought into the field through the 10 mm port. To date, in our experience, the aforementioned steps can be accomplished with 30 to 40 minutes.

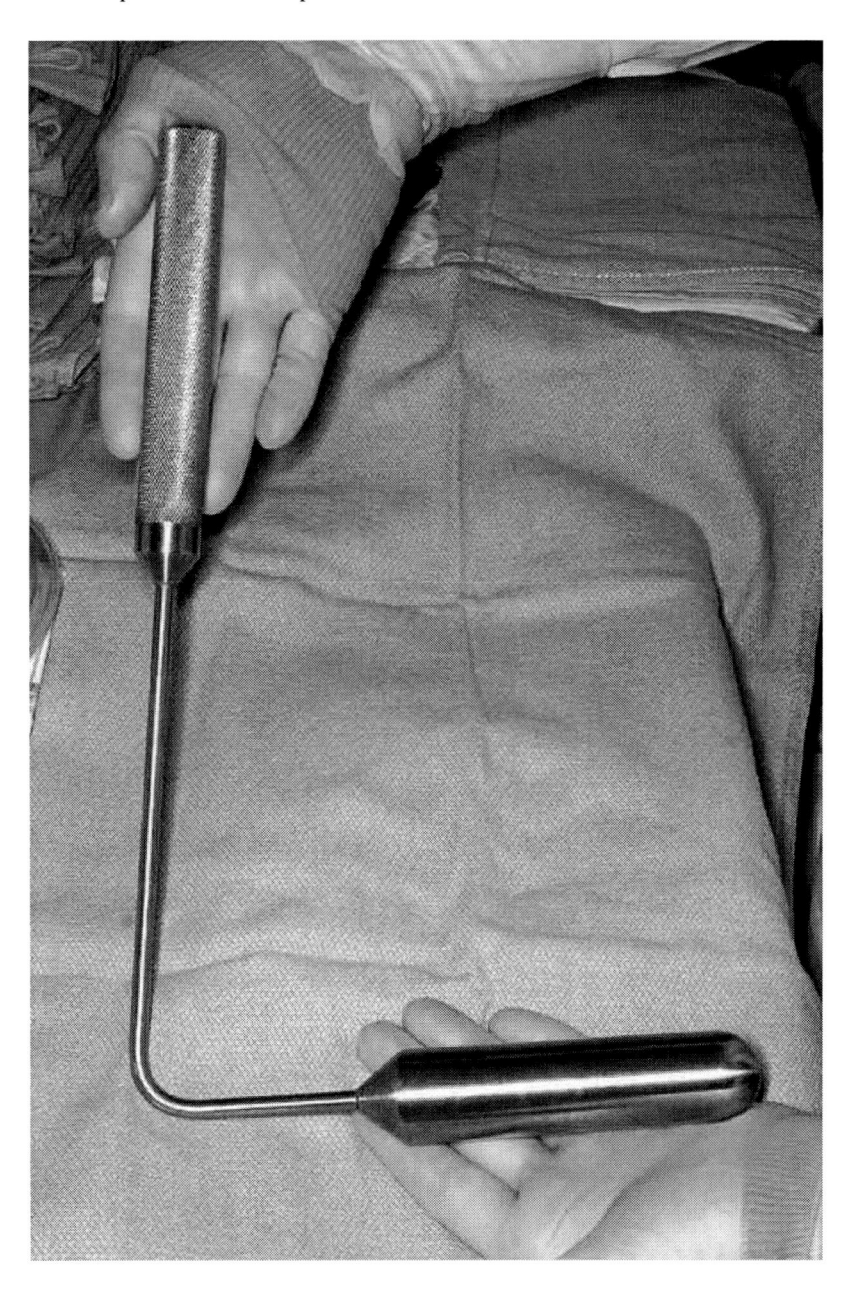

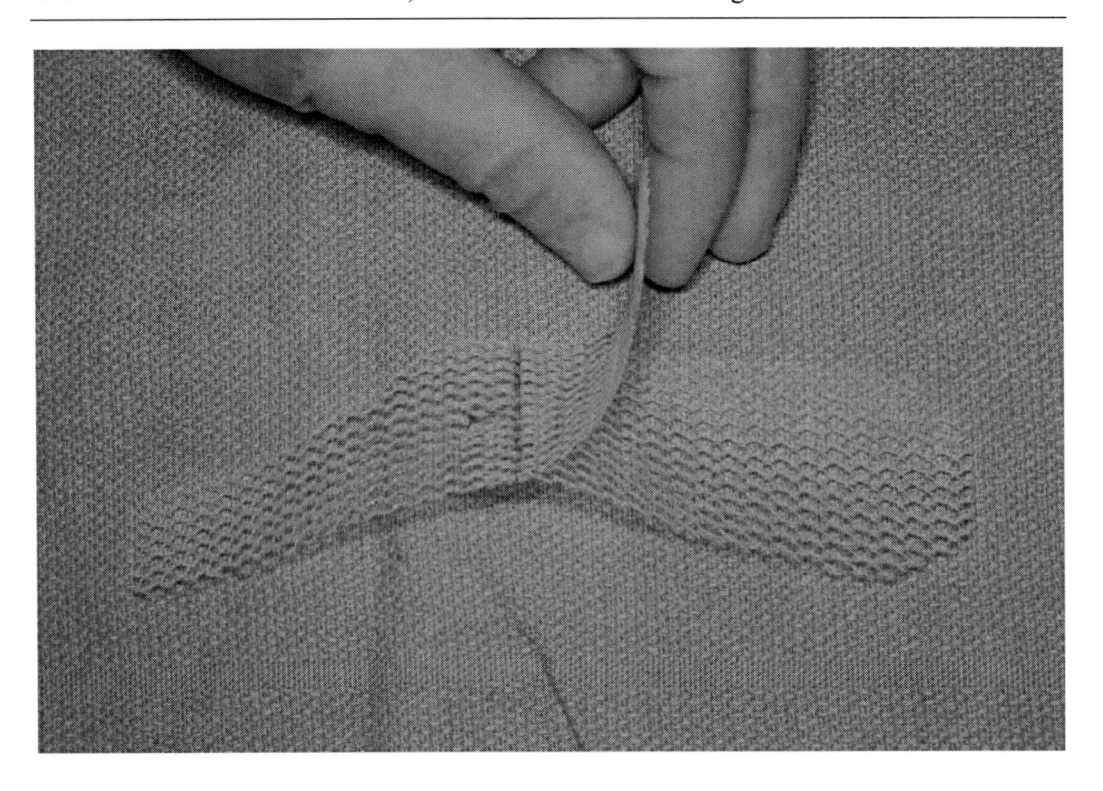

The robot is now docked with the base positioned at the foot of the bed. The main reason to utilize the robot at this point in time is to facilitate and greatly reduce the operative time needed for suturing of the graft to the vagina and the sacrum. The Y-shaped graft is inserted via a port. The graft is then robotically sutured using 1.0 Gore-Tex. The 30 degree lens and vaginal retractor maximize exposure for placement of the sutures. We have found that placing the posterior sutures first, as they are more difficult, followed by suturing the anterior portion of the Y-graft reduces the difficulty of the process. The tail end of the graft is then sutured to the sacral promontory using three to four interrupted sutures with careful attention to avoid any undo tension on the vagina. We also perform a standard Halban's culdoplasty with plication of the uterosacral ligaments to further aid in the prevention of recurrent vaginal prolapse. The posterior peritoneum is then closed to completely retroperitonealize the graft.

RESULTS

At our institution, we have performed robotic-assisted laparoscopic sacrocolpopexy on twenty-five patients for the treatment of high grade, symptomatic vaginal vault prolapse over that past 24 months. Mean age is 66 (47-82) years. Ten patients of the twenty-five patients (40%) underwent concurrent a concurrent anti-incontinence procedure at the time of the prolapse repair to treat concurrent stress urinary incontinence. Mean total operative time was 3.2 (2.25-4.75) hours. Initially, the "skin-to-skin" time was 4.75 hours. However, with experience and utilizing multiple various time saving steps, we are now routinely completing the case under two and a half hours.

One patient had to be converted to an open procedure secondary to unfavorable anatomy. All but one patient were discharged from the hospital after an overnight stay; one patient left on postoperative day #2. All patients were dismissed on oral pain medication. Ten of the patients have reported they only required non-steroidal antiinflammatory medication for control of their pain. One patient had persistent vaginal bleeding for 2 days post operatively, a complication related to the anti-incontinence portion of the case not the prolapse repair. Her hemoglobin remained stable with no further sequelae.

COMPLICATIONS

Complications were limited to mild port site infections in two patients, which resolved with oral antibiotic therapy. One patient developed recurrent grade 3 rectocele, but had no evidence of cystocele or enterocele. One patient developed an small erosion of the synthetic cuff into the vagina 6 months following the procedure. This was easily managed with an outpatient, transvaginal excision. Significant incontinence (>1pad/day) was present in 2 patients. All 25 patients reported being satisfied with the outcome of their surgery and 24/25 would recommend it to a friend. The one patient who did not recommend the procedure was the solitary patient who was converted to an open procedure.

Limitations of Robotic-Assisted Sacrocolpopexy

One of the obvious limitations with this procedure is the learning curve associated with laparoscopy itself. Clearly, the technical aspect of laparoscopy requires advanced training, however, with the addition of robotics, the technical difficulty of the procedure is actually reduced. Individuals with basic laparoscopy skills usually are able to master the procedure when it is combined with robotics. However, the advantage of the robot does come with a price tag attached. Currently, the da Vinci Robotic system can be purchased for roughly $1 million. It is true the device cuts down on operative time but for many facilities, the price tag may prohibit its purchase. In larger institutions, the device is used in many other surgical specialties, thereby, saving considerable operative time, and thereby, making the purchase price more palatable.

CONCLUSION

We feel, and the data supports, that transabdominal sacrocolpopexy is the most durable and effective treatment of post-hysterectomy vaginal vault prolapse. However, not every patient is a candidate for this procedure due to age, concurrent medical conditions or concerns regarding postoperative recovery time. We also feel that the advantage of a robotic-assisted laparoscopic sacrocolpopexy accomplishes the identical repair as that of the open transabdominal technique. The morbidity associated with that of the open procedure is greatly reduced and the hospital stay has been reduced from 2-5 days with the open procedure, down to one day with the laparoscopic repair.[26,27] Also, based upon early, short-term results, it appears that the durability of the repair will be the same as with the open procedure. Potentially, many more women will be able to be offered the strongest repair for prolapse while still keeping the morbidity to a minimum. As long-term results become available we will better be able to determine the durability of this repair.

Relative contraindications would be the same for most laparoscopic procedures including patients with prior abdominal surgeries and those with morbid obesity. Clearly, longer follow-up is needed; however, the robotic-assisted laparoscopic sacrocolpopexy described in this report may be an ideal approach to the surgery repair of vaginal vault prolapse.

THE FUTURE OF ROBOTICS IN GYNECOLOGY

Though the robotics experience is early, the potential for robotics in this surgical specialty is significant. Clearly, there are limitations to robotics, however, since many gynecologic surgeons feel comfortable with the use of laparoscopy the potential to transfer those skill to robotics is clearly present and the benefit to patients potentially dramatic.

REFERENCES

1. Beste, TM, Nelson KH, Daucher JA. Total laparoscopic hysterectomy utilizing a robotic surgical system. *Journal of the Society of Laparoendoscopic Surgeons* 2005. Jan-Mar;9(1):13-5.

2. DiMarco DS, Chow GK, Gettman MT, Elliott DS, "Robotic-assisted laparoscopic sacrocolpopexy for treatment of vaginal vault prolapse." *Urology* February 2004. 63(2): 373-376.

1. Elliott DS, Frank I, DiMarco DS, Chow GK,: "Gynecological use of robotically assisted laparoscopy: sacrocolpopexy for the treatment of high-grade vaginal vault prolapse. *American Journal of Surgery,* 2004,188 (Suppl to October 2004) 52S-56S.

2. Jenkins TR. Laparoscopic supracervical hysterectomy. *American Journal of Obstetrics and Gynecology* 2004. Dec;191(6):1875-84.

3. Yu CK, Cutner A, Mould T, Olaitan A. Total laparoscopic hysterectomy as a primary surgical treatment for endometrial cancer in morbidly obese women. *British Journal of Obstetrics and Gynecology* 2005. Jan 112(1):115-117.

4. Barakat RR. Laparoscopically assisted surgical staging for endometrial cancer. *International Journal of Gynecologic Cancer* 2005. Mar-Apr 15(2):407.

5. Subair O, Omojole F, Mistry N, Morgan H. Trainees and the management of ectopic pregnancy. *Journal of Obstetrics and Gynaecolog*. 2004. Oct 24(7):811-2.

6. Marchionni M, Bracco GL, Checcucci V, Carabaneanu A, Coccia EM, Mecacci F, Scarselli G. True incidence of vaginal vault prolapse. Thirteen years of experience. *Journal of Reproductive Medicine* 1999. 44(8):679-84.

7. Dwyer PL, Lee ETC, Hay DM. Obesity and urinary incontinence in women. *British Journal Obstetrics and Gynaecology* 1988. 95(1):91-6.

8. Virtanen HS, Makinen JI. Retrospective analysis of 711 patients operated on for pelvic relaxation in 1983-1989. International Journal Gynecology Obstetrics 1993. 42(2):109-15.

9. Olsen A, Smith V, Bergstrom J, Colling J, Clark A. Epidemiology of surgically managed pelvic organ prolapse and urinary incontinence. *Obstetrics Gynecology* 1997. Apr 89(4):501-6.

10. Addison WA, Timmons MC: Abdominal Approach to Vaginal Eversion. *Clinical Obstetrics and Gynecology* 1993. 36(4) 995-1004.

11. Timmons MC, Addison WA, Addison SB, Cavenar MG: Abdominal sacral colpopexy in 163 women with posthysterectomy vaginal vault prolapse and enterocele. Journal Reproductive Medecine 1992. Apr 37(4):323-327.

12. Cundiff GW, Harris RL, Coates K, Low VHS, Bump RC, Addison WA: Abdominal sacral colpoperineopexy: A new approach for correction of posterior compartment defects and perineal descent associated with vaginal vault prolapse. *American Journal Obstetrics and Gynecology* 1997. Dec 177(6):1345-1353.

13. Snyder TE, Krantz KE: Abdominal-retroperitoneal sacral colpopexy for the correction of vaginal prolapse. *Obstetrics and Gynecology* 1991. Jun 77(6):944-949.

14. Menefee SA, Miller KF, Wall LL: Results of abdominal sacral colpopexy using polyester mesh in the treatment of posthysterectomy vaginal vault prolapse and enterocele. *Obstetrics and Gynecology* 1999. Sept 54(9):563-565.

15. Reddy K, Malik TG., Short-term and long-term follow-up of abdominal sacrocolpopexy for vaginal vault prolapse: initial experience in a district general hospital. *Journal of Obstetrics and Gynaecol.* 2002. Sep 22(5):532-6

16. Addison WA, Timmons MC, Wall LL, Livengood CH: Failed abdominal sacral colpopexy: observations and recommendations. *Obstetrics and Gynecology* 1989. Sep74(3 pt 2):480-483.

17. Addison WA, Timmons MC: Abdominal sacral colpopexy for the treatment of vaginal vault prolapse with enterocele. In: Te Linde's Operative Gynecology, Eighth Ed. John A. Rock and John D. Thompson Ed. Lippincott-Raven Publishers, Philadelphia, 1997. pp1030-37.

18. Webb MJ, Aronson MP, Ferguson LK, Lee RA. Posthysterectomy vaginal vault prolapse: primary repair in 693 patients. *Obstetrics and Gynecology* 1998. 92(2):281-5.

19. Podratz LK, Ferguson VR, Lee RA, Symmonds RE: Abdominal sacral colpopexy for posthysterectomy vaginal vault descensus. *Obstetrics and Gynecology* 1995. Oct 50(10):719-720.

20. Karram M, Goldwasser S, Kleeman S, Steele A, Vassallo B, Walsh P. High uterosacral vaginal vault suspension with fascial reconstruction for vaginal repair of enterocele and vaginal vault prolapse. *American Journal of Obstetrics and Gynecology* 2001.185(6):1339-42; discussion 42-3.

21. Benson JT, Lucente V, McClellan E. Vaginal versus abdominal reconstructive surgery for the treatment of pelvic support defects: a prospective randomized study with long-term outcome evaluation. *American Journal of Obstetrics and Gynecology* 1996.175(6):1418-21; discussion 21-2.

22. Ostrzenski A. Laparoscopic colposuspension for total vaginal prolapse. *International Journal of Gynaecology and Obstetrics* 1996.55(2):147-52.

23. Cosson M, Rajabally R, Bogaert E, Querleu D, Crepin G. Laparoscopic sacrocolpopexy, hysterectomy, and burch colposuspension: feasibility and short-term complications of 77 procedures. *Journal of the Society of Laparoendoscopic Surgeons* 2002.6(2):115-9.

24. Cosson M, Bogaert E, Narducci F, Querleu D, Crepin G. Laparoscopic sacral colpopexy: short-term results and complications in 83 patients. *Journal de Gynecologie Obstetrique et Biologie de la Reproduction* (Paris). 2000. Dec 29(8):746-750.

25. Montironi PL, Petruzzelli P, Di Noto C, Gibbone C, De Sanctis C, Fedele M. Combined vaginal and laparoscopic surgical treatment of genito-urinary prolapse. *Minerva Ginecologica* (Italy) 2000. Jul-Aug 52(7-8):283-8.

In: Robotics in Surgery: History, Current and Future Applications ISBN 1-60021-386-3
Editor: Russell A. Faust, pp. 147-172 © 2007 Nova Science Publishers, Inc.

Chapter 9

ROBOTIC APPLICATIONS IN NEUROSURGERY

Lucia Zamorano[1], Qinghang Li[2] and Richard Rhiew[2]

[1]Harper University Hospital, Detroit Medical Center,
Farmington Hills, MI USA
[2]Neurological Surgery Department, Wayne State University, Detroit, MI, USA

INTRODUCTION

Revolutionary advances in computer and information technologies are widely applying into modern medical world. Using image guided, computer assisted interactive surgical navigation procedures are quite common in many medical centers. With the development of computer assisted surgery, the appearance of medical robotic system is the next step for precise conversion of the preoperative surgical plan, derived from the navigation system, into surgical action. Medical robots are extensions of computer systems that allow programmed physical interaction with the environment in the medical field. They have tremendous potential for improving the precision and capabilities of physicians when performing surgical procedures. Medical robotic systems are playing an increasing role in different image-guided surgical procedures. The key advantages are that robots can effectively position, orient, and manipulate surgical tools in 3D space with a high level of accuracy. Several medical robots or robotic arms have been reported for clinical applications [1]. However, the application of robotics to medicine is still in an early stage, and many questions remain open regarding their effectiveness, safety, and cost. Unlike the area of industrial robotics, which grew rapidly during the 1970s and 1980s, only a few clinical application of robotics exist until now. Even it is believed the benefits of medical robotics will become increasingly clear, and this will lead to a continued rise in their use, there are only few commercial companies selling medical robots and the total number installed is extremely small. The market will most likely continue to grow slowly.

An author from Czech, Kapek, was the first user of the term 'robot'. According to the Robotic Institute of America, a robot is "a reprogrammable, multifunctional manipulator designed to move materials, parts, tools, or other specialized devices through various programmed motions for the performance of a variety of tasks." A robotic system, however, is more than a mechanical manipulator. These robots consist of nearly rigid links that are connected with joints that allow relative motion from one link to another. Attached to the end of the links is the robot hand, usually referred to as the end-effector. The robot is controlled by a computer system that is used to move the end-effector to any desired point and orientation within its workspace. Jo Engelberger, one of the robot patriarchs, said, "You know one when you see one!" and this may yet prove to be the most appropriate definition for the use of robots in surgery. The development of minimally invasive surgery and introduction of medical imaging techniques (virtual reality) is a paradigm shift for surgical application of medical robots for reproducibility and improved precision in surgical procedures. Neurosurgery saw the first clinical application of robotics, and continues to be an important test case for robotic technology[1]. More than 3000 patients that have undergone robotic brain surgery. Robotic surgery differs from computer-assisted surgery by the fact that instead of a surgeon performing the operation it is performed by a computerized robot. The robots are much more precise and performs with more delicacy and precision than a human ever possibly could, and they cause less damage to the brain, but at present they cannot replace the surgeons. They can also help doctors visualize what would normally be impossible, and they ultimately are economical because fewer staff is required for the surgery, and patients spend less time in hospital following surgery [1]. Several other medical robotics review articles with a focus on surgical procedures have been written [2-7]. Davies describes the history of surgical robotics and gives one classification for the types of robot systems studied by researchers [2]. Taylor discusses several taxonomies for surgical robotics and presents a different classification [3]. Troccaz and Delnondedieu give a historical review and describe passive, semiactive, and active robotic systems [4]. Howe and Matsuoka provide an overview of applications in image-based procedures, orthopedic surgery, and neurosurgery, among others [5]. Cleary and Nguyen give a detail introduction of medical robotics in different applications [6]. According to our own experience, we also introduced some medical robotic systems that were used for clinical neurosurgery [7]. This article highlights the state of the art of medical robotics engaged in neurosurgical procedures. In this chapter, we will focus on robots that play an active role during a surgical intervention. These systems are not meant to replace the physician, but rather to augment the capabilities of the physician as a surgical tool. This chapter is not intended to be comprehensive, but rather to give an overview of the field, with a focus on key historical developments and current work.

HISTORICAL REVIEW

The first recorded medical application of a robot was in 1985. This robot was a simple positioning device to orient a needle for biopsy of the brain. The robot used was a PUMA 560 industrial robot [1]. The procedure was performed well but the safety issues concerning the operation of the robot prevented this work from continuing. Currently, there are several commercial ventures and a handful of research laboratories active in the field of medical robotics. These early research efforts have led to some commercial products. The future of robotics in the operating theatre is best illustrated by the work at Grenoble University Hospital, which has built the NeuroMate robot of Integrated Surgical Systems, as described later in this chapter. **Table 1** provides a chronology of developments in the robotic neurosurgery literature.

Table 1. Chronological Advances of Robotics in Neurosurgery

1987
Benabid AL, Cinquin P, Lavalle S, Le Bas JF, Demongeot J, de Rougemont J. Computer-driven robot for stereotactic surgery connected to CT scan and magnetic resonance imaging. Technological design and preliminary results. Appl Neurophysiol. 1987;50(1-6):153-4.
Young RF. Application of robotics to stereotactic neurosurgery. Neurol Res. 1987 Jun;9(2):123-8.
1988
Kwoh YS, Hou J, Jonckheere EA, Hayati S. A robot with improved absolute positioning accuracy for CT guided stereotactic brain surgery. IEEE Trans Biomed Eng. 1988 Feb;35(2):153-60.
1990
Koyama H, Uchida T, Funakubo H, Takakura K, Fankhauser H. Development of a new microsurgical robot for stereotactic neurosurgery. Stereotact Funct Neurosurg. 1990;54-55:462-7.
Glauser D, Flury P, Durr P, Funakubo H, Burckhardt CW, Favre J, Schnyder P, Fankhauser H. Configuration of a robot dedicated to stereotactic surgery. Stereotact Funct Neurosurg. 1990;54-55:468-70.
1991
Drake JM, Joy M, Goldenberg A, Kreindler D. Computer- and robot-assisted resection of thalamic astrocytomas in children. Neurosurgery. 1991 Jul;29(1):27-33.
1992
Benabid AL, Lavallee S, Hoffmann D, Cinquin P, Demongeot J, Danel F. Potential use of robots in endoscopic neurosurgery. Acta Neurochir Suppl (Wien). 1992;54:93-7.
1994
Fankhauser H, Glauser D, Flury P, Piguet Y, Epitaux M, Favre J, Meuli RA. Robot for CT-guided stereotactic neurosurgery. Stereotact Funct Neurosurg. 1994;63(1-4):93-8.
1995
Giorgi C, Eisenberg H, Costi G, Gallo E, Garibotto G, Casolino DS. Robot-assisted microscope for neurosurgery. J Image Guid Surg. 1995;1(3):158-63.
Glauser D, Fankhauser H, Epitaux M, Hefti JL, Jaccottet A. Neurosurgical robot Minerva: first results and current developments. J Image Guid Surg. 1995;1(5):266-72.
1997
Schweikard A, Adler JR. Robotic radiosurgery with noncylindrical collimators. Comput Aided Surg. 1997;2(2):124-34.
Zamorano L, Matter A, Saenz A, Buciuc R, Diaz F. Interactive image-guided resection of cerebral cavernous malformations. Comput Aided Surg. 1997;2(6):327-32.
Andrews R, Mah R, Galvagni A, Guerrero M, Papasin R, Wallace M, Winters J. Robotic multimodality stereotactic brain tissue identification: work in progress. Stereotact Funct Neurosurg. 1997;68(1-4 Pt 1):72-9.
1998
Wapler M, Stallkamp J, Weisener T, Urban V. Motion feedback as a navigation aid in robot assisted neurosurgery. Stud Health Technol Inform. 1998;50:215-9.
Hefti JL, Epitaux M, Glauser D, Fankhauser H. Robotic three-dimensional positioning of a stimulation electrode in the brain. Comput Aided Surg. 1998;3(1):1-10.

Table 1. Chronological Advances of Robotics in Neurosurgery (Continued)

1999
Tseng CS, Chung CW, Chen HH, Wang SS, Tseng HM. Development of a robotic navigation system for neurosurgery. Stud Health Technol Inform. 1999;62:358-9.
Wapler M, Braucker M, Durr M, Hiller A, Stallkamp J, Urban V. A voice-controlled robotic assistant for neuroendoscopy. Stud Health Technol Inform. 1999;62:384-7.
2000
Schweikard A, Glosser G, Bodduluri M, Murphy MJ, Adler JR. Robotic motion compensation for respiratory movement during radiosurgery. Comput Aided Surg. 2000;5(4):263-77.
Giorgi C, Sala R, Riva D, Cossu A, Eisenberg H. Robotics in child neurosurgery. Childs Nerv Syst. 2000 Nov;16(10-11):832-4.
Radetzky A, Rudolph M, Starkie S, Davies B, Auer LM. ROBO-SIM: a simulator for minimally invasive neurosurgery using an active manipulator. Stud Health Technol Inform. 2000;77:1165-9.
2001
Chang SD, Adler JR. Robotics and radiosurgery--the cyberknife. Stereotact Funct Neurosurg. 2001;76(3-4):204-8.
2002
Quinn AM. CyberKnife: a robotic radiosurgery system. Clin J Oncol Nurs. 2002 May-Jun;6(3):149, 156.
Koyama J, Hongo K, Kakizawa Y, Goto T, Kobayashi S. Endoscopic telerobotics for neurosurgery: preliminary study for optimal distance between an object lens and a target. Neurol Res. 2002 Jun;24(4):373-6.
Li QH, Zamorano L, Pandya A, Perez R, Gong J, Diaz F. The application accuracy of the NeuroMate robot--A quantitative comparison with frameless and frame-based surgical localization systems. Comput Aided Surg. 2002;7(2):90-8.
Cleary K, Stoianovici D, Patriciu A, Mazilu D, Lindisch D, Watson V. Robotically assisted nerve and facet blocks: a cadaveric study. Acad Radiol. 2002 Jul;9(7):821-5.
Hongo K, Kobayashi S, Kakizawa Y, Koyama J, Goto T, Okudera H, Kan K, Fujie MG, Iseki H, Takakura K. NeuRobot: telecontrolled micromanipulator system for minimally invasive microneurosurgery-preliminary results. Neurosurgery. 2002 Oct;51(4):985-8; discussion 988.
Zimmermann M, Krishnan R, Raabe A, Seifert V. Robot-assisted navigated neuroendoscopy. Neurosurgery. 2002 Dec;51(6):1446-51; discussion 1451-2.
2003
Goto T, Hongo K, Koyama J, Kobayashi S. Feasibility of using the potassium titanyl phosphate laser with micromanipulators in robotic neurosurgery: a preliminary study in the rat. J Neurosurg. 2003 Jan;98(1):131-5.
Chang SD, Main W, Martin DP, Gibbs IC, Heilbrun MP.
An analysis of the accuracy of the CyberKnife: a robotic frameless stereotactic radiosurgical system. Neurosurgery. 2003 Jan;52(1):140-6; discussion 146-7.
Federspil PA, Geisthoff UW, Henrich D, Plinkert PK. Development of the first force-controlled robot for otoneurosurgery. Laryngoscope. 2003 Mar;113(3):465-71.
Willems PW, Noordmans HJ, Ramos LM, Taphoorn MJ, Berkelbach van der Sprenkel JW, Viergever MA, Tulleken CA. Clinical evaluation of stereotactic brain biopsies with an MKM-mounted instrument holder. Acta Neurochir (Wien). 2003 Oct;145(10):889-97; discussion 897.
Goto T, Hongo K, Kakizawa Y, Muraoka H, Miyairi Y, Tanaka Y, Kobayashi S. Clinical application of robotic telemanipulation system in neurosurgery. Case report. J Neurosurg. 2003 Dec;99(6):1082-4.

Table 1. Chronological Advances of Robotics in Neurosurgery (Continued)

2003	
	Varma TR, Eldridge PR, Forster A, Fox S, Fletcher N, Steiger M, Littlechild P, Byrne P, Sinnott A, Tyler K, Flintham S. Use of the NeuroMate stereotactic robot in a frameless mode for movement disorder surgery. Stereotact Funct Neurosurg. 2003;80(1-4):132-5.
2004	
	Nimsky Ch, Rachinger J, Iro H, Fahlbusch R. Adaptation of a hexapod-based robotic system for extended endoscope-assisted transsphenoidal skull base surgery. Minim Invasive Neurosurg. 2004 Feb;47(1):41-6.
	Louw DF, Fielding T, McBeth PB, Gregoris D, Newhook P, Sutherland GR. Surgical robotics: a review and neurosurgical prototype development. Neurosurgery. 2004 Mar;54(3):525-36; discussion 536-7.
	Zimmermann M, Krishnan R, Raabe A, Seifert V. Robot-assisted navigated endoscopic ventriculostomy: implementation of a new technology and first clinical results. Acta Neurochir (Wien). 2004 Jul;146(7):697-704. Epub 2004 May 17.
	Psarros TG, Mickey B, Gall K, Gilio J, Delp J, White C, Drees J, Willis M, Pistemmna D, Giller CA. Image-guided robotic radiosurgery in a rat glioma model. Minim Invasive Neurosurg. 2004 Oct;47(5):266-72.
2005	
	Mendez I, Hill R, Clarke D, Kolyvas G. Robotic long-distance telementoring in neurosurgery. Neurosurgery. 2005 Mar;56(3):434-40; discussion 434-40.

WHY A ROBOT?

Initial experimentation with surgical robotics consisted largely of adaptations of existing robot technology from the industrial sector. Humans and machines are complementary rather than competitive, with one another. Human superiority stems from qualities such as flexibility, adaptability, judgement and hand-eye coordination. Human shortcomings include fatigability, memory limitations, inability to simultaneously process large amount of data, tremor and tissue susceptible to injury. Robot superiority includes the ability to accurately position and reposition instruments, absence of tremor, uniform and controlled application of force, stamina, strength, and the ability to process vast quantities of data simultaneously. The challenge is that they are limited by their lack of judgment, suboptimal spatial coordination, poor adaptability, and susceptibility to malfunction. The primary goal in adapting robots for neurosurgery is to enhance and standardize care so that all patients receive the same excellent level of care. Development of this new tool should be viewed as a reflection of human development, a measure of human progress, and the ability to transform this challenge into the reproducible and routine. Robots offer a wide array of benefits in the surgical field in terms of:

- Repeatable tool position and trajectory
- Steady motion
- Ability to react rapidly to changes in force level
- Remote operation
- Ability to remain poised in a fixed position
- Greater three-dimensional spatial accuracy

- More reliable system design
- Ability to achieve much greater precision

CLASSIFICATION

There are several ways to classify the use of robots in medicine. Taylor stresses the role of robots as tools that can work cooperatively with physicians to carry out surgical interventions, and identifies five classes of systems: 1) intern replacements, 2) tele surgical systems, 3) navigational aids, 4) precise positioning systems, and 5) precise path systems [8]. Other classifications of surgical robotics are based on the intrinsic complexity of the robotic technology and safety. One classification divides surgical robots in active and passive systems based on the type of robot control: surgeon vs computer. A passive mechanism is one where the surgeon provides the physical energy to drive the surgical tool; an active mechanism is one where motion is achieved using non-human powered devices and in general involves a computer. Active mechanisms, by definition, have a degree of autonomy, although the surgeon must at least be able to monitor the complete process and intervene if the procedure is not going according to plan. Some devices will move from being passive to active within a single procedure. Several medical robotic systems have combined both active and passive mechanisms.

Another classification is based on the intrinsic safety of the device. An intrinsically safe design is a mechanism that has physically restricted motion so that all possible movements are safe.

The following are the various types of surgical robots being used today. The use is based on the type of interaction the surgeon has with the system:

- Active systems, which perform part of the surgical intervention autonomously. An example is ROBODOC (Integrated Surgical Systems Inc.).
- Semi-active systems that provide mechanical guidance for carrying out a surgical procedure (predetermined environment) e.g. NeuroMate. More recently, this class has been enlarged to include programmable devices, which provide the same type of interaction, renamed as synergistic systems.
- Passive systems, which provide information that allow a surgeon to compare the real task being executed with the planned task. Image-based navigation systems provide this functionality.
- Finally, Teleoperated master-slave systems allow the execution of orders transmitted by the surgeon to a slave robot, at a distance – whether in the same operating room or trans-global.

THE NEUROSURGICAL APPLICATIONS OF ROBOTS

Neurosurgery is a key area of application of medical robotics. The main reasons are: (i) the brain is firmly held in a solid container allowing fixation of devices to hold it in position during the procedure; (ii) the anatomical topology is fairly stable, corresponding to a rather well known functional somatotopy; (iii) brain imaging has been the most progressive field during the last decades, combining several modalities; (iv) the brain is the organ where the highest precision is required for surgical procedures; (v) stereotactic procedures have opened the way for numerical approaches through minimally invasive routes. We highlight here the currently available robotassisted neurosurgical applications and tasks performed:

Robot-assisted neurosurgical tasks

Typical neurosurgical tasks being robotized include instrument positioning and micropositioning, trajectory planning and precise needle insertion, free motion allowing the instrument to be arbitrarily positioned and oriented, motion in a constrained region, motion and force scaling, and soft tissue cutting and destructing, among many other tasks.

Positioning

Robot-assisted positioning overcomes the human hand's tremor and fatigue. Robots developed for instrument position include NeuroMate [9], Minerva [10] and IMARL [11]. Certain surgical manoeuvers, such as microsurgery or stereotactic electrode placement, demand micro-positioning with micrometer accuracy.

Precise needle insertion and biopsy

A compact robotic system called MINI-RCM for precise needle insertion under surgical guidance is reported. Several systems are available for robotic assistance with biopsies such as the NeuroMate, as described separately [7, 9, 11-13].

Instrument holding and moving

Tiresome and strenuous, but simple, tasks such as retractor fixation, light and camera positioning, and suction control are all easily robotized. Robot-assisted holding is also seen with the recent CyberKnife from Accuray [14] where the end effector is a Linac.

Motion and force scaling

Modern neurosurgery has reached a point where the scale of the operative field is so small that even skilled surgeons are reaching the limits of their dexterity. A telemanipulator RAMS (Robot-Assisted Microsurgery) scales down the surgeon's hand motion and filters tremor. Using RAMS, the surgeon holds a master input handle, similar to a surgical instrument to command the motions of the robot instrument. The surgeon's hand motions are then transferred in real-time through a computer system, where they are processed to control the robot's motion. Sensor signals from the instrument are monitored and modified by the computer. This process miniaturizes the surgeon's movement at the tissue level and prevents an incorrect movement or tremor associated with anxiety, fatigue, or age. In addition, forces sensed through the surgical instruments can also be amplified [15].

Force control

Force control is critical when performing tasks such as brain retraction. Continuous contact must be maintained without damaging the retracted tissue. Robotic retraction may present a superior alternative to human retraction by minimizing the forces exerted on tissues [16].

Soft tissue cutting and ablation

PUMA 200, a robotic system that controls high intensity, focused ultrasound destruction of subcortical lesions, has been described [17, 18]. Robotic assisted identification of tissues can improve brain tumor excision [12]. Both robots and stereotactic frames are capable of localizing targets and delivering low-energy interstitial irradiation, such as the photoelectron.

High load-bearing capacity

Robots are capable of supporting and guiding heavy objects such as an x-ray source or linear accelerator (approximately 150 kg) (CyberKnife from Accuray) [14].

Improved safety margin in delivery of radiotherapy

Robots are able to compensate for the motion by tracking the target. The CyberKnife currently employs such technology with an improved safety margin by reducing erroneous extralesional radiation delivery to adjacent normal tissues [14].

Object grasping

Systems are available in which two robotic "fingers" are capable of grasping objects as small as 2 pm in size [19].

Bone drilling & bolting

The Fraunhofer research scientists (Germany) have developed a special prototype 'Rolled' for spinal column operations which can drill and insert bolts. It incorporates a force and torque sensor in order to precisely monitor the drilling and bolting process. Sensors record the forces that are active in drilling and bolting and check whether they are within the specified limits [20].

Robot-assisted neurosurgical applications

Key neurosurgical applications include stereotactic neurosurgery, robotized microscopes, endoscopic neurosurgery, tumor resection, radiosurgery and telepresence.

Stereotactic neurosurgery

CT guided stereotactic brain surgery was one of the first robotic-assisted applications in surgery. The use of a PUMA 260 robot for stereotactic surgery offers an arbitrary trajectory at an arbitrary location within its working areas [1]. NeuroMate has been used in over 3000 patients. It provides a fast and easy method for trajectory modifications [9]. Another robot, Minerva, is used for three-dimensional positioning of a stimulation electrode [10]. The IMARL robotic navigation system can be applied for treatment of Parkinson's disease and biopsy of brain tumors [11]. The development of a needle insertion manipulator, as reported by Masamune *et al.*, has both a safe mechanical design and the capacity for being sterilized [21]. Fankhauser *et al.* reported a robot, which performs an automatic penetration of the skin, skull, and meninges, and is able to handle two stereotactic instruments for depth electrodes and biopsy [13]. Robotic multimodal stereotactic brain tissue identification, which is addressed in Andrews *et al.*, can improve procedures such as stereotactic brain biopsy, functional and implantation neurosurgery, and brain tumor excision [12].

Robotized neurosurgical microscopes

Multi-coordinate manipulator (MKM) from Zeiss facilitates the localization and minimizes manipulation, as described in the next section [22]. The actuated robotic microscope, SURGISCOPE enables the neurosurgeon to have at the same time a microscope, a pointing device, and a tool for automatic maneuverability in the brain [2]. A robotic arm connected to a neurosur cal operative microscope is presented in Giorgi *et al.* [23].

Endoscopic neurosurgery

Robot-assisted endoscopic neurosurgery solutions, where a voice-controlled system is used, are presented in Benabid [24] and in Wapler [25]. Zimmermann et al. also reported their experience using robot-assisted navigated neuroendoscopy [39].

Tumor resection

A robotic-based high-intensity-focused ultrasound system for the destruction of subcortical lesions is reported by Davies *et al.* [17]. Systems designed by Drake *et al.*, Andrews *et al.*, and Kelly *et al.* can improve brain tumor excision [12, 18, 26]. The robot performs image-guided resection, combining 3D reconstruction of the tumor volume, computer-oriented stereotactic microscope, projection of the tumor margins into the eyepieces of the microscope, and joy-stick-manoeuvered laser beam for tumor vaporization [26]. The NeuRobot is a telecontrolled microscopic micromanipulator system designed for tumor excision, as reported by Goto *et al.* [27]. The MKM and Surgiscope have also this software capabilities.

Radiosurgery

The CyberKnife robotic system allows a linear accelerator to be arbitrarily positioned in a 6 degrees-of-freedom (DoF) orientation. Image guided robotic radiosurgery utilizing a Fanuc manipulator has also been described [14].

Telepresence

The Integrated Remote Neurosurgical System (IRNS) as described in Kassell *et al.*, is a remotely operated neurosurgical microscope with high speed communications and a surgeon-accessible user interface [28].

Neurosurgical robotic systems

This section describes a few robotic devices currently being used in various neurosurgical procedures to reach the anatomy of interest while minimizing collateral damage.

Multi-coordinate Manipulator (MKM)

Frameless navigation devices have recently undergone evaluation to the point where they are being used more efficiently in the clinical setting. Most of the current systems utilize some form of mechanical arm to correlate registered points in space to the patient's image in the computer terminal. However, the articulated arm can be cumbersome and is an additional obstacle in the surgical field. In response to some of these difficulties inherent with frameless stereotaxy, the MKM (Mehrkoordinaten Manipulator; Multicoordinate manipulator) robotic microscope system (Carl Zeiss, Oberkochen, Germany) was developed. Essentially it is an optically based system in which the CT and/or MRI data are superimposed three-dimensionally onto the surgical field as seen through the microscope using heads-up display technology and it is specifically designed for image-guided procedures in neurosurgery [22].

The MKM robotic microscope system consists of (a) a surgical microscope, (b) robotic carrier system, and (c) a computer workstation that integrates the microscope with the robotic system (Figure 1). The surgical microscope is a standard OPMI ES (Zeiss OPMI-ES, Carl Zeiss, New York NY, USA), with a 1:6 ratio zoom system. The microscope has an auto focus feature with a digitally encoded zoom that selects the true focal plane. Also featured is a continuously variable focus length from 200 to 400 mm, illuminated by a xenon lamp. The robotic carrier is motor-driven along six axes; by translational motion to different positions in space, pivot motion about a point in the focal plane of the microscope, and pivot motion about any point on the optical axis outside the focal plane of the microscope.

This system is equipped with a sturdy motorized base that allows easy relocation of the system through a drive shaft. The surgical microscope and the robotic system are integrated by a portable computer workstation in the operative suite (see Figure 1). A voice-recognition system activates important functions of the microscope and robotic system. For example, by using the microphone installed on the microscope, the surgeon can use voice commands to adjust the focus (i.e., "auto focus," "focus-defocus"), or position the microscope to different preset positions (i.e., "standby," "surgical position," "surgical trajectory," etc.). The MKM robotic microscope system also has a data-superimposing monitor that projects the target contour and volume, as well as navigational information for the stereotactic procedure according to the surgical plan. Projections can also be oriented to the surgeon's perspective, making them intuitively easy to follow because of the head-up display. A very useful feature of the MKM robotic microscope is the ability to "preview" the surgery using focus defocus, to bring perspective to the surgeon's eye view at different depths. In theory, during neuronavigation, the microscope's actual focal point serves as a virtual probe; therefore, no external pointing devices are needed.

The surgical procedure

To use the MKM robotic microscope the following steps are required: image data acquisition, surgical planning, intraoperative registration, and intraoperative navigation by the robotic microscope during the surgical procedure.

Image data acquisition

The imaging modalities of computed tomography (CT), magnetic resonance imaging (MRI), and positron emission tomography (PET) have been widely used for image-guided neurosurgery. In order to use them for navigation, these images need to be registered with one another (multi-modality image registration) and with physical space (image-to-surgical space registration). Stereotactic frame systems and fiducial markers are usually used for registration. The MKM robotic microscope system can be used with both frame-based and frameless techniques. Both CT and MRI data are transferred directly to the computer workstation in the surgical suite.

Surgical planning

The primary objective of surgical planning is to simulate and optimize the surgical approach. Surgical planning is performed using the Stereotactic Treatment Plan (STP) software (Leibinger-Fischer, Freiburg, Germany). After registering the CT and MRI, the surgeon defines the target and other "volumes of interest" by manually delineating. This marks the contour of the lesion and other structures that the surgeon wants to identify intraoperatively.

Once a target has been defined, the surgeon defines the optimal trajectory. The approach can be a simple straight line (straight trajectory) or a more complex nonlinear approach along a curved line (curved trajectory). While conventional stereotaxis provides a straight approach, the MKM robotic microscope allows more complex curved approaches, allowing access to deep targets using trans-sulcal approaches. Both straight-line and curved approaches can be defined using computer visualization and manipulation tools. Information on multiple alternative trajectories can be stored in the computer memory.

Intraoperative registration

In the operative suite, the surgical procedure starts by matching the patient' image in the intraoperative space (intraoperative registration) by selecting reference points using the robotic microscope. Although the MKM robotic microscope system can define as many as 20 reference points, usually 3 or 4 points are sufficient. For intraoperative registration, the microscope is moved to the reference point (e.g., a fiducial marker) that was selected in pre-surgical planning. A visible cross is used to center the reference point in the microscope's field of view, with both focal distance and auto focus at maximal magnification. After the coordinates of all reference points have been stored, the system automatically loads the coordinates of the entry point from the computer workstation and performs a landmark test to analyze whether the system is correctly matched with the coordinate system of the patient.

Intraoperative guidance and navigation

At the beginning of the surgical procedure, "standby" and the "surgical" positions are defined. The standby position is a defined position outside the surgical field to which the microscope can be moved at any time during the procedure. In the standby position, the robotic microscope will not interfere with the surgeon's movements during open craniotomies. The surgical position is used during the procedure to access the surgical field. The microscope can be moved from the standby position to the surgical position by a voice command whenever necessary (Figure 2).

During surgery, the ability to remotely control the microscope position, the continuous display of contours from the surgeon's perspective, and the continuous display of the center of the focal point allow for true navigation and guidance. The data-superimposing monitor projects data from the workstation into the right eyepiece while the field of the surgery remains fully visible (Figure 3).

The integration of the robotic system with the microscope also introduces a "key-hole feature" that consists of a pivot movement of the microscope with different focal lengths, allowing one to explore large cavities through a simple burr-hole.

Clinical experience

Our initial reported clinical experience included 24 image-guided procedures using the MKM robotic microscope. The cases include surgery for primary brain tumors (18), cavernous angiomas (2), third ventricular colloid cyst (1), arteriovenous malformation (1), and metastatic lesions (2). Surgical approaches included 3 intraventricular, 7 frontal, 3 deep parietal, 1 midline interhemispheric, 2 posterior fossa, 6 deep temporal, and 1 spinal lumbar posterior approach. In each case, computer assisted surgical planning was used to identify neighboring vital structures and to contour these structures with the pathology, to assist the surgeon in their identification and preservation. All results were clinically satisfactory. Postoperative CT and MRI studies showed total or subtotal resection [29].

Accuracy

In all cases, a second type of localizing technology was available; i.e., stereotactic ring or infrared digitizer. Localization of the entry was accurate in all cases. However, in some instances localization was lost because of movements of the patient. The dural opening and the superficial part of the surgery were clearly performed with accurate navigation. However, at the deeper levels it was difficult to achieve an exact focus for display of the contours, resulting in a loss of accuracy.

Advantages of the MKM robotic system

Image guided craniotomy can be performed without a localizing arch and aiming tools.
During the approach to deep, complex lesions, the MKM robotic microscope enables guidance with the best possible trajectory without the need to follow a straight line (conventional stereotaxis requires a straight trajectory).
During surgical exposure and resection of skull-base tumors, the MKM robotic microscope provides intraoperative visualization of the tumor geometry, allowing the surgeon to maintain orientation even with irregularly shaped tumors [30].

Disadvantages of the MKM robotic system

An important disadvantage encountered with the surgical robotic microscope is that it requires a fixed position of the patient in relation to the microscope and robot base. A sudden movement of the patient could disrupt an accurate intraoperative localization. For deep lesions, the main limitation of the MKM is its inability to precisely determine the accurate depth to display the contours. In deep portions of the brain it is difficult to use the focal point as the virtual probe. To overcome these limitations we interfaced the MKM with an infrared system allowing dynamic reference [29] and complementarities between the two systems. The MKM is bigger than a normal surgical microscope and occupies more space in the surgical suite.

NEUROMATE

NeuroMateTM (Integrated Surgical Systems, Inc., Davis, CA), is an image-guided, computer-controlled robotic system originally developed by Benabid et al. [7, 9, 31-33] The current version (Figure 4) is a commercial product that has been licensed by Integrated Surgical Systems (Davis, CA), and is FDA approved. NeuroMate includes a five-degree-of-freedom robotic arm and a PC-based kinematic positioning software system. The visualization software (VoXimTM, IVS Software Engineering) allows precise image-based planning and visualization of multiple trajectories. During surgery, the system can interactively and effectively position, orient, and manipulate surgical tools in 3D space.

The major clinical applications of NeuroMate include: (a) tumor biopsies, (b) stereoelectroencephalographic investigations of patients with epilepsy, and (c) midline stereotactic neurosurgery and functional neurosurgery of the basal ganglia. A typical clinical procedure consists of an initial data acquisition step, followed by data transfer to the control computer, and then the procedure itself The NeuroMate can be used with a frame or in frameless conditions. In the frameless mode images are acquired with an implantable base that allows insertion of different helicopter-shaped non co-planar devices. They include CT and MRI localizers that provide markers (which can be clearly identified in the image) that define the points of commonality between the image and the real space. These markers are first located and digitized in the image using the VoXim software. The same base can be used with an intraoperative localizer device that has sonic emitters. A similar complementary helicopter is mounted in the distal effector of the robot that consists of microphones. The intraoperative registration is made using this sonic system. (see Figure 5). The ultrasound receiver and transmitter system mounted on the robot and patient capture the same points as marked in the image space. The ultrasound system collects position data from which the system can compute the patient registration parameters. After the capture process, a registration is done to match the image space with the patient space.

The defined trajectory is used to command the robot to position a mechanical guide, which is aligned with this trajectory. The robot is then fixed in this position and the physician uses this guide to introduce a surgical tool such as a drill, probe, or electrode. The use of a laser probe for surgical guidance is also an important tool.

Advantages of NeuroMate surgical robotics

Experience with NeuroMate showed that surgical robots can reduce human error and can also save time in procedures involving multiple targets and biopsies. The results suggested that NeuroMate could extend human capabilities by assisting with microsurgical tasks at an acceptable spatial resolution. In addition, given a well known phenomenon of human tiring and loss of attention over time, robotic assistance may be beneficial in lengthy microsurgical procedures. Our evaluation on cost benefits and safety showed that the robotic arm could effectively provide the surgeon with complete control of the surgical field making the system passive, that is, guided at all times by a surgeon, increases its safety. The study results indicated that a the robotic arm not only performs as a surgical tool holder, but also increases surgical safety, resulting in improved efficiency and cost savings to the institution. This type of robotic arm may prove to be highly useful for holding, supporting, and stabilizing a variety of conventional and surgical devices such as biopsy needles and drills. It also has the potential to draw a contour on the skull surface for optimized craniotomy based on preoperative planning data. We experienced that from the qualitative perspective there are several advantages in using a robotic system. In effect, many surgical plans demand the realization of precise manipulation of instruments involving high positioning and orientation accuracy in the 3D patient space. Infrared navigators (now in common use) can only indicate how the instruments are being manipulated in the image space. This guidance, though useful, does not help the surgeon in positioning and orienting the tools during complex manipulations, which limits the accuracy of the procedures to the surgeon's dexterity. To circumvent these difficulties, robotized solutions in conjunction with the CAD/CAM concept have been applied to the implementation of imageguided surgery. NeuroMate can efficiently position, orient, steadily hold, and manipulate tools in 3D space with a high level of accuracy comparable to that of the most accurate standard neurosurgery techniques. The obvious advantages include efficient intraoperative registration, optimal localization for biopsy, accurate shaping of craniotomy, and the use of multiple trajectories to define margins of resection. Figure 6 shows the NeuroMate medical robotic system in the surgical environment.

Limitations and suggested improvements

We performed the first clinical application of NeuroMate in the USA in 1999. Preliminary testing and early clinical experiences with NeuroMate demonstrated the promising advantages of robotic surgery and identified the most important directions for improvement. Among all the advantages with NeuroMate, we concluded that further development of the software and hardware of the NeuroMate system, along with better ergonomics, was needed to improve its usability and practically to bring it to clinical application. One of the main limitations with NeuroMate is that it is so bulky and obtrusive in operating room. It also prevents patient movement during the surgical procedure, which sometimes is needed for better accessibility to the surgical site. It can hold limited surgical tools such as a needle or an electrode and has just 5 DoF. There is a need for a robotic manipulator with 7 DoF to act as a robotic assistant for the surgeon. Further potential developments also include robotic drawing of the optimized craniotomy. Although NeuroMate can be effective in biopsy, further development is needed for the use of robotics in open surgery. We also need to pursue the integration of robotics with free-hand techniques such as augmented reality and robotic augmentation.

DISCUSSION AND FUTURE DIRECTIONS

The field of surgical robotics is still in its infancy, and we are just at the beginning of this era. Only a handful of commercial companies exist, and the number of medical robots sold each year is very small. Part of the reason for this is that the medical environment is a very complex one, and the introduction of new technology is difficult. In addition, the completion of a medical robotics project requires a partnership between engineers and clinicians that is not easy to establish. The technological challenges and research areas for medical robotics include both the development of system components and the development of systems as a whole [6]. Research is needed in: (a) Safety, (b) System accuracy, (c) System architecture, (d) Software design, (e) Mechanical design, (f) Imaging-compatible designs, and (g) User interface. For medical robotic systems, the development of application test beds is critical to move the field forward. These test beds can also serve to improve the dialog between engineers and clinicians. However, at least in the United States, it is difficult to get funding to develop these test beds. Governmental funding agencies such as NIH or NSF will usually not fund such efforts, as they are geared more towards basic research than applied research and development, while manufacturers are usually not interested because the environment and investment payback for medical robotics is uncertain. The regulatory issues for medical robotics have not been fully explored, although several systems have received FDA approval. Also, the litigious nature of American society makes full clinical use of robots a risky venture. These factors remain obstacles to advancing the field. In the following sections, each of the seven system components listed above are briefly discussed.

Safety issues

"DO NO HARM" is a fundamental principle in any surgeon's training, and surgeons are naturally very concerned about the safety of the application of medical robotics in the operating room. Safety issues have been extensively discussed by Davies [2, 34] and Elder [35]. According to Davies, medical robotics differ from industrial robotics in that medical robots must operate in cooperation with people to be fully effective. Safety measures that can be taken include the use of redundant sensors, the design of special-purpose robots whose capabilities are tailored to the task at hand and the use of fail-safe techniques so that if the robot does fail it can be removed and the procedure can be completed by the surgeon. Other challenging safety issues for medical robotics in surgery are the need for sterilization to minimize the risk of infection.

Davies also presents a hierarchical scheme for the host of tools available to surgeons, ranging from hand-held tools to a fully powered autonomous robot. As the hierarchy moves towards autonomous robots, the surgeon is less and less in control, and more dependent on the mechanical and software systems of the robot.

Safety can be accomplished using mechanical constraints. Other alternatives are programmable constraints, which are inherently not as safe, but are more flexible. The idea is to dynamically constrain the range of possible motions [4, 36] based on the task to be accomplished. For example, there are important differences in the constraints necessary for trajectory procedure such as holding a needle biopsy versus a complex surgical resection.

Accuracy and repeatability

Accuracy is a very important issue in computer-assisted surgery. A recent AANS survey of 250 neurosurgeons disclosed that surgeons had little tolerance for error (12 mm accuracy in general, and 2-3 mm for spinal and orthopedic applications). All elements of visualization, registration, and tracking must be accurate and precise, with special attention given to errors associated with intraoperative tissue deformation [37].

A medical robot's precision is normally measured in two ways, namely repeatability and accuracy. Repeatability measures the error that occurs when the robot attempts to return to the same point in space. Accuracy is measured as the error that occurs when the robot attempts to reach a designated target. Robots have excellent repeatability, on the order of 0.1 mm [38]. However, their accuracy is much poorer, such that the tool position may be as much as 5-6 cm and 4-5 degrees away from its intended position and orientation. These inaccuracies are due to a number of factors, including manipulator design, control errors, and external sensing errors. Although controllers and sensors can be improved and noisy data filtered, there is not much that can be done about the manipulator design. Drake et al. did a comparison of accuracy between the PUMA robotic system and the ISG viewing wand. They reported that the repeatability of the PUMA 200 robotic system is approximately 0.05 mm and accuracy is no more than 2 mm [18]. For the ISG Viewing Wand, two standard deviations of error is ± 0.66 mm. The accuracy of the PUMA and viewing wand is almost equivalent. However, in computer assisted neurosurgery, there are a number of other sources of error that are greater than those of the robotic pointer: the errors must be accounted for are associated with image acquisition and processing and with the patients. The authors did a comparison of the application accuracy between the NeuroMate robotic system and other routinely used surgical navigation systems [37]. The results have shown that the accuracy of the frame based NeuroMate robot is comparable to (if not better than, in some cases) that of standard localizing systems, whether they are frame-based or infrared tracked. The frameless robot configuration is a little less accurate, but is within an acceptable standard of accuracy of 2 mm. From the qualitative perspective, there are several advantages in using a robotic system. In effect, many surgical plans demand the realization of precise manipulation of instruments involving high positioning and orientation accuracy in the 3D patient space. Infrared navigators (now in common use) can only indicate how the instruments are being manipulated in the image space. This guidance, though useful, does not help the surgeon in positioning and orienting the tools during complex manipulations, which limits the accuracy of the procedure to the surgeon's dexterity. In addition, we found that the frame based robotic solution is statistically better than frame-based infrared navigation. Frame-based approaches can result in human errors, are cumbersome to use, and are limited in terms of what instruments can be mounted. To circumvent these difficulties, robotized solutions in conjunction with the CAD/CAM concept have been applied to the implementation of image guided surgery. NeuroMate can efficiently position, orient, steadily hold, and manipulate tools in 3D space with a high level of accuracy comparable to that of the most accurate standard neurosurgery techniques. The obvious advantages include efficient intraoperative registration, optimal localization for biopsy, accurate shaping of craniotomy, and the use of multiple trajectories to define margins of resection. Our goal is to further develop the use of robotics in open surgery and to pursue the integration of robotics with free-hand techniques such as infrared image guidance, and visualization techniques such as augmented reality. Robotic neurosurgery is a new and promising field of challenge in this century.

System architecture

For medical robotics to evolve as its own field, and for the cost and difficulty of developing prototype systems to decrease, the establishment of system architecture would be an enabling step. The systems architecture should emphasize modularity (as noted by Taylor in the design of the Steady-Hand robot, which emphasizes modularity in mechanical design), control system electronics, and software [8]. The architecture design for neurosurgery has to be focused on the required access and manipulation of tools, accuracy of position, and force level control. High safety standards must be applied because the robot system is to operate in close proximity with the patient. A potential hazard is a "runaway" joint. Selecting a suitable manipulator configuration can reduce the risk. The following criteria need to be considered during the design of a medical robotic system:

- At the working site, tool motion should be achieved by moving a minimum number of joints.
- The facility for tool and end-effector position should be deduced simply by visual inspection of joint positions.
- By manual override, the tool and end-effector should be extracted and withdrawn from the working site safely by moving one joint at a time.
- The patient should be outside of the workspace available to the manipulator when the end-effector is moved to the working site.

In summary, safety is the most important issue for system architecture design.

Software design

The development of a software environment for medical robotics, possibly including an appropriate real-time operating system, is a significant challenge. The software portion is a very important component in the system to control the robot's motion. The design of software must follow the standards of system design. Many researchers developing medical robotics systems base their software development on commercially available software packages that may not be suitable for the surgical environment. However, the low cost and widespread availability of these software packages makes their use attractive, and there are steps that can be taken (such as watchdog timers, backup systems, and error recovery procedures) to make these systems more reliable. Still, it is believed that, along with the system architecture mentioned above, a robust software environment geared to the medical environment would be a substantial contribution. Although this software environment would still need to be customized for different surgical procedures, researchers would at least have a starting point for their development work. The needs of the surgeon must be considered at all times to design systems that are appropriate for current operating theatres.

Mechanical design

In addition to better software design, novel mechanical designs are needed to improve the utility of robotics in medical procedures. The mechanical portion of a robot is composed of a base, links, actuators, and an end-effector. As noted in the historical review in this paper, the first recorded medical application of a robot was for biopsy of the brain, using a standard PUMA industrial robot. Although some other researchers have described the use of industrial robots for medical tasks, it is the belief of these authors and others (for example Davies [2]) that special-purpose mechanical designs are more appropriate for most applications. In particular, these designs should be safer, as they can be designed specifically for the medical environment and customized for different medical procedures. However, it should be noted that special-purpose designs will not enjoy the same econonues of scale as more general designs, and another solution may be to develop more general-purpose medical robots with specialized end-effectors. One point that needs to be carefully considered is the chosen end-effector such as an ultrasound or infrared sensing system which may have influence on the application accuracy [37].

Imaging-compatible systems

With the increasing popularity of image-guided interventions, robotic systems are required that can work within the constraints of various imaging modalities such as CT and MRI. While these systems are, for the most part, still under the direct control of the physician, in the future they will be increasingly linked to these imaging modalities. In this review, some systems were noted that fall within this category, such as the MRI-compatible manipulator of Masamune et al. [21] and the CT integrated robot Minerva [10].

User interface

One question that arises in the development of all medical robotics systems concerns the user interface. What is a suitable user interface for a medical robot?

Should the robot be given a commanded path or volume and then autonomously carry out the task? Is a joystick or pushbutton interface appropriate, or would the physician rather manipulate the tool directly with the assistance of the robot? Is force feedback required for a high-fidelity user interface? These are all questions that require further investigation by the medical robotics community. The answer certainly will vary, depending on the medical task for which the robot is designed. It seems that medical robots will, at least initially, be more accepted by physicians if the physicians feel that they are still in control of the entire procedure. The present user interface includes:

- A joystick or pushbutton. The surgeon can control the medical robot by hand.
- Voice control. The surgeon can control the medical robot by voice command.
- A foot panel. The surgeon can control the medical robot by foot.

Current research: preserving the essence

Augmenting the capabilities of surgeons by robots has a great potential to improve precision and accuracy in the treatment of lesions, and therefore, enhance the outcomes of all kinds of surgery. Research demonstrates that most robotic systems used with computer assisted surgery (CAS) have been focused on precise placement of a needle for tumor biopsies or machining 3D surfaces in orthopedic applications. In these cases the robot typically follows preprogrammed trajectories, which are defined during a planning phase utilizing preoperative imaging data from MRI, CT or ultrasound sources. Other robotic systems, such as Intuitive Surgical's da Vinci, have successfully enhanced the surgeon's dexterity in laparoscopic and cardiac procedures. But the field of medical robotics is still in its infancy; there is no integration between robotic manipulators and the enormous advances in CAS to optimally use multiple and complex modalities of a patient's pre-operative and intraoperative data to assist the surgeon. This important gap is preventing CAS from taking advantage of robotic manipulators' capabilities. There is a critical need for an adequate marriage of CAS to advanced robotic manipulators in a way that the surgeon can benefit from the assistance of both systems and control the manipulator while having direct access to the surgical field. The gap is an important problem that prevents a potentially great improvement in surgical precision and accuracy. This problem is more important in critically located lesions in organs such as the brain and heart, where lesions are surrounded by vital structures that must be avoided. The surgeon must narrowly access critical sites and react to the structure shifts that may invalidate the preoperative medical images and surgical plans. Our long-term goal is to develop more powerful and precise technologies with broad applicability to the field of surgery. This is consistent with the mission of our laboratory, which is to research, develop and use state of the art software, hardware, and visualization techniques to optimize surgical outcomes. Our overall objective is to develop a highly dexterous and precise robotic manipulator and its interface with our surgical CAS navigation system. The central hypothesis is that integration of advanced CAS and the robotic micromanipulator which will be conducted by our unique multidisciplinary team of advanced surgeons and expert micromanipulator developers, will bring the field of surgery into a new dimension and will enable surgeons to successfully perform procedures that can only be imagined today. We intend to develop an integrated system with a single interface to switch between planning, navigation, and robotic mode enabling the surgeon to have direct access to the surgical field and control of the integrated system. Our current objective is to fully define the problem, address the major feasibility issues and the issues associated with the design and construction of a prototype of the robotic manipulator for CAS. In an initial phase, we will perform studies based on the platform that will be obtained by integrating an existing 7-DoF Master-Slave Robotic Surgical system developed at SRI with the CAS navigation system developed at

Wayne State University. The rationale that underlies the project is that, once feasibility for the proposed computer-assisted robotic manipulator has been established by this first phase, the pieces will be in place to design and develop new and innovative instrumentation that is expected to increase the precision of many kinds of surgery dramatically; and even enable surgeons to perform novel interventions. Though we intend to develop the proposed manipulator for application to brain surgery, the system is expected to have broad applicability in different surgical procedures, from tumor surgery in other body locations to complex transplants or trauma surgery.

The future market for medical robotics and computer assisted surgery

Computers, working in tandem with a variety of microprocessor-enabled equipment and instruments, support and facilitate the work of the surgeon and have brought a level of safety and precision to surgery that would have been inconceivable just a few years ago. These computers, electronic equipment, and instruments are referred to collectively as medical robotics and computer assisted surgery (MRCAS) or, more dramatically, "the Operating Room of the Future". MRCAS is used in a growing number of operating rooms around the world, largely as a result of the popularity of minimally invasive surgical (MIS) techniques. The need to perform delicate surgical procedures, safely, in tight spaces where the surgeon cannot see directly, has created a growing market for devices that act as extensions of the surgeon's eyes and hands: remote imaging, data processing arid feedback, and robotics.

The task of controlling a large number of motors, taking into account sensory feedback from a number of different sources, can be achieved only by using computer technology. It is at this stage that the surgeon does become more of an observer than a controller. This level of technology will then necessitate a clear understanding of all the safety issues.

The fixture of these applications relies mainly on technical progress in informatics, about image recognition to adapt the pre-planning to the actual surgical situation, to correct brain shifts (for instance), about image fusion, integrated knowledge such as brain atlases, as well as virtual reality.

According to a soon-to-be-released report from Business Communications Company, Inc. (www. bccresearch.com) RB-182 Medical Robotics and Computer Assisted Surgery Market, the U.S. market for medical robotics and computer-assisted surgical equipment grew from $105 million in 1999 to an estimated $245 million in 2002, at an AAGR (average annual growth rate) of 32.6%. The market is projected to grow at an AAGR of 22.4% over the next five years, reaching $673 million by 2007.

Surgical navigation systems are the largest product segment of the U.S. MRCAS market, although their share of the market is projected to decline from 61.2% in 2002 to 52.0% in 2007. Surgical robots are the fastest growing U.S market segment, with a projected AAGR of almost 35% between 2002-2007. At this rate, sales of surgical robots are projected to grow from $50 million in 2002 to $220 million in 2007, making them the second largest segment of the market.

In terms of surgical applications, neurosurgical applications account for the bulk of the U.S. MRCAS market, i.e. 57.1% in 2002. However, endoscopic surgical applications are the fastest-growing application segment, and are expected to gain significant market share at the expense of neurosurgery by 2007, when endoscopic applications will account for 21.6% of the market.

The global market for MRCAS was an estimated $433 million in 2002 and is projected to exceed $1.1 billion by 2007, at an AAGR of 21.6%. The U.S. thus accounted for an estimated 56.6% of global MRCAS sales in 2002, a percentage that is projected to increase to 58.4% by 2007. Europe was the second largest regional MRCAS market in 2002, with estimated sales of $108 million (25% of the global market), followed by Japan with $44 million (10%) and other countries with a total of $36 million (8%). Other countries, including Asia-Pacific market other than Japan, Latin America and the Middle East, are the fastest-growing regional market with a projected 20022007 growth rate of 25.0% annually. These markets collectively are expected to pass Japan in importance by 2007.

CONCLUSIONS

The use of robots in medicine clearly offers great promise. We are just in the initial stages of the application of robotics to medicine, and much more work remains to be done. In particular, the development of more test beds is required for different medical procedures so that more experience with the technology and its integration into clinical practice can be gained. The issues of cost, safety, and patient outcomes also need to be considered. Although there have been some modestly successful commercial medical robots in the neurosurgery, such as NeuroMate and MKM, they still are not completely adopted by the neurosurgeon community.

The full benefits of medical robots in neurosurgery will not appear until more integrated systems are developed, in which the robots are linked to the imaging modalities or to the patient anatomy directly. There must be an increased effort towards compatibility of software, image standards, planning software, and end effectors. The ideal should be to have all image modalities converging in a unique planning system, from which various procedures could be dispatched toward various effectors (microscopes, stereotactic robot, tool holder, radiosurgical generator, etc), which would act on the brain of the patient, independent of the disease which is inside it. This link will highlight the potential advantages of robots, such as the ability to follow respiratory motion, and enable physicians to successfully complete procedures that can only be imagined today. We must not forget the essence of things; that is, the patient must be treated in the best possible manner, not just in a possible manner. Medical robotics has tremendous potential for improving the precision and capabilities of surgical procedures.

REFERENCES

1. Kwoh YS, Hou J, Jonckheere EA, Hayati S. A robot with improved absolute positioning accuracy for CT guided stereotactic brain surgery. *IEEE Transactions on Biomedical Engineering* 1988 Feb; 35(2):153–60.

2. Davies B. A review of robotics in surgery. Proceedings of the Institution of Mechanical Engineers [H].2000; 214:129-40.

3. Taylor RH. Robots as surgical assistants: where we are, whether we are tending, and how to get there. In: *Proceedings of the 6th Conference on Artificial Intelligence in Medicine Europe* (AIME 97) Grenoble, France, 1997:3–11.

4. Troccaz J, Delnondedieu Y. Robots in Surgery. In: proceedings of *IARP Workshop on Medical Robots*, Vienna, Austria, 1996.

5. Howe RD, Matsuoka Y. Robotics for surgery. *Annual Review of Biomedical Engineering* 1999; 1:211–40. Review.

6. Cleary K and Nguyen C. State of the Art in Surgical Robotics: Clinical Applications and Technology Challenges. *Computer Aided Surgery* 2001; 6(6):312–28. Review.

7. Zamorano L, Li Q, Jain S, Kaur G: Robotics in neurosurgery: state of the art and future technological challenges. *International Journal.of Medical Robotics and Computer Assisted Surgery* 2004:1(1):7-22.

8. Taylor RH, Jenson P, Whitcomb L, Barnes A, Kumar R, Stoianovici D, Gupta P, Wang ZX, deJuan E, Kavoussi L. A steady-hand robotic system for microsurgical augmentation. *International Journal of Robotics Research* 1999; 18:1201–10.

9. Benabid AL, Cinquin P, Lavalle´e S, Le Bas JF, Demongeot J, de Rougemont J. Computer-driven robot for stereotactic surgery connected to CT scan and magnetic resonance imaging. Technological design and preliminary results. *Applied Neurophysiology* 1987; 50:153–4.

10. Burckhart CW, Flury P, Glauser D. Stereotactic brain surgery. *IEEE Engineering Medicine and Biology* 1995; 14:314–7.

11. Tseng CS, Chung CW, Chen HH, Wang SS, Tseng HM. Development of a robotic navigation system for neurosurgery. *Studies in Health Technolopgy and Informatics* 1999; 62:358–9.

12. Andrews R, Mah R, Galvagni A, Guerrero M, Papasin R, Wallace M, Winters J. Robotic multimodality stereotactic brain tissue identification: Work in progress. *Stereotactic and Functional Neurosurgery* 1997; 68(1–4 Pt 1):72–9.

13. Fankhauser H, Glauser D, Flury P, Piguet Y, Epitaux M, Favre J, Meuli RA. Robot for CT guided stereotactic neurosurgery. *Stereotactic and Functional Neurosurgery* 1994; 63(1–4):93–8.

14. Adler JR Jr, Murphy MJ, Chang SD, Hancock SL. Image guided robotic radiosurgery. *Neurosurgery* 1999; 44(6):1299–307.

15. Das H, Zak H, Johnson J, Crouch J, Frambach D. Evaluation of a telerobotic system to assist surgeons in microsurgery. *Computer Aided Surgery* 1999; 4(1):15–25.

16. Hein A, Lueth TC, Bier J, Hommel G. A robotics retractor hook holder. In: Lemke Hu, Vannier MW, Inamura K, Farman AG, editors. *Computer Assisted Radiology and Surgery CARS'99*. North Holland, Elsevier 1999;823–7.

17. Davies BL, Chauhan S, Lowe MJS K: A robotic approach to HIFU based neurosurgery. In: Wells WM, Colchester A, Delp S, editors. *Medical Image Computing and Computer-Assisted Intervention MICCAI'98 Lecture Notes in Computer Science*. Springer: Berlin, 1998;1496:386–96.

18. Drake JM, Joy M, Goldenberg A, Kriendler D. Computer- and robotassisted resection of thalamic astrocytomas in children. *Neurosurgery*. 1991 Jul; 29(1):27–33.

19. Tanikawa T, Arai T, Masuda T. Development of a micro manipulation system with two-finger micro hand. *Proceedings of Intelligent Robots and Systems Conference IROS'96*. 1996;2:981–7. doi:10.1109/IROS.1996.571063.

20. Birgit Niesing. Robots for spine surgery. *Fraunhofer magazine*. 2001;2:46–7.

21. Masamune K, Kobayashi E, Masutani Y, Suzuki M, Dohi T, Iseki H, Takakura K. Development of an MRI-compatible needle insertion manipulator for stereotactic neurosurgery. *Journal of Image Guided Surgery* 1995; 1(4):242–8.

22. Kiya N, Dureza C, Fukushima T, Maroon JC. Computer navigational microscope for minimally invasive neurosurgery. *Minimally Invasive Neurosurgery* 1997 Sep; 40(3):110–5.

23. Giorgi C, Eisenberg H, Costi G, Gallo E, Garibotto G, Casolino DS. Robot-assisted microscope for neurosurgery. *Journal of Image Guided Surgery* 1995; 1(3):158–63.

24. Benabid AL, Lavallee S, Hoffman D, Cinquin P, Demongeot J, Danel F. Potential use of robots in endoscopic neurosurgery. *Acta Neurochirurgica* Suppl. (Wien) 1992;54:93–7.

25. Wapler M, Braucker M, Durr M, Hiller A, Stallkamp J, Urban V. A voice-controlled robotic assistant for neuroendoscopy. *Studies in Health Technology and Informatics* 1999; 62:384–7.

26. Kelly PJ, Kall BA, Goerss S, Earnest F 4th. Computer-assisted stereotaxic laser resection of intra-axial brain neoplasms. *Journal of Neurosurgery* 1986 Mar; 64(3):427–39.

27. Goto T, Hongo K, Kakizawa Y, Muraoka H, Miyairi Y, Tanaka Y, et al. Clinical application of robotic telemanipulation system in neurosurgery. Case report. *Journal of Neurosurgery* 2003 Dec; 99(6):1082–4.

28. Kassell NF, Downs JH 3rd, Graves BS. Telepresence in Neurosurgery: The integrated remote neurosurgical system. *Studies in Health Technology Informatics* 1997;39:411–9.

29. Zamorano L, Vinas FC, Buciuc R, Jiang Z, Diaz F. Advanced neurosurgical navigation using a robotic microscope integrated with an infrared-guided neurosurgery. In: Tamaki N, editor. *Computer-Assisted Neurosurgery*. Tokyo: Springer Verlag; 1997; 43–55.

30. Nakamura M, Tamaki N, Tamura S, Suzuki H, Ehara K. Navigational surgery of skull base and other vital area lesions using the Mehrkoordinaten Manipulator (MKM) System. In: Tamaki N editor. *Computer- Assisted Neurosurgery*. Tokyo: Springer Verlag. 1997; 190–203.

31. Lavallee S. A new system for computer assisted neurosurgery. *Proceedings of the Eleventh IEEE Engineering in Medicine and Biology Conference*, 1989:926–7.

32. Lavallee S, Troccaz J, Gaborit L, Cinquin P, Benabid AL, Hoffmann D. Image-guided operating robot: a clinical application in stereotactic neurosurgery. In: Taylor RH, Lavallee S, Burdea GS, Mosges R, editors. *Computer-Integrated Surgery: Technology and Clinical Applications*. Cambridge, MA: MIT Press, 1996:343–51.

33. Benabid AL, Hoffmann D, Ashraff A, Koudsie A, Bas JFL. Robotic guidance in advanced imaging environments. In: Alexander E III, Maciunas RJ, editors: *Advanced Neurosurgical Navigation*. New York: Thieme Medical Publishers, Inc. 1999:571–83.

34. Davies B. A discussion of safety issues for medical robots. In: Taylor RH, editor. *Computer-Integrated Surgery: Technology and Clinical Applications*. Cambridge, MA: MIT Press. 1996:287–96.

35. Elder MC, Knight JC. Specifying user interfaces for safety-critical medical systems. In: *Medical Robotics and Computer Assisted Surgery*. New York: Wiley-Liss, 1995:148–55.

36. Schneider O, Troccaz J. A six-degree of freedom arm with dynamic constraints (PADyC): work in progress. *Computer Aided Surgery* 2001; 6:340–51.

37. Li Q, Zamorano L, Pandya A, Perez R, Gong J and Diaz F. The Application Accuracy of the NeuroMate Robot—A Quantitative Comparison with Frameless and Frame-Based Surgical Localization Systems. *Computer Aided Surgery* 2002; 7:90–8.

38. Groover MP, Weiss M, Nagel N, Odrey NG. *Industrial Robotics: Technology, Programming, and Application*. New York: McGraw- Hill. 1986.

39. Zimmermann M, Krishnan R, Raabe A, Seifert V: Robot-assisted navigated neuroendoscopy. *Neurosurgery* 2002 Dec; 51(6):1446-51; discussion 1451-2.

In: Robotics in Surgery: History, Current and Future Applications ISBN 1-60021-386-3
Editor: Russell A. Faust, pp. 173-184 © 2007 Nova Science Publishers, Inc.

Chapter 10

APPLICATION OF ROBOTICS TO CARDIOTHORACIC SURGERY

Sumit Bose
Department of Biomedical Engineering
Johns Hopkins University
Baltimore, Maryland

David D. Yuh
Division of Cardiac Surgery
Johns Hopkins Hospital
Baltimore, Maryland

Abstract

The application of robotic platforms to cardiothoracic surgery has lagged somewhat behind other surgical specialties due in large part to the relatively confined and rigid anatomic cavity, microsurgical requirements, and potential complications from inadvertent tissue injury and prolonged intervals on cardiopulmonary bypass. Nevertheless, robotic assistance has proved useful in performing several minimally-invasive cardiac operations, including mitral valve repair, atrial septal defect closures, epicardial biventricular lead placement, and coronary artery bypass. Future applications towards radiofrequency ablation for atrial fibrillation and laser transmyocardial revascularization are under development.

Early outcomes studies of robot-assisted minimally-invasive cardiac operations have indicated that shorter hospitalizations, reduced pain, fewer wound complications, and less postoperative disability can be anticipated. Nevertheless, the learning curve for robotic surgery is steep and does require new skill sets not otherwise employed in conventional cardiac surgery.

The tactile demands of cardiac surgery have also stimulated research interest in conferring force feedback (i.e., "haptics") capabilities to surgical robotic systems. Moreover, the digital control systems inherent in surgical robotic platforms may facilitate accurate objective modes of assessing technical competence in surgical trainees as an adjunct to surgical simulation systems.

INTRODUCTION

Technological advancements are rapidly replacing traditional methods of surgery with complex and modern techniques. The conventional approaches to performing cardiac surgery generally involve a median sternotomy which provides optimal access to all cardiac structures and vessels. However, disfigurement and pain is associated with this incision. As a result, over the years, less invasive and traumatic approaches to cardiothoracic surgery have been developed, including the use of digital robotic systems.

The da Vinci Surgical System (Intuitive Surgical, Sunnyvale, CA) is currently being applied to cardiothoracic operations. This surgical system is made up of a surgeon console, computer telemetry and control system, two robotic surgical arms and a two-camera robotic endoscope (**Figure 1**). Commands delivered from the master console precisely control endoscopic instruments actuated by robotic manipulator arms. The surgeon's hand motions are relayed to a computer processor, which digitizes the instructions and conveys the information to the robotic manipulators.

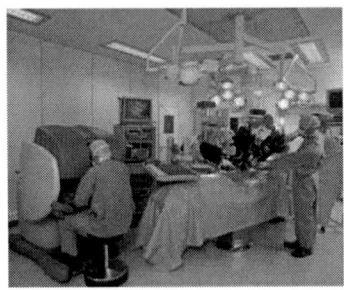

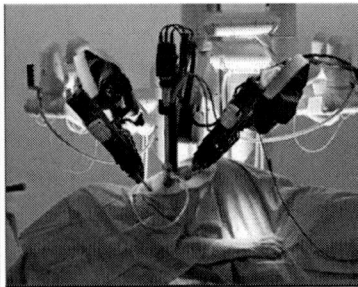

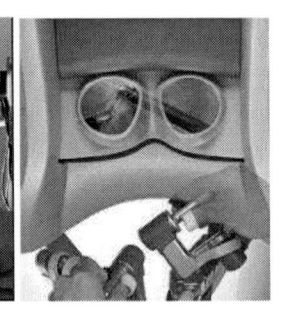

Figure 1. The da Vinci Surgical System (Inuitive, Inc., Sunnyvale, CA). Operating room setup with surgeon seated at control console (left panel). The da Vinci robot consisting of two manipulation arms and one camera arm (middle panel). The surgeon's console with three-dimensional endoscopic viewer and hand controls (right panel). Photos courtesy of Intuitive Surgical, Sunnyvale, CA.

Digitized control systems confer substantial benefits. The da Vinci's computer controller is capable of filtering high-frequency motion signals, thereby eliminating surgical tremor.[1] The computer interface also enhances dexterity by converting macroscopic movements at the surgeon's console into precise instrument maneuvers inside the patient, otherwise referred to as "motion-scaling". The da Vinci system possesses a three-dimensional, two-camera optical system which preserve depth perception, a significant advantage over conventional two-dimensional endoscopes. Surgical robotic systems also generally permit "indexing", or the ability to move instruments in any direction beyond the surgeon's comfort zone. For instance, the robot hand controls are like a computer mouse, where the mouse can be picked up and moved to a comfortable position when the edge of the mouse pad is reached. Similarly, with the da Vinci system, a foot pedal on the master console is depressed, the hand controls are brought to a comfortable position and the foot pedal is released to continue.[1]

Robotic systems allow surgeons to perform complex operations in anatomic spaces with limited access.[1] Operations that have been performed on patients with robotic systems like the da Vinci Surgical System have achieved clinical success in terms of safety and efficacy. The use of robotics in cardiothoracic surgery has led to shorter hospital stays, reduced incisional pain, and fewer wound complications and infections. Therefore, the advantages and future potential of robotics certainly warrant continued use and further development of this technology.

ROBOTICS IN CARDIOTHORACIC SURGERY

Brief History

Historically, the earliest technological instruments developed for minimally-invasive surgery were retraction devices and laparoscopic camera holders. As time progressed, robot-held retractors became available that were manually positioned and controlled by humans. In 1994, AESOP became the first FDA-approved surgical robot. AESOP was a voice-controlled endoscopic camera positioner, capable of being used with an endoscope of any size. Since then, AESOP has been incorporated into a modern robotic system now in clinical use, known as Zeus. AESOP and Zeus were developed by Computer Motion (CMI, Goleta, CA), which merged with Intuitive Surgical (ISI, Sunnyvale, CA) in June 2003. Intuitive Surgical created the da Vinci Robotic System, the first FDA-approved robot for use in laparoscopic procedures.[1] The first intracardiac procedure was performed in 1997 using a prototype of the da Vinci Robotic System. In December 2003, Chitwood and colleagues performed a robotic mitral valve repair, the first such minimally invasive cardiac procedure in the United States. Soon thereafter in 2001, a totally endoscopic technique was used to perform a robot-assisted atrial septal defect repair.[2]

Technical Challenges

There are some limitations that are prevalent in using cutting-edge technology like robotics in cardiothoracic surgery. Mastering robot-assisted cardiothoracic surgery requires a steep "learning curve". Surgeons, physician assistants and the operating room staff are required to undergo several hours of laboratory practice prior to clinically applying this technique. An important topic of discussion is whether there is a way of deciding when a surgeon is cognitively and technically competent enough to perform surgeries on patients using a robotic system. Furthermore, there is speculation on what is the best way to teach robotic surgery to cardiothoracic surgeons-in-training and surgeons only experienced in traditional open surgical procedures.

CURRENT ROBOTIC CARDIAC SURGICAL APPLICATIONS

Mitral Valve Repair

Minimally-invasive mitral valve repairs are facilitated by robotic telemanipulation and three-dimensional videoscopy. This approach requires peripheral arterial and venous cannulation, transthoracic aortic crossclamping and antegrade cardioplegia.[3] The mitral valve can be accessed via a transpleural approach through a small right thoracotomy (**Figure 2**).

The right lung of the patient is deflated and a small 4 to 5-cm mini-thoracotomy is created through the fourth or fifth intercostal space and the pericardium is opened and suspended. The right (or left) femoral artery and vein are cannulated and cardiopulmonary bypass is initiated. A transthoracic aortic crossclamp is applied and antegrade cardioplegia is delivered to arrest the heart.[4] At this point, a left atriotomy is performed and an atrial retractor is used to elevate the interatrial septum to expose the mitral valve. The da Vinci videoscope is directed toward the mitral valve through the mini-thoracotomy incision. Two more incisions are made in the chest wall for the placement of the left and right robotic arms. The left arm instrumentation port is created in the second or third intercostal space and the right arm port incision is made in the fifth or sixth intercostal space. The robotic instruments are placed through these two ports to access the left atriotomy.[3] From here on, standard operating techniques are used for mitral valve repair. After the valve is repaired, the robotic instrument arms are removed from the patient and the left atriotomy is closed.[4]

Thusfar, compared to conventional techniques, robot-assisted mitral valve repairs have resulted in low operative mortality rates, reduced blood product transfusions, and reduced hospitalization times[3].

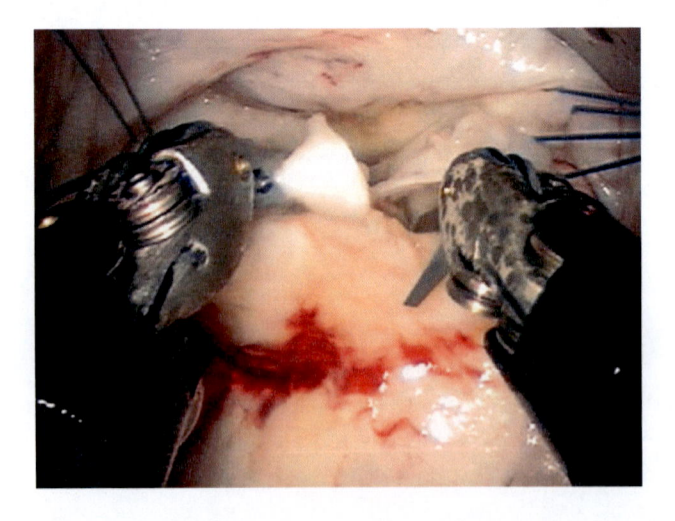

Figure 2. Posterior trapezoidal resection of mitral valve leaflet with the da Vinci surgical robotic system. Reproduced with permission from Chitwood WR, Nifong LW, Elbeery JE, et al. Robotic mitral valve repair: trapezoidal resection and prosthetic annuloplasty with the da Vinci surgical system. J Thorac Cardiovasc Surg 2000; 120: 1171-1172.

Atrial Septal Defect Closure

The first completely endoscopic atrial septal defect (ASD) repair with robotic technology was performed in the United States in July 2001.[2] According to a study done by Morgan and associates, robotic techniques can improve the postoperative quality of life in patients who undergo ASD repair.[5] With the robotic approach, the patient is positioned in a modified left lateral decubitus position, with the pelvis relatively flat and the right arm either suspended above the head or tucked at the side.[2] Four right transpleural incisions are created. Upon establishing selective left lung ventilation with right lung deflation, a 12-mm size incision is made along the fourth intercostal space in the midclavicular line of the right chest. This port is used to insert the videoscopic camera. Two 8-mm size incisions are made in the third and sixth intercostal spaces in the anterior axillary line on each side of the camera port. A fourth incision 15-mm in size is required in the fourth intercostal space of the posterior axillary line. This incision serves as a "working port" and is used for the delivery of sutures, suction, etc. In order to initiate cardiopulmonary bypass (CPB), bicaval venous drainage is established via internal jugular and femoral vein cannulas. Arterial perfusion is delivered with a 21 Fr. endoaortic balloon cannula placed through the femoral artery.[5] After CPB is initiated, antegrade cardioplegia is delivered and a right atriotomy is performed exposing the ASD. Using anatomical landmarks, the ASD is identified and closed with the double layer primary suture or patch closure technique. The atriotomy is closed and the patient is taken off CPB.[2]

A study examining the quality of life after robot-assisted ASD repair reports that patients report an excellent quality of life 30 days postoperatively. The quality of life assessment measures were significantly higher for patients who had a robot-assisted ASD repair when compared to patients who underwent a conventional sternotomy or thoracotomy for this operation. Furthermore, the study illustrates that robotic ASD repair is superior to non-thoracosopic techniques in terms of patients' bodily pain, physical role, social function, emotional role, vitality and mental health. The robotic approach toward ASD repair decreases the invasiveness of intracardiac procedures and avoids the operative trauma in patients undergoing cardiac surgery.[5]

Totally Endoscopic Coronary Artery Bypass Grafting (TECAB)

Minimally invasive surgical techniques are continuously evolving with the aid of the da Vinci Surgical System. Totally endoscopic coronary artery bypass grafting (TECAB) is a newly developed closed chest procedure that has been used on patients with coronary artery disease. Traditionally, CABG is performed via a median sternotomy. The wound complications, pain, and disfigurement associated with sternotomy have been generally accepted due to exceptional postoperative outcomes.[4]

TECAB represents an attempt to perform minimally-invasive coronary revascularization with reduced risks and enhanced patient benefits. The first TECAB was performed by Loulmet and colleagues in 1998.[4] Similar to other robot-assisted operations, a TECAB procedure requires general anesthesia and single lung ventilation. Both radial arteries are cannulated for monitoring of the endoaortic balloon occlusion catheter. The patient is placed in a supine position with the left side of the chest elevated about 30° to 40°. The videoscope is inserted through a port created in the left fifth intercostal space close to the anterior axillary line. The left and right robotic arms are delivered into the left chest through ports placed in the third and seventh intercostal spaces. At this point, the left chest cavity is insufflated with warm CO_2 (37°C) to ensure sufficient working space.

In general, the left internal thoracic artery (LITA) to left anterior descending coronary artery (LAD) anastomosis is performed with TECAB. The LITA is mobilized and its branches are cauterized using low-energy electrocautery. After systematic heparinization, cardiopulmonary bypass (CPB) is initiated. An endoscopic pericardiotomy is performed and the target vessel is identified. In order to carry out the LITA-LAD anastomosis, a 6 to 7-mm arteriotomy is performed and the LITA is anastomosed end-to-side using a 7–0 polypropylene suture (**Figure 3**).[6]

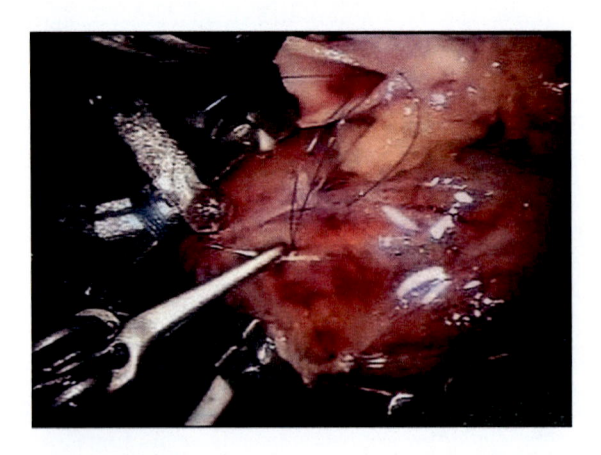

Figure 3. Totally endoscopic coronary artery bypass techniques. The left internal mammary artery (LIMA) is harvested as a pedicle by the da Vinci robotic system. An anastomosis is created between the LIMA and the left anterior descending aorta. Note the stabilization device. Reproduced with permission from Mohr FW, Falk V, Diegler A, et al. Computer enhanced "robotic" cardiac surgery: experience in 148 patients. *J Thorac Cardiovasc Surg* 2001; 121(5): 842-853.

Despite its promise, TECAB is associated with a steep learning curve, longer operative times, and conversion rates.[6] These issues need to be resolved with improved target vessel identification modalities, stabilization devices, cardioplegia delivery systems, and both distal and proximal anastomotic devices. Favorably, Mohr and colleagues have described that they successfully completed TECAB procedures on 22 out of 27 patients under arrested conditions with a patency rate of 94.5%, determined by angiography at three months' follow-up. Furthermore, TECAB appears to be a convenient way of performing coronary anastomoses in regions that are hard to access through direct CABG.[4] Hope remains that TECAB will achieve widespread application.

"Hybrid" Procedures (Combined Robotic and Catheter-Based)

Recently, TECAB has been combined with catheter based coronary intervention. In these "hybrid" procedures, the left internal mammary artery (LIMA) is grafted to the left anterior descending artery (LAD) in conjunction with catheter-based angioplasty and stenting of other coronary vessels.[7]

Although hybrird procedures have only been performed on a select number of patients, the postoperative results of this combined procedure have been impressive. Hybridized coronary revascularization appears to be a reasonable minimally-invasive approach in the treatment of multivessel coronary artery disease.

Left Ventricular Epicardial Lead Placement for Biventricular Pacing

Secondary to intraventricular conduction delays, approximately 30% of heart failure patients suffer from ventricular dysynchrony. The arrhythmic contraction pattern of the left and right ventricles impairs the already depressed cardiac contractility in patients with idiopathic and ischemic cardiomyopathies.[8] Scientific trials have demonstrated that ventricular resynchronization with biventricular pacing improves the ventricular function of the heart, improving exercise capacity and quality of life.[8] In most cases, biventricular pacing systems are placed percutaneously, however the left ventricular coronary sinus lead cannot be placed this way in approximately 15% of cases due to anomalous coronary venous anatomy or other technical reasons. Robot-assisted epicardial lead placement is a minimally invasive approach towards placing the left ventricular lead in such cases. Traditionally, a left thoracotomy approach would otherwise be used.

This procedure performed under general anesthesia and requires selective right lung ventilation. The patient is placed in a full posterolateral thoracotomy position (right side down) and secured to the operating table. A 10-mm incision is made on the left seventh intercostal space just anterior to the scapular line space for placing the endoscopic camera inside the patient. In order to gain access to the heart, two additional 8-mm incisions, which serve as the instrumentation ports are created in the left fifth and ninth intercostal spaces along the scapular tip line. Another 10-mm incision is created posterior to the camera port to serve as a delivery entrance for instruments and accessories. The left chest is insufflated with 8 to 10 mm Hg of CO_2 in order to create more working space between the heart and the chest wall. Using the da Vinci system, the pericardium is opened posterior to the phrenic nerve. Sometimes retraction sutures are used by surgeons to achieve better anatomical exposure. At this point, the obtuse marginal (OM) vessels are identified for epicardial lead placement. A pacing lead is introduced by the assistant surgeon through the working port. The epicardial lead is placed on the left ventricular surface with either the screw-in technique or suture fixation, leaving the proximal end of the lead outside the chest (**Figure 4**).[4, 8]

It has been determined that the region in the proximity of the second or third OM vessels in the posterobasal area is most favorable for epicardial lead placement. This region can be identified by using a temporary pacing wire to map the ventricular electrogram and determining the latest area of activation in relation to the patient's QRS complex. After the pacing lead is attached to the left ventricular surface, it is tested for voltage threshold and resistance. A second epicardial lead is also placed in the same region of the left ventricular surface as a backup. The pericardium is closed over the two leads for permanent fixation.[8] Both the leads are retrieved from the chest either via the right arm or working port and tunneled to and parked within a counter incision made in the left axilla. A single 19 Fr. soft plastic drain is placed in the chest through the left arm port for air and fluid evacuation and removed prior to the completion of the surgery. The ports are removed from the patient and all incisions are closed.[4]

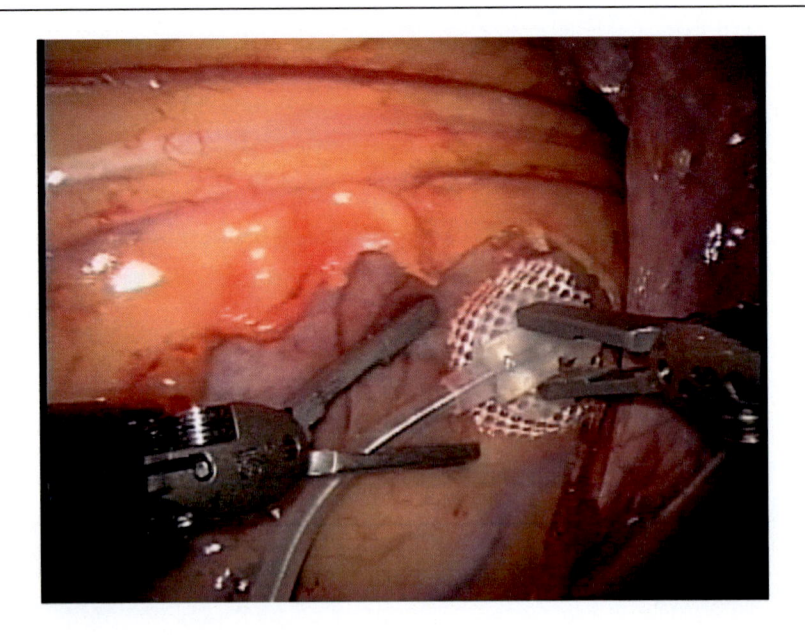

Figure 4. Robot-assisted epicardial biventricular lead placement as viewed by operating surgeon through da Vinci master console. Reproduced with permission from Rose EA, Gelijns AC, Moskowitz AJ et al. Long-term use of a left ventricular assist device for end-stage heart failure. NEJM 2001; 20:1435-1443.

In the second phase of this operation, the patient is redraped and positioned in a supine position. In most cases, the patient already has a biventricular pacing generator placed in the left subclavicular pocket. This pocket is reopened and the pacing device is removed from the pocket. The leads are delivered to the pocket and retested for threshold voltage and resistance. The best lead is connected to the generator and the second lead is capped and tacked to the pectoralis fascia for backup use in the future. The biventricular pacing device is reinserted into the pocket, the device is reprogrammed, and the incision is closed.[8]

FUTURE ROBOTIC CARDIAC SURGICAL APPLICATIONS

Transmyocardial Revascularization

In recent years, coronary artery bypass grafting (CABG) has become the standard technique to cure angina in patients with ischemic heart disease.[4] However, there is a subset of patients with intractable angina due to diffuse, small-vessel coronary disease which is not amenable to percutaneous coronary intervention or CABG. Transmyocardial revascularization (TMR) is a therapeutic operation for this group of "no-option" patients that aims to increase the delivery of oxygenated blood into ischemic myocardial regions. Currently, TMR is performed via a median sternotomy or left thoracotomy. Allen and colleagues have demonstrated long term angina relief and longer survival times after open TMR procedures in no-option patients.[9] We have developed a minimally-invasive approach to TMR using the da Vinci system. This technique uses the da Vinci Surgical System combined with a prototype flexible fiberoptic Holmium:Yttrium-Aluminum-Garnet (Ho:YAG) laser TMR device (CardioGenesis Corporation, Foothill Ranch, CA). We have reported off pump totally endoscopic TMR in canine subjects, evaluating the risks and benefits associated with this new technique.[9]

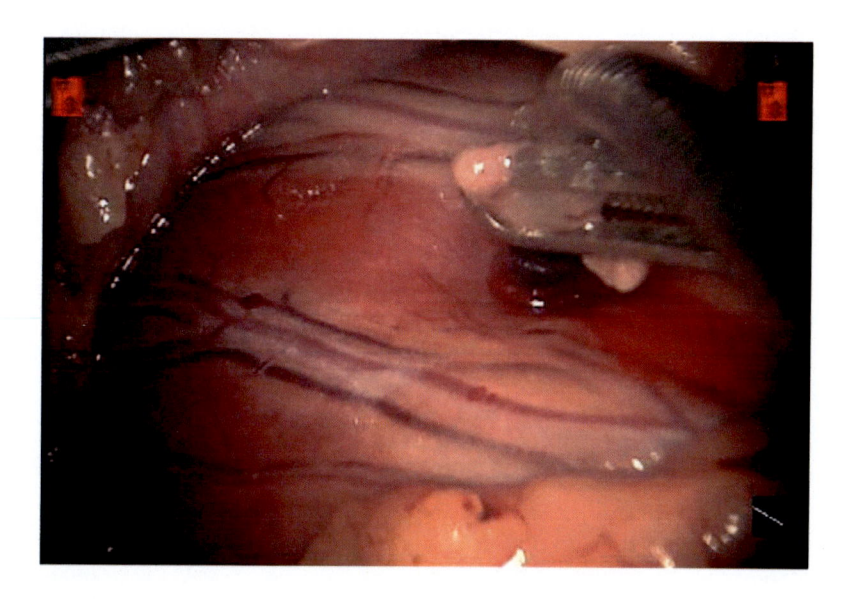

Figure 5. Surgeon's views through da Vinci master console of robot-assisted, endoscopic transmyocardial revascularization. The fiberoptic laser probe is positioned on the epicardial surface using the da Vinci instrumentation.

Robot-assisted TMR is conducted under general anesthesia. The subject is positioned in a modified right lateral decubitus position and put on selective right lung ventilation. Similar to other robot-assisted operations, four left transpleural chest incisions are created. A videoscope is inserted into the left thoracic cavity through a 12-mm port in the seventh intercostal space along the midscapular line. Two 5-mm incisions are made for the left and right robotic arms in the fifth and ninth intercostal spaces along the posterior scapular line. A 5-mm working port incision is also made in the seventh intercostal space, about 4 cm posterior to the videoscopic port. Two transverse pericardiotomies placed 1 to 2 cm anterior and posterior to the left phrenic nerve are performed using the da Vinci instrumentation. A modified prototype of the SoloGrip III TMR Ho:YAG laser handpeiece (TMR2000; CardioGenesis Corporation) fitted with a 1-mm CardioGenesis CrystalFlex Fiberoptic probe is introduced into the left thoracic cavity through the 5-mm working port. This fiberoptic probe is grasped by the DeBakery forceps and positioned on the epicardial surface with the da Vinci system (**Figure 5**). The tableside surgeon advances the CrystalFlex fiber with the handheld SoloGrip and discharges the laser pulses. The intensity of the pulses is 7 watts, which is delivered at a repetition rate of 5 Hz with a pulse width of 200 μsec ($\pm 25\%$). Based on preoperative evaluation of the ischemic regions, TMR channels are created in the beating heart through the apical, anterior, anterolateral, posterobasal, posterolateral and inferior walls of the left ventricle. The density of channels is maintained approximately at 1 channel/cm^2. Transmural penetration is detected by the tableside surgeon via auditory feedback or by transesophageal echocardiography.[4,9]

In our initial experience with robotic TMR, we encountered no instances of epicardial vessel laceration. For each channel created, a perpendicular angle of attack to the epicardial plane was achieved due to easy maneuvering of the flexible probe ensured by the da Vinci instruments. Totally endoscopic robot-assisted TMR is capable of creating channels to all left ventricular regions without port relocation or instrument exchanges. The da Vinci surgical robot provides good dexterity and excellent visualization, which greatly reduces the risk of inadvertant injury when performing TMR. Clinical studies are underway to determine the safety and efficacy of this approach.

Radiofrequency Ablation for Atrial Fibrillation

The surgical Maze operation, first performed in 1988, set the standards for surgical treatment of atrial fibrillation. This procedure uses the cut-and-sew technique to interrupt irregular conduction pathways that cause atrial fibrillation. Although the Maze III procedure has been successful, it is rather complex and invasive. In recent years, less invasive ways of surgically treating atrial fibrillation using various ablative techniques have been explored.[4] Totally endoscopic robot-guided pulmonary veins ablation is one such method that is carried out using the da Vinci system. This minimally invasive operation is performed through the right chest and requires general anesthesia and left single lung ventilation. The patient is placed in a supine position and port accesses for the right and left robotic arms are created in the second and fourth intercostal spaces along the anterior axillary line. CO_2 insufflation is administered and the pericardium is incised approximately 1 cm anterior to the right phrenic nerve. The pericardial folds between the superior vena cava (SVC) and the right upper pulmonary vein and between the inferior vena cava (IVC) and the right lower pulmonary vein are dissected.[11] A microwave ablation device like the Flex 10TM probe (Afx Inc., Fremont, CA) is used to encircle all four pulmonary veins by way of the transverse and oblique sinuses. Upon determining the proper orientation of the microwave energy probe beneath the left atrial appendage, a circular lesion, also known as a "box lesion" is produced in order to create a continuous epicardial ablation line. In addition, the microwave device is used to create another lesion along the interatrial groove to connect the two ends of the epicardial lesion.[4,11] Despite the fact that these surgical techniques for atrial fibrillation are in their preliminary stages, robot-assisted approaches have proven feasible and have produced favorable outcomes thusfar.

FUTURE DIRECTIONS

Haptic Feedback

Although robot-assisted approaches are being applied to complex cardiothoracic procedures, prolonged operative times, difficulty in performing force-sensitive operations, and the severe consequences of technical error remain. The absence of force feedback, also referred to as "haptic" feedback, is an important limitation in performing cardiac operations.

Sutures breakage and delicate tissue injuries can occur from excessive applied forces. These errors can lead to prolonged cardiopulmonary bypass and cardiac ischemic (crossclamp) durations, irreversible injury to cardiac structures, serious hemorrhage, and even death. The risk of severe complications like these might be reduced by implementing haptic feedback in robot-assisted surgery.

Presently, surgeons use visual cues such as tissue deformation to estimate applied force.[11] It has been suggested that haptic feedback in the form of sensory substitution can facilitate the performance of dexterous surgical tasks.[11] We have reported that the amount of force applied to various grades of fine polypropylene suture was more consistent and showed less deviation during robot-assisted knot tying in the presence of sensory substitution. Compared to the manual techniques, applied mean tension was greater for each suture type when robotic manipulation was used in combination with haptic feedback.[11]

Motion Recognition for Surgical Training

Robotic technology has provided an avenue to accurately measure the surgical skills of trainees. A proposed evaluation method employs statistical models of motion recognition. Exploiting the computer interface inherent in robotic surgical systems, a statistical signal recognition model can be applied to the obtained telemetric data to objectively quantify surgical dexterity.

One statistical signal model that can be designed to recognize real world processes is known as the "Hidden Markov Model" (HMM). This stochastic model is based on the idea that complex processes can be broken down into a series of small steps, which in turn can be modeled using single component signals. The assumption made in the HMM is that each of the component signals can be characterized as a parametric random process and that the parameters of this stochastic process can be precisely determined. Motion related parametric data can be acquired from several repetitions of a robot-assisted surgical task-models performed by an expert surgeon. Data from the expert performance of each task-model can be used to build a series of HMMs representing the ideal sequence of motions necessary to successfully and safely perform robot-assisted operations.

REFERENCES

1. Kant AJ, Klien MD and Langenburg SE. Robotics in pediatric surgery: perspectives for imaging. *Pediatric Radiology* 2004; 34(6): 4454-61.

2. Argenziano M, Oz MC, Kohmoto T, Morgan J, Dimitui J, Mongero L, Beck J, Smith CR. Totally endoscopic atrial septal defect repair with robotic assistance. *Circulation* 2003 Sep 9; 108[Supp 1]: II191-4.

3. Chitwood WR Jr. Current status of endoscopic and robotic mitral valve surgery. *Annals of Thoracic Surgery* 2005; 79: S2248-S2253.

4. Yuh DD. New surgery for congestive heart failure. In: Baughman K, Baumgartner WA, eds. *Treatment of Advanced Heart Disease*. New York, NY, Marcel Dekker. (in press).

5. Morgan JA, Peacock JC, Kohmoto T, Garrido MJ, Schanzer, BM, Kherani AR, Vigilance, DW, Cheema, FH, Kaplan S, Smith, CR, Oz MC, Argenziano M. Robotic techniques improve quality of life in patients undergoing atrial septal defect repair. *Annals of Thoracic Surgery* 2004; 77(4): 1328-33.

6. Dogan S, Aybek T, Andressen E, Byhahn C, Mierdl S, Westphal K, Matheis G, Moritz A, Wimmer-Greinecker G. Totally endoscopic coronary artery bypass grafting on cardiopulmonary bypass with robotically enhanced telemanipulation: report of forty-five cases. *Journal of Thoracic and Cardiovascular Surgery*. 2002; 123: 1125-31.

7. Bonatti J, Schachner T, Bonaros N, Laufer G, Kolbitsch C, Margreiter J, Jonetzko P, Pachinger O, Fredrich G. Robotic totally endoscopic coronary artery bypass and catheter based coronary intervention in one operative session. *Annals of Thoracic Surgery*. 2005; 79: 2138-41.

8. DeRose JJ, Ashton RC, Belsley S, Swistel DG, Vloka M, Ehlert F, Sackner-Bernstein J, Hillel Z, Steinberg JS. Robotically assisted left ventricular epicardial lead implantation for biventricular pacing. *Journal of the American College of Cardiology* 2003; 41(8): 1414-9.

9. Yuh DD, Simon BA, Fernandez A, Bustamante A, Ramey N, Baumgartner WA. Totally endoscopic robot-assisted transmyocardial revascularization. *Journal of the Thoracic and Cardiovascular Surgery* 2005; 130(1): 120-4.

10. Gerosa G, Bianco R, Buja G, diMarco F. Totally endoscopic robotic-guided pulmonary veins ablation: an alternative method for the treatment of atrial fibrillation. *European Journal of Cardio-Thoracic Surgery*. 2004 Aug; 26(2): 450-2.

11. Bethea BT, Okamura AM, Kitagawa M, Fitton TP, Cattaneo SM, Gott VL, Baumgartner WA, Yuh DD. Application of haptic feedback to robotic surgery. *Journal of Laparoendoscopic and Advanced Surgical Techniques* 2004; 14(3): 191-5.

Chapter 11

ROBOTICS TECHNOLOGY IN PEDIATRIC GENERAL AND THORACIC SURGERY

Mustafa H. Kabeer, Vinh T. Lam and David L. Gibbs
Children's Hospital of Orange County, Orange, CA USA

INTRODUCTION

Minimally invasive surgery (MIS) began with peritoneoscopy and became routine in the 1990's with laparoscopic cholecystectomy being the driving force for this surgical revolution. The advent of automated insufflation devices and high resolution 3 chip charge coupling device (CCD) cameras made this a useful and routine approach. Surgeons are constantly evaluating these MIS techniques and developing new ones so that their patients may benefit from smaller incisions, less pain, quicker recovery and shorter hospital stay. These benefits come at the cost of less dexterity for the operating surgeon, uncomfortable positioning, counter-intuitive movement, loss of 3D vision, and tremor magnification. The early fears that these less invasive procedures were not as safe and did not have good outcomes have been put to rest. Almost every form of laparoscopic and thoracoscopic procedure has been shown to have some benefit over its open procedural counterpart.

Pediatric surgeons rapidly embraced minimally invasive surgery in the treatment of their young patients. Laparoscopic cholecystectomy, appendectomy and Nissen fundoplication have become routine at many centers. Since then, many now perform laparoscopic pyloromyotomy and pullthrough for imperforate anus as well as thoracoscopic approaches for pulmonary decortication and biopsies. Other operations involving delicate tissue manipulation or complex suturing such as repair of tracheoesophageal fistula, pulmonary lobectomy, portoenterostomy or excision of choledochal cyst are performed by a select few surgeons with exceptional skills but cannot be done on a regular basis with predictable outcomes by most surgeons.

Many surgeons still do not perform many of the basic minimally invasive procedures on a routine basis. Physician comfort with new techniques and hospital support for implementing new technologies play large roles in performing minimally invasive surgeries. These procedures require relearning an operation and performing it under awkward circumstances which can make them difficult. With MIS, we are no longer able to place our hands into the body cavity, thus sacrificing dexterity and control. Surgeons had to use counter intuitive movement, go from the normal 3D view to a 2 D view on the television screen and often times assumed uncomfortable positions for extended lengths of time which can increase tremor.

Such technological change involves learning the new technology, dedicating time to become familiar and master these new techniques and taking new and additional calculated risk until it becomes routine. As a result, many surgeons still perform few minimally invasive procedures and certainly, the highly complex procedures are for many completely out of reach. Pediatric surgeons have the additional difficulty of carrying out these procedures in patients with smaller cavities which allow even less visibility and require manipulation of tissues which are smaller, more delicate and more susceptible to injury. This has made it difficult for children to benefit fully from advances in MIS technology.

The advent of robotics has improved visualization and dexterity and regained ergonomic positioning for the surgeon. It also reintroduced 3D visualization with the use of special scopes. Surgical robots enhance human capacity rather than replace it. They do not autonomously perform operations but are more like tele-manipulators controlled by computers that enhance a human surgeon's actions performed at a console. Robotics technology will allow us to perform microsurgery in tiny spaces without tremor allowing more precise movement.

The challenge for the future of pediatric surgery is really in trying to do more complex operations in a less invasive manner in more consistent and uniform ways. Surgical robotics technology may help achieve the goal of making minimally invasive techniques more available since it corrects for many of the deficiencies with conventional laparoscopy and thoracoscopy.

HISTORY

Robotic surgery began in 1998 with the introduction of da Vinci (Intuitive Surgical, Sunnyvale, CA) and Zeus (Computer Motion, Goleta, CA). Adult robotic surgery was off to a robust start with applications in general surgery and cardiac surgery. Soon afterwards, it found a stronghold in urology with its application for radical prostatectomy.

Initial application in pediatric surgery was sparse and random. Black from Stanford and Le Bret from Paris had performed PDA ligation in children with the use of Zeus.[1] Gutt et al. from Germany utilized robotics for several general surgical procedures in children and found it to be safe, feasible and comparable to laparoscopy.[2,3]

Much of the benefit from adult medicine is not quickly translated into care for pediatrics. The Children's Hospital of Michigan (CHM) took the initiative to start the first pediatric surgical robotics program specifically designated to utilizing robotics, conducting research and developing new technology for the benefit of children.[4] A concerted effort was undertaken by physicians, administrators, and engineers under the leadership of Drs. Klein and Lyman. Auner and colleagues, from the School of Engineering, and Klein, Kabeer, Langenburg, and Lelli, from the Department of Pediatric Surgery, were instrumental in making this successful from the technical and clinical aspects. We began investigating the possible impact of robotic surgery for the pediatric population, the extent of its use and the possibilities for future development. We evaluated robotics technology for use in the clinical arena as well as developing instruments to facilitate force feedback (haptics) and smaller 3D scopes. Soon after initiation of the program, CHM had started doing various procedures such as cholecystectomy, fundoplication, diaphragmatic hernia repair and Heller myotomy.[5,6] Since that time, many other notable children's hospitals have begun incorporating this technology into their practice of pediatric surgery and in the training of their fellows.

ROBOTICS TECHNOLOGY

Robotics technology allows for a transition from traditional laparoscopy and thoracoscopy by allowing refinement of function. With conventional MIS, surgeons have limited range of motion and no wrist articulation. Surgeon tremor is magnified due to the distance of the effector tip from the point of control as well as the surgeon standing in awkward positions while controlling the instrument. Movement of instruments is also opposite to the intended movement due to the fulcrum effect requiring the surgeon to move the instrument to the right if the tip is to move to the left. Finally, 3D vision is given up for a television monitor providing only 2D views.

Robotic surgery retains the benefit of MIS such as smaller incisions, less pain, quicker recovery, and fewer wound complications and corrects many existing problems. It allows for 3D view, full wrist articulation, intuitive movement and better ergonomic position. It can also filter tremor and allow for motion scaling.

The specific benefits of Zeus and daVinci are noteworthy but should be taken in the context that Zeus is no longer manufactured. Zeus is an open platform system allowing a wider variety of smaller diameter instruments to be utilized in the robotic arms, has modular arms that fit on the table and can move with patient position. It also has a smaller distance from the wrist articulation to the instrument tip allowing it to work in a smaller 3D space. Da Vinci allows the best life like 3D view with true separation of right and left eye views and allows for more range of motion with fluid movement of the instrument tips.

The disadvantages of da Vinci include initial equipment costs, upkeep costs, and the replacement of reusable instruments. There is also increased set up time and increased training of personnel involved. Zeus disadvantages are related more to its 3D visualization which is achieved by alternating left and right views with the use of polarized light whereas daVinci utilizes separate right and left eye views giving true 3D. This true 3D is achieved at the cost of utilizing a large 12 mm dual scope which is not ideal for pediatric surgery and not usable for neonatal surgery. The instruments are also 8mm and can only be used 10 x before requiring replacement. The daVinci can function with a 5mm scope but is only 2D. Five millimeter instruments are available but they do not have the same quality grasp or movement and need a larger volume of space for articulation within the cavity.

Safety measures are built-in and reliable. The intracorporeal movement is only as safe as the surgeon. Large scale unobserved movements can cause significant injury. Extracorporeal movement of the instrument holders and robotic arms is limited and once in position may occasionally bump into adjacent arms, instruments or the assistant. These types of external collisions are minor and have caused no injury to the patient. The computer tracks all hand movements at the console and samples position at over 1300 times per second. As a result, instrument tips correctly reflect hand movement of the operating surgeon with high fidelity. The instruments and the robotics technology have never been cited as a reason for injury to a patient. In the event that prompt conversion to an open procedure is required, the instrument and surgical cart can easily and quickly be disengaged and moved away. A report documenting two conversions due to bleeding during splenectomy were uneventful and neither patient required blood transfusion.[7]

ROBOTICS SETUP

The use of the da Vinci requires positioning and draping of the instrument arms as well as positioning of the console. The console, the robotics cart and the endoscopic cart are connected to each other with cables. The patient is then brought into the room and undergoes anesthesia. The patient is positioned and the table then turned so that the robotics cart can be positioned, allowing enough space for the arms to unfold and extend out over the patient. It may be useful to elevate small children on foam pads to allow for enough space for the robotic arms so they do not collide with the bed.[7] The patient is prepped and draped with sterile sheets and the ports are put into place. The camera is first utilized in the 30 degree up position to watch the abdominal wall as the incisions and the trocars are placed. Next, the robotics cart is brought to the bedside. We leave enough space free near the head and pad it with foam. It is worth noting that the equipment is large and intrusive and can block the ability of the anesthesiologist to quickly check on the endotracheal tube.[8] In general, the robotics cart with the instrument arms is positioned so that the procedure is done with the arms facing inward to the cart and the endoscope looking inward or towards the robotics cart. The robotic arms are positioned and connected onto the trocars. The inner aspect of the trocar is again examined with the camera to make sure that the black bar on the trocar is just on the inner aspect of the cavity. Next, the instruments are placed into the arms and watched as they enter the body cavity to the site of surgery. Once the instruments are in place, the camera is again positioned in the 30 degree down position. Care must be taken to keep the camera lens and housing warmed with wash cloths to decrease fogging of the lens upon entry into the warmer body cavity. The operating surgeon then sits at the console and the assistant stays at the bedside to change instruments, perform retraction or place sutures through the assistant port. More recently, there is a fourth arm which can also be positioned via a separate port which can then be used for retraction. The fourth arm can be activated via a toggle switch and moved and then stabilized when the toggle is turned over to the other instrument arm. The procedure is then performed. Takedown of the instruments involves removing the instruments, disconnecting the robotic arms from the trocars and then removing the trocars. Finally, the incisions are closed. In case of emergency, the instruments and arms can be quickly removed and the unit is wheeled away from the table. With practice, this takes minimal time and often is done in a few seconds.

CLINICAL EXPERIENCE

Any procedure that can currently be performed with minimally invasive techniques may also be performed with robotics technology given the constraints of requiring slightly more body surface area for port placement. The benefit would be most notable in more complex cases especially those requiring suturing.

Over the last 18 months, we have performed 39 robotic assisted cases: 34 Nissen fundoplications, 1 Heller myotomy, 1 splenectomy, 1 resection of posterior mediastinal mass and 2 pulmonary lobectomies. We also had one child with malrotation in whom correction was attempted with robotic assistance. The patient had significant gaseous bowel distention that precluded any visualization or dissection. This was converted to an open procedure. Cases performed with robot assistance at other institutions have included repair of diaphragmatic hernia, pyloroplasty, repair of TEF, excision of choledochal cyst, and even a Kasai portoenterostomy.

All of the descriptions will be provided for the use of da Vinci. It should be noted that port placement and size of patients can vary when using the Zeus system.

PATIENT SELECTION

Preoperative workup is specific to each disease process and is the same as for a minimally invasive or open procedure. Our patients were at least 10 kg. This limit was established due to the size of the instruments (8mm) and the scope (12mm.). Smaller patients may be selected as long as there is enough surface are on the body to allow for at least 10cm between ports. Smaller patients may be used if one uses the 5mm instruments or the 2D 5mm scope. We believe that the 5mm instruments currently being offered do not perform as well as the 8mm instruments in regard to movement and grasp and the benefit of 3D is lost with the smaller 2D scope. As a result, we currently perform minimally invasive procedures on children less than 10 kg without robotic assistance. Finally, we obtain full informed consent.

OPERATIVE PREPARATION

All procedures are performed in a dedicated robotics room to allow for adequate space for instrumentation. The surgical cart, monitor and console are positioned and prepared with sterile drapes before the patient arrives in the room. Once the patient is anesthetized, the table is positioned in the manner it will be needed for the entire case. Table position cannot be changed once the robotic arms are attached at the trocar sites without disconnecting the arms, detaching the surgical cart and rebooting the computer. Subsequently, the patient is prepped and draped in a sterile fashion. The trocars are placed in sequential manner. The first is the 12mm trocar allowing entry of the scope. The remaining trocars are placed under direct visualization. The surgical cart is then positioned over the patient in such a manner that the operative site is inbetween the robotic arms and the surgical cart. (Fig. 1) The instruments are inserted and directed to the operative site under direct visualization.

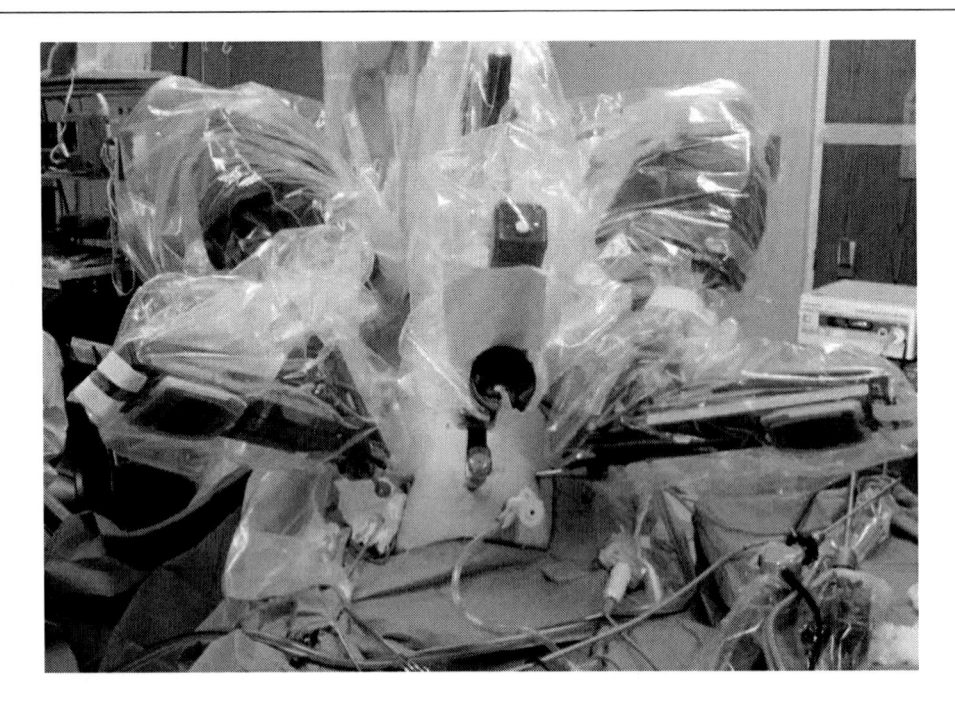

Figure 1. The da Vinci system is positioned during a robot assisted Nissen fundoplication. The surgical cart is placed at the head of the patient and the arms come over the top and attach at the trocars. The right and left arms are on the sides and the middle arm holds the scope. The instrument arms come in at a position such that the operative site is between the port entry and the surgical cart.

ROBOT ASSISTED FUNDOPLICATION

The patient is positioned at the end of the bed with arms tucked at the side and legs in low lithotomy. The bed is raised and placed in reverse Trendelenburg position.

The trocar placements for fundoplication are similar to those for laparoscopic fundoplication except that the liver retractor is placed via a 5mm Apple trocar in the right upper quadrant further lateral and superior to the right upper quadrant trocar for the left robotic arm. (Fig. 2 A, B) This allows for significantly fewer external collisions. The left hand instrument is a Cadiere forceps and the right hand instruments change from harmonic scalpel to hook cautery and then a needle holder. Dissection starts with division of short gastric vessels followed by the gastrohepatic ligament using the harmonic scalpel. A combination of hook cautery and harmonic scalpel are used to define the crus and take down the phrenoesophageal ligament. A 10cm penrose drain is passed around the esophagus and sutured together to itself to allow for easy grasping and retraction.(Fig. 3) Repair of the hiatal hernia and the fundoplication are performed using 2-0 Ethibond sutures and calibrating with a Bougie dilator. The sutures for the repair are 12-14 cm in length to allow for intracorporeal knot tying.(Fig. 4) Upon completion, the scope is used to visualize removal of the liver retractor. The instruments and trocars are removed and the sites are closed.

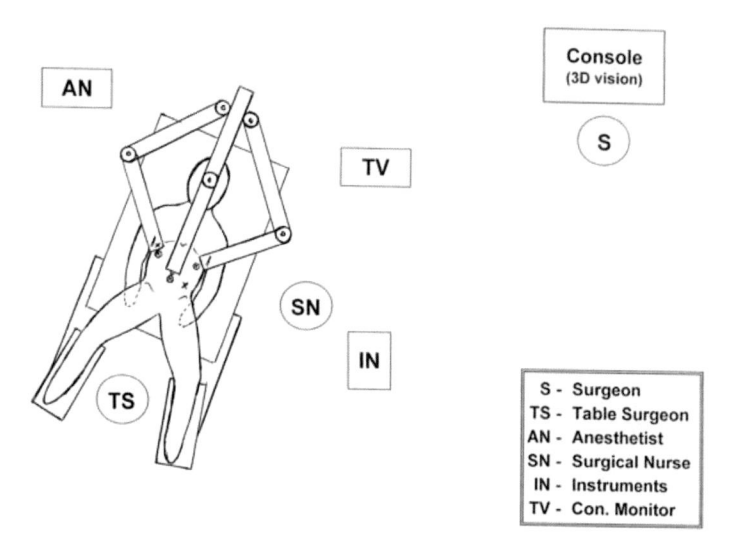

Robotics Technology in Pediatric General and Thoracic Surgery 191

Figure 2A. Schematic depicting the port sites for a Nissen fundoplication and positions of the patient, surgical cart and robotic arms. There are five ports: infraumbilical 12 mm incision for the scope, two 8 mm incisions for the robotic arms in the right and left upper quadrant, a 5mm Apple trocar inferior to the costal margin and lateral and superior to the right upper quadrant incision to be used for the liver retractor and a 5 mm Step Innerdyne trocar in the left lateral or left lower abdomen as the accessory port.

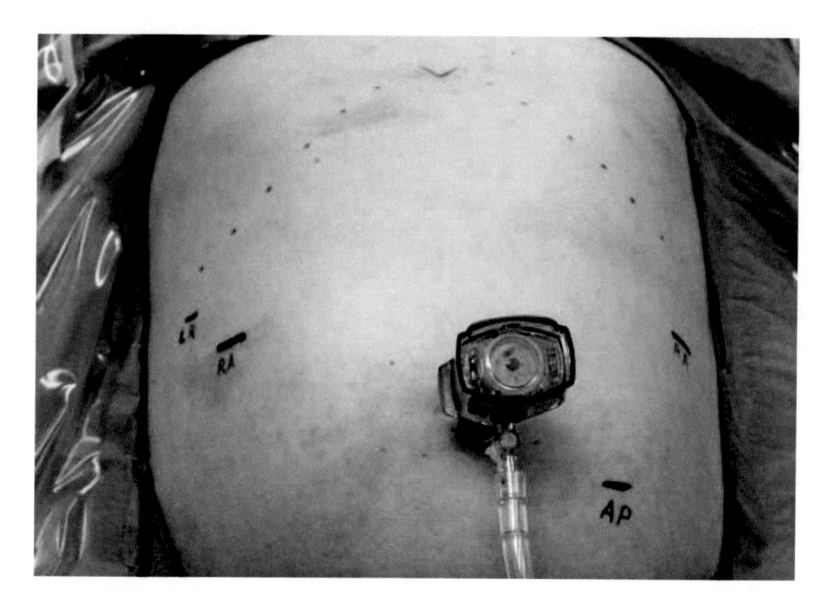

Figure 2B. A photograph of the port positions for a robot assisted Nissen fundoplication. A 10-12 Ethicon trocar is placed through the infraumbilical incision, RA seen in the right and left upper abdomen is the site for Robotic Arm, LR in the right upper quadrant is for Liver Retractor and AP seen in the left lower abdomen is for Accessory Port.

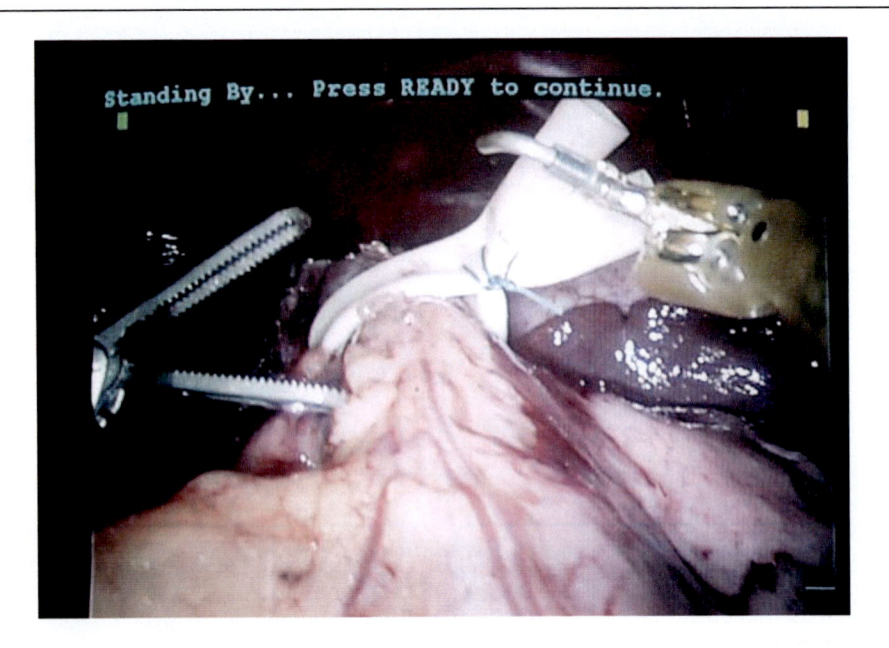

Figure 3. An intraoperative photograph revealing the tips of the Cadiere forceps held on the left side and the hook cautery at the right side. A 10 cm penrose drain is sutured to itself after being passed around the esophagus. This allows for quick and easy retraction of the esophagus during repair of the hiatal hernia and the fundoplication. It is sutured to itself so it can be released but not have the penrose fall out of place.

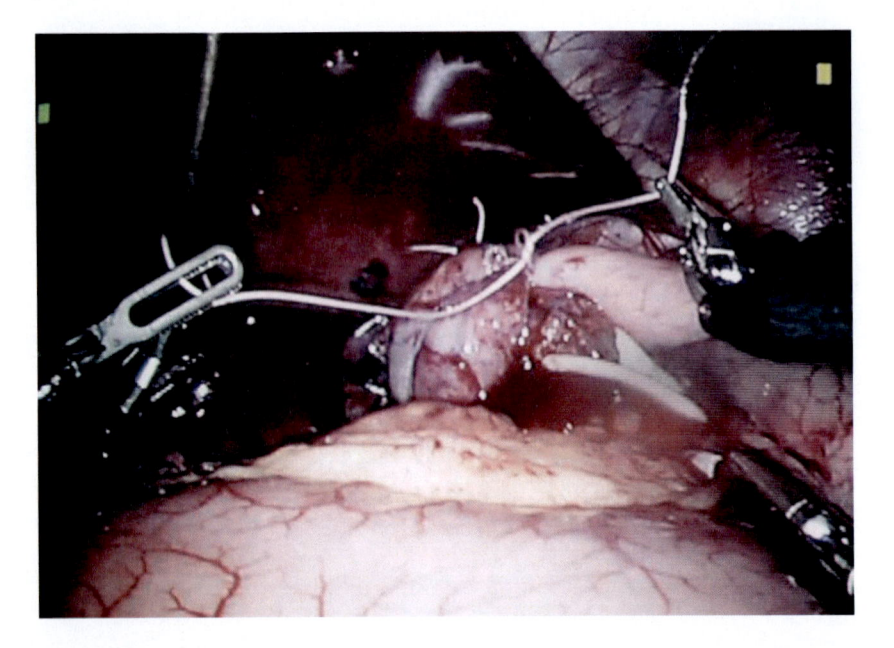

Figure 4. An intraoperative photograph revealing the tips of the Cadiere forceps held on the left side and the needle holder seen at the right side. The two instruments are performing an intracorporeal knot on the last stitch during the fundoplication.

HELLER MYOTOMY

The Heller myotomy is performed with similar positioning of the patient as a fundoplication. (Fig. 2A,B) The ports are placed in a similar manner and careful selection of port placement is crucial such that the scope and instruments are able to reach into the mediastinum as the esophageal myotomy progresses. Once the crus is defined and the esophagus is mobilized, the myotomy is started on the anterior gastric wall approximately 2 cm below the GE junction and extended up along the anterior esophageal wall for 6-8 cm. The myotomy is started with the bovie cautery on the thicker gastric wall and then blunt separation as it progresses upward using a Cadiere forceps in both hands. A lighted endoscope in the esophagus can be useful during the dissection. Judicious use of the hook cautery is also helpful prior to blunt dissection.

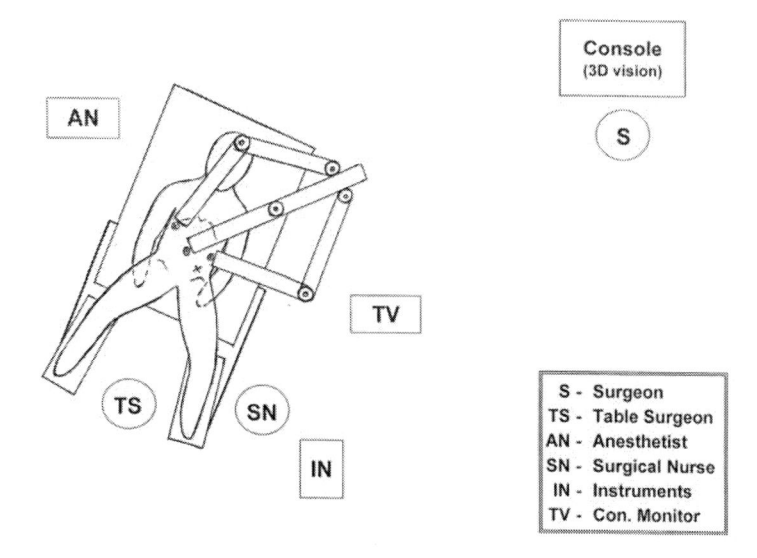

Figure 5. Schematic depicting the port sites for a splenectomy. The port positions are similar to those for a Nissen fundoplication with the exception of the left upper quadrant port being placed lower on the abdomen. A liver retractor is not shown but would be very useful. The spleen is brought out through the left lower quadrant accessory port incision.

SPLENECTOMY

Splenectomy can be performed with a variety of port and patient positions. Patients may be placed in lithotomy with varying degrees of either bed rotation to the right or having a roll in the left flank to allow for 30 degree rotation. The patient may even be placed in a right lateral decubitus position. Our preferred position is lithotomy position with subsequent rotation of the bed and placement of a rolled towel under the left flank. The ports are placed in the umbilicus, one in the midepigastrium, one between the previous two at the midline and one in the left lower quadrant. Alternatively, the ports can be placed similar to a fundoplication with the exception of the left upper quadrant port being placed lower in the abdomen so the instrument does not enter immediately on top of the spleen. (Fig. 5) Liver retraction can be of significant help during the case. A Cadiere forceps is used as the left hand instrument and a harmonic scalpel is placed in the right hand. Short gastric vessels are divided and the hilar vessels are delineated with care. Once a blunt grasper is passed underneath the vessels so that a window is created posteriorly, an endovascular GIA stapler can then be passed to divide the splenic vessels. The attachments are taken down with a harmonic scalpel and hook cautery as the case progresses but is best to not take them down completely till the splenic vessels have been divided. This allows the spleen to stay in position during the manipulation. The spleen is placed in a large endopouch and then brought out through the left lower quadrant incision after morselization.

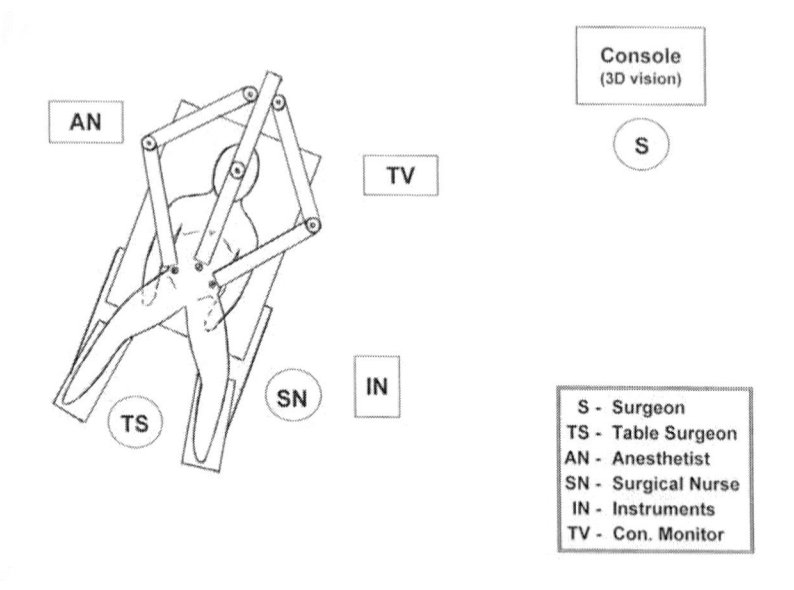

Figure 6. Schematic depicting the port sites for a Ladd procedure. This requires three ports. The scope enters through an infraumbilical incision, the two robotic arms enter via a left lower and right lower quadrant incision.

LADD PROCEDURE

We have performed eight Ladd procedures laparoscopically. The robot assisted Ladd procedure was quickly converted to an open procedure due to extensive gaseous distention of the bowel. This precluded good visualization and thus was not attempted with conventional laparoscopy either. The port placement is the same as for conventional laparoscopic approach with the scope being placed through an infraumbilical incision and the right and left arms being placed through a right lower and left lower quadrant port. (Fig. 6)

MEDIASTINAL MASS

The description is intended for operation of posterior mediastinal masses. The patient is placed in lateral decubitus position. Patients may need to be placed in different positions, even prone, for anterior mediastinal masses. The ports are positioned so that the mass is opposite the scope. The ports for the robotic arms are placed 10 cm away from the scope.(Fig. 7) An accessory port is placed to allow for a fan retractor to keep the lung away from the field of view. (Fig. 8) The mass is then taken down with hook cautery or harmonic scalpel after the parietal pleura is opened. (Fig. 9) The excised mass is placed in an endopouch and brought out through the accessory port. (Fig. 10) The chest tube is directed posteriorly and towards the apex under direct visualization through an existing port site.

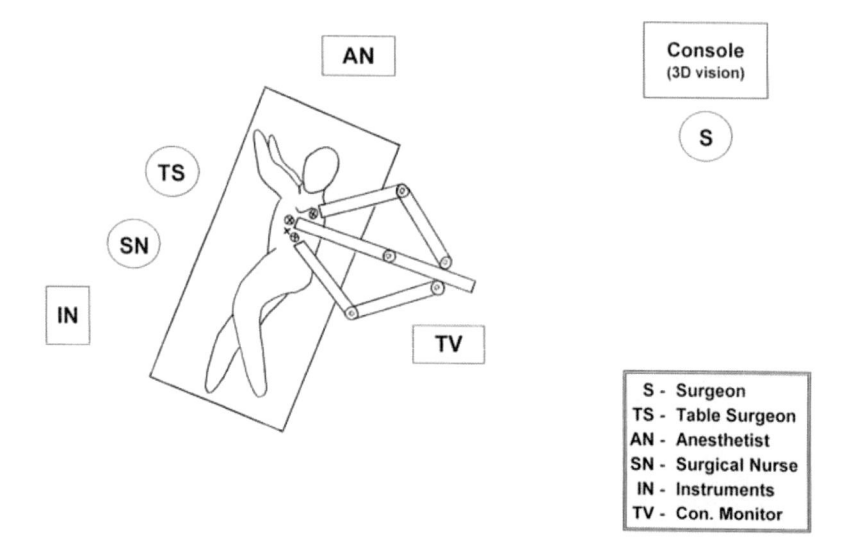

Figure 7. Schematic depicting a patient in right lateral decubitus position with a 12 mm incision at the anterior axillary line at the 5th rib space, the left arm entering through a 4th rib space incision posterior to the scapula, the right arm entering the chest through a 7th rib space incision in the posterior axillary line, and an accessory port through a 5 mm Step Innerdyne trochar at the 6th rib space in the anterior axillary line. The surgical cart is positioned at the side of the table such that the mass is between the port of entry and the surgical cart.

PULMONARY RESECTION

After the patient is anesthetized with a double lumen endotracheal tube, an arterial line, a central line, a Foley catheter and a thoracic epidural catheter are placed. The patient is placed in lateral decubitus position. The ports are placed and the lung is dissected to isolate pulmonary vessels and the lobar bronchus. (Fig. 11A,B) The vessels can be tied and then divided with an endovascular GIA stapler, Ligasure or after applying Ligaclips.(Fig. 12 A,B) The bronchus is also skeletonized and then divided with an endovascular GIA stapler. Upon completion, a chest tube is placed under direct visualization.

One pulmonary resection involved a left upper lobectomy for congenital cystic adenomatoid malformation and another a right lower lobectomy for intralobar pulmonary sequestration.(Fig. 13)

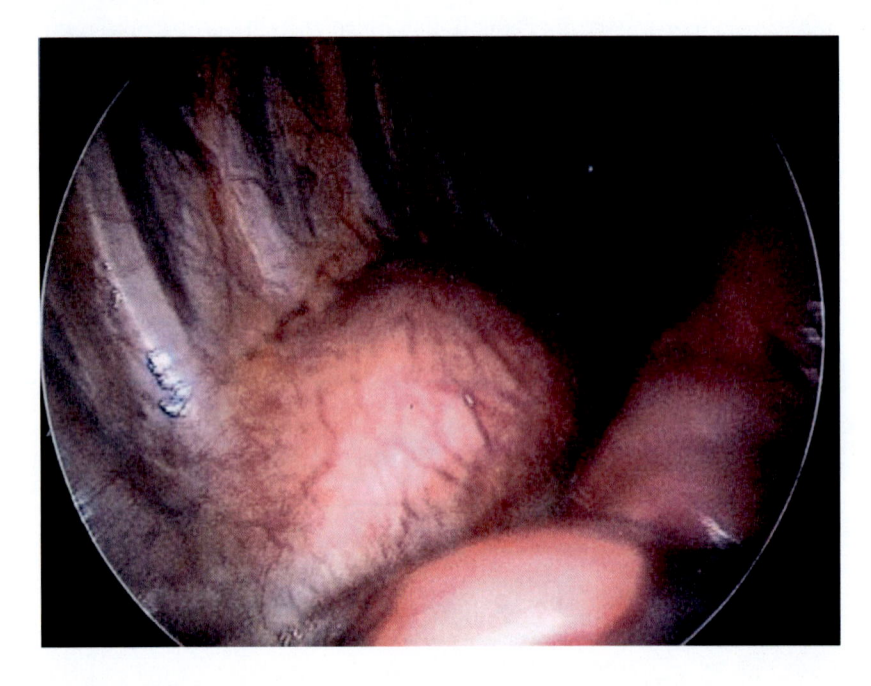

Figure 8. Intraoperative view of a 5 cm mass in the paravertebral thoracic space in a 8 yr old child. The lung is seen in the peripheral edges.

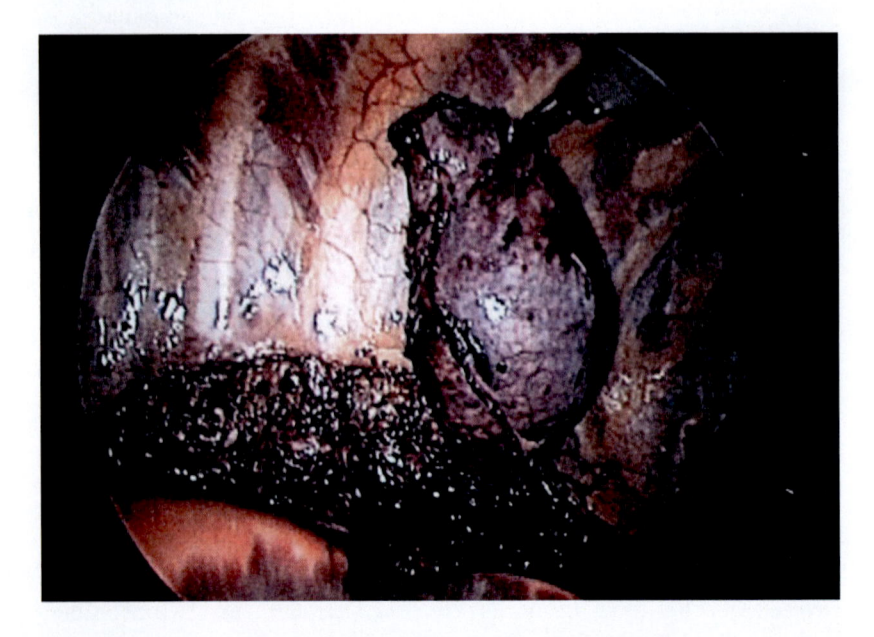

Figure 9. Intraoperative view of the mass after it is excised out of the space.

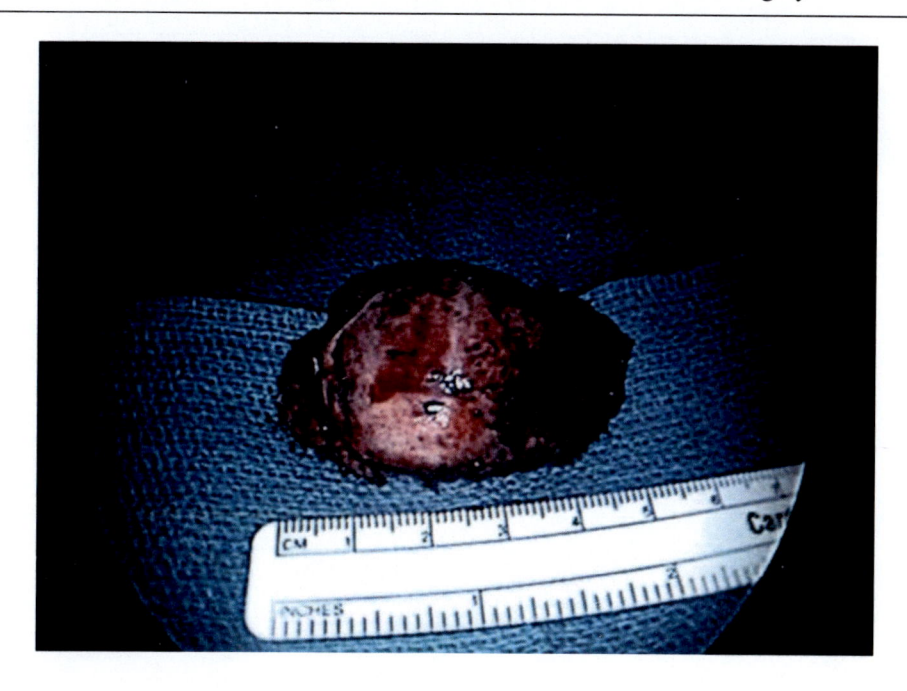

Figure 10. Intraoperative view of the mass after it is pulled out of the thoracic cavity.

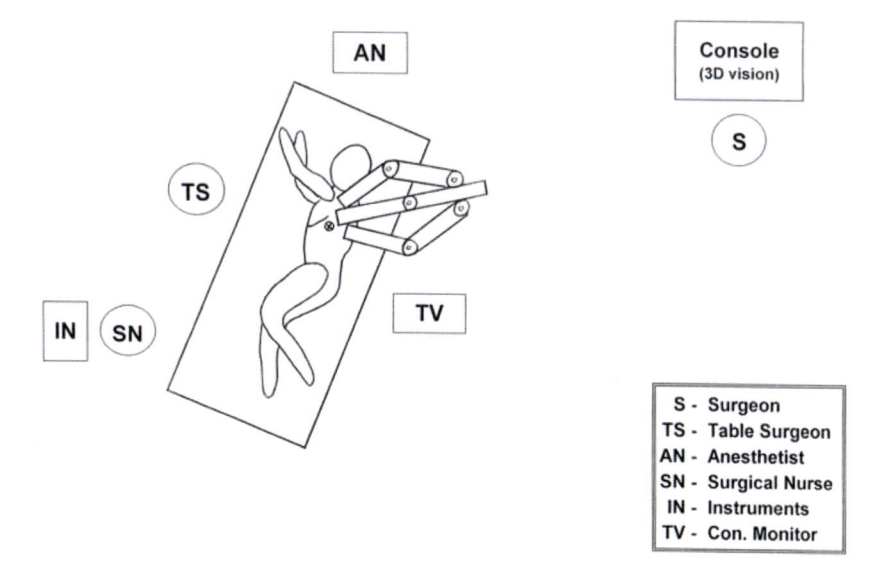

Figure 11A. Schematic depicting a patient in right lateral decubitus position with a 12 mm trochar at the position and two 8mm ports for the robotic arms.

198   Mustafa H. Kabeer, Vinh T. Lam and David L. Gibbs

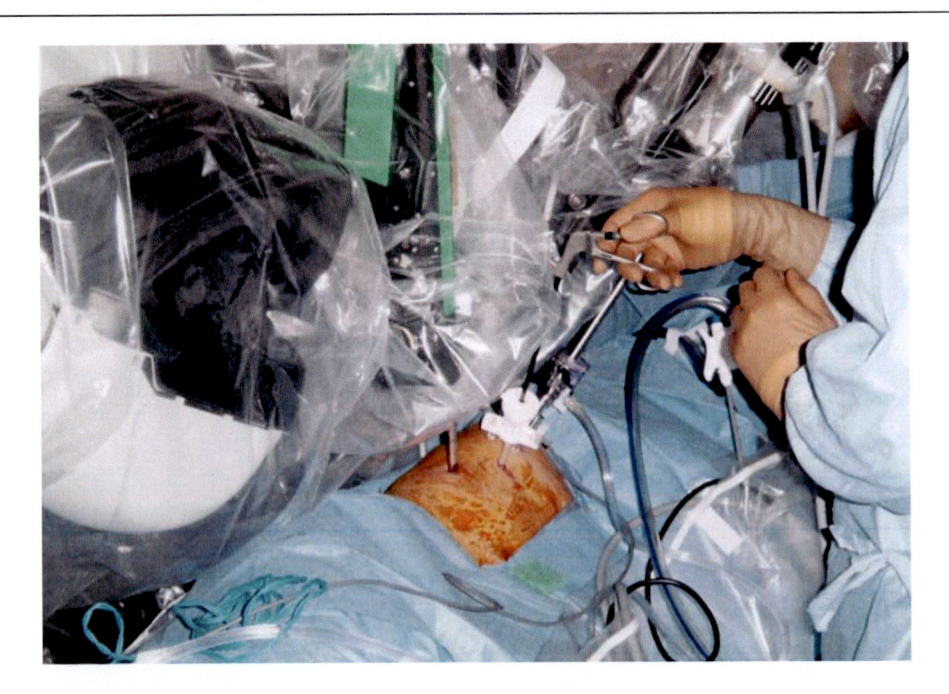

Figure 11B. Intraoperative photograph of external port placements during a right lower lobe pulmonary resection for intralobar pulmonary sequestration.

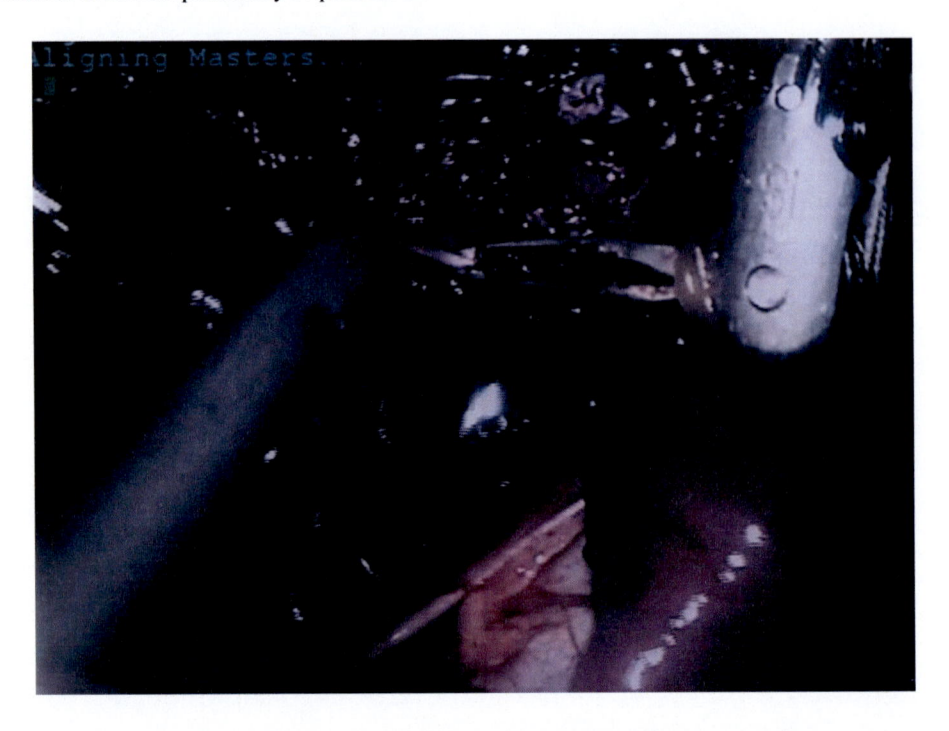

Figure 12A. Intraoperative photograph of a Cadiere grasper in the left hand and a Maryland dissector in the right hand holding onto a pulmonary arterial branch to the right lower lobe.

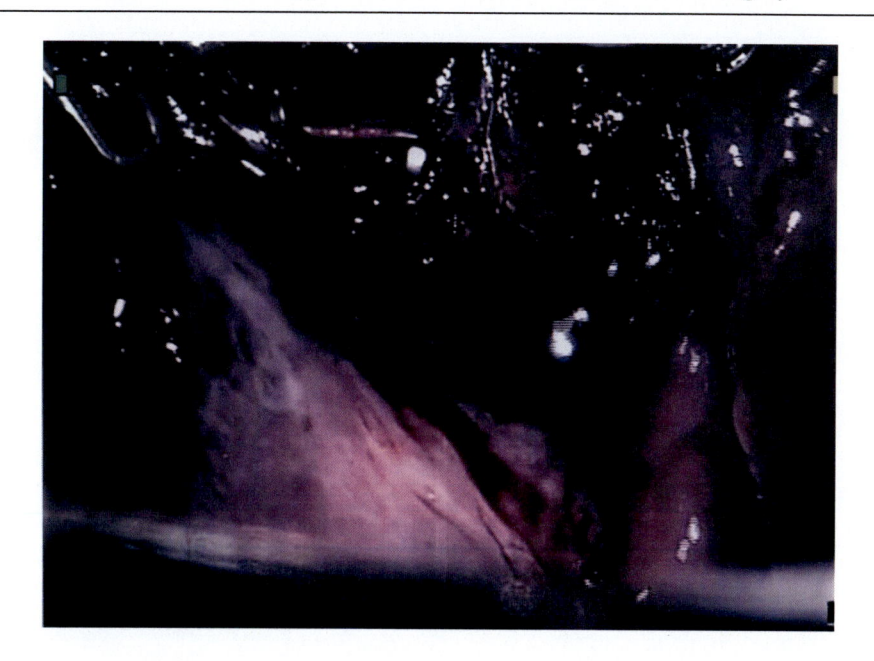

Robotics Technology in Pediatric General and Thoracic Surgery 199

Figure 12B. Intraoperative photograph of Ligaclips being applied proximally and distally on the dissected pulmonary arterial branch to the right lower lobe. The ligaclips are seen in the left mid upper portion of the photograph.

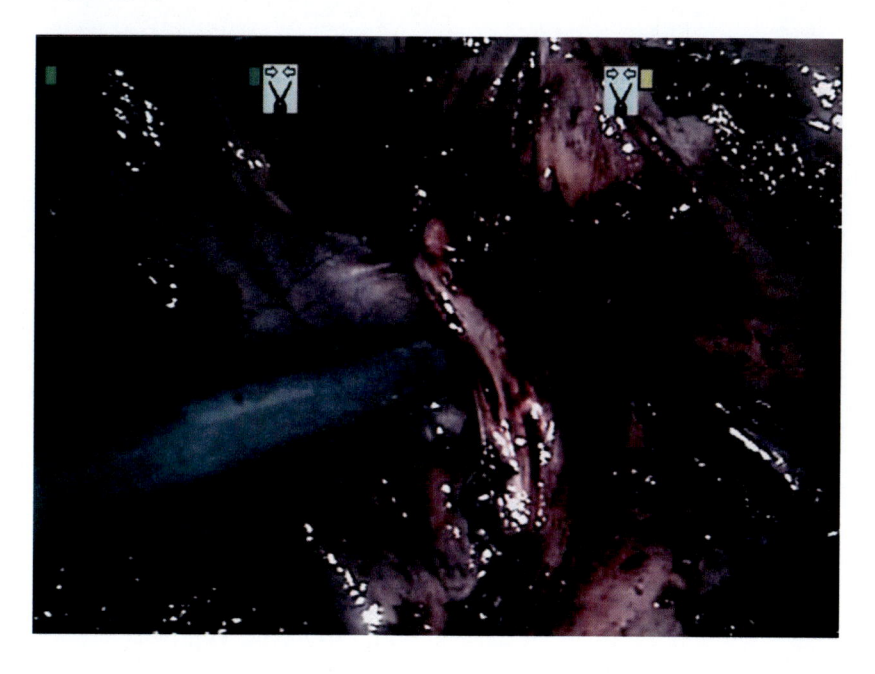

Figure 13. Intraoperative photograph of the Cadiere grasper passing behind the systemic arterial supply to the intralobar sequestration.

OUTCOMES

High definition magnified 3D views of the operative field and articulating instruments allowing precise suture placement in any direction may translate into better surgery and better outcomes. The technology is still too young to have long term data on outcomes. We believe that the biggest benefit from this technology will be in better long term outcomes since traditional minimally invasive surgery already provides improved short term outcomes such as less pain, shorter length of stay and quicker recovery.

In our series, we had one patient with fundoplication requiring a repeat trip to the operating room due to a paraesophageal hernia soon after surgery. It may have been due to repair of the hiatal hernia over a large bougie dilator. In order to avoid swallowing difficulty postoperatively, a large dilator was utilized since he was a large patient. He had a long standing history of retching and began to do so immediately after surgery. This was not a complication of robotic surgery. There was an additional patient who intermittently has retching and difficulty swallowing but has been evaluated and found to have an intact fundoplication. There have been no recurrent hiatal hernias or problems with ongoing reflux in the remainder of the patients after fundoplication. No other patients having other types of procedures have reported any problems.

Surgeons need to continuously search for ways of doing things that will improve the lives of our young patients. The negative attitudes toward laparoscopic cholecystectomy took time to disappear and all new technologies will undergo such testing.

Despite optimism about the benefits of robotics technology, it is not yet clear that it has a definite place in pediatric surgery. Many centers are becoming facile with routine operations raising hope that surgeons will then begin to test this technology in more difficult operations. Eventually the difficult and complex operations will also become routine and safe to perform in very little children with minimal invasion.

CURRENT CLINICAL RESEARCH-ROBOTICS APPLICATIONS

There have been several animal models for the study of pediatric surgical disorders. Some complex procedures have been attempted on animal models such as repair of biliary atresia with a Kasai portoenterostomy and repair of tracheoesophageal fistula (TEF) with an esophago-esophageal anastamosis. Hollands began some noteworthy experiments studying the possibility of complex suturing utilizing the Zeus system on such operations.[9,10] Lorincz et al. from CHM also performed studies on pigs to simulate the Kasai operation for biliary atresia. The mean operating time was 330 minutes and five of eight survived to one month having normal gastrointestinal function and no jaundice.[11] An esophageal atresia model requiring an esophageal anastamosis was also performed on pigs with five of seven surviving to one month with a mean operating time of 120 minutes. All survivors were eating well. It was noted that the Zeus system seemed critical in working in such small volume cavities.[6] Knight et al. and Aaronson et al. also showed feasibility of utilizing robotics in treating fetal disorders such as in utero repair of myelomeningocoele.[12,13]

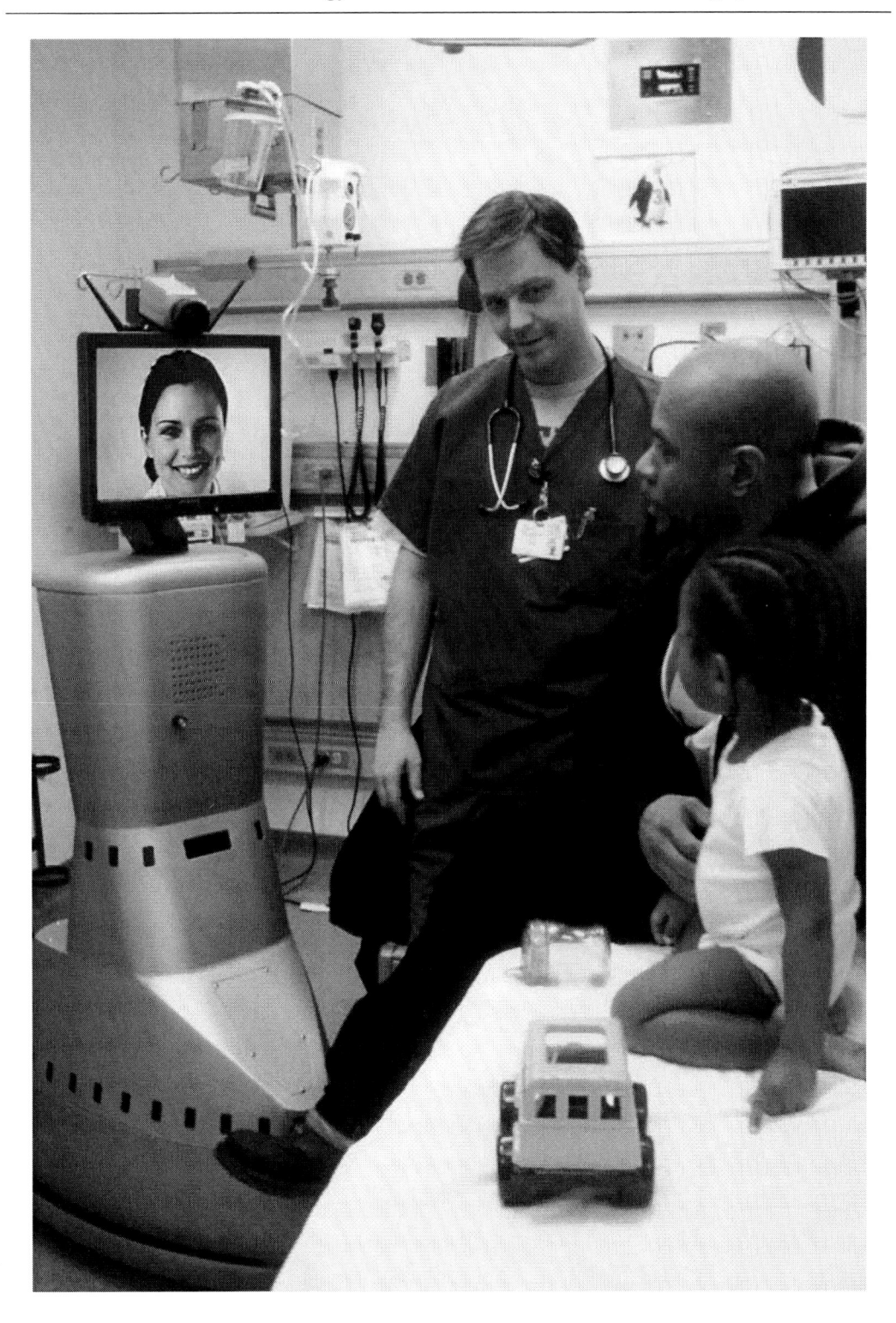

Figure 14. A robot showing the picture of the physician controlling the robot and the interaction between the physician and the patient, her father and the nurse in the room.

FUTURE DEVELOPMENTS

The field of robotics technology will have to undergo much more change in the next few years. The console can be built into the room. The surgical cart or individual robotic arms can be suspended on booms thus allowing easier maneuverability or have docking positions on the bed to allow for changes in bed position during an operation. This technology will also have to become less expensive to allow for more widespread use. Teaching can also be improved if there is a learning console which allows for the resident to perform an operation in concert with an attending surgeon providing guidance from the teacher's console. The biggest hurdle for full incorporation into pediatric surgery will be the availability of reliable and fully functional 5mm instruments with high fidelity. The large 3D 12 mm scope also needs to be re-engineered to allow downsizing to 5mm and still allow crisp separation and true 3D. Virtual reality and haptics are currently under development in various labs and will eventually become incorporated. It may also be useful to have the operating surgeon have individual right and left eye views simultaneously but separately channeled into a goggle head set which can give the sense of 3D viewing currently allowed via the console but in a manner that still preserves peripheral vision.

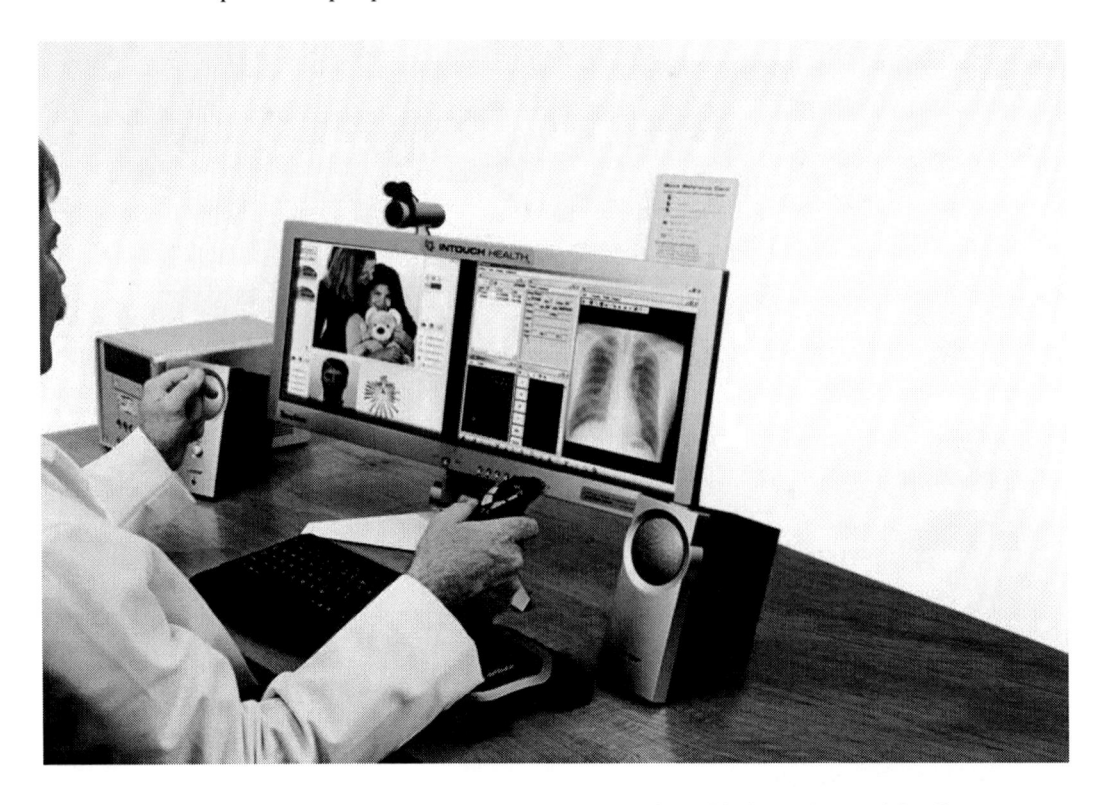

Figure 15. The control station which allows live video interaction with the patient and family.

Telemedicine will also become incorporated into the field of robotics. There exist current systems which allow interactions remotely for consultation. Technology for remote interactions with patients is currently available but underutilized. The system has two components comprised of a freely navigating robot which has direct interaction with the patient (Fig. 14) and the control station which is employed by the physician to maneuver the robot and have direct interaction with the patient and family.(Fig. 15)

REFERENCES

1. Le Bret E, Papadatos S, Folliguet T. Interruption of patent ductus arteriosus in children: robotically assisted versus videothoracoscopic surgery. *Journal of Thoracic and Cardiovascular Surgery* 2002;123:973-6.

2. Gutt CN, Markus B, Kim ZG, Meininger D, Brinkmann L, Heller K. Early experiences of robotic surgery in children. *Surgical Endoscopy*, 2002; 16:1083-6.

3. Heller K, Gutt C, Schaeff B, Beyer PA, Markus B. Use of the robot system da Vinci for laparoscopic repair of gastroesophageal reflux in children. *European Journal of Pediatric Surgery* 2002;12:239-42.

4. Langenburg S, Kabeer M, Knight C, Fleischmann L, Auner G, Lyman W, Klein M. Surgical Robotics: Creating a New Program. *Pediatric Endoscopy and Innovative Technique* 2003; 7(4):415-9.

5. Knight CG, Lorincz A, Gidell KM, Lelli J, Klein MD, Langenburg SE. Computer-assisted robot-enhanced laparoscopic fundoplication in children. *Journal of Pediatric Surgery* 2004; 39:864-6.

6. Lorincz A, Langenburg S, Klein M. Robotics and the pediatric surgeon. *Current Opinions in Pediatrics* 2003;15:262-6.

7. Luebbe B, Woo R, Wolf S, Irish M. Robotically assisted minimally invasive surgery in a pediatric population: initial experience, technical considerations, and description of the daVinci Surgical System. *Pediatric Endosurgery and Innovative Techniques* 2003;7:385-402.

8. Mariano ER, Furukawa L, Woo R, Albanese CT, Brock-Utne JG, Anesthetic concerns for robot-assisted laparoscopy in an infant. *Anesthesia and Analgesia* 2004; 99:1665-7.

9. Hollands CM, Dixey LN. Robotic-assisted esophagoesophagostomy. *Journal of Pediatric Surgery* 2002; 37;983-5.

10. Hollands CM, Dixey LN, Torma MJ. Technical assessment of procine enteroenterostomy performed with Zeus robotic technology. *Journal of Pediatric Surgery*. 2001; 36:1231-3.

11. Lorincz A, Knight CG, Langenburg SE, Rabah R, Gidell K, Dawe E, Grant S, Klein MD. Robotic-assisted minimally invasive Kasai portoenterostomy: a survival porcine study. *Surgical Endoscopy* 2004; 18:1136-9.

12. Lorincz A, Knight CG, Kant AJ, Langenburg SE, Rabah R, Gidell K, Dawe E, Klein MD, McLorie G. Applying the Zeus robotic surgical system to fetal sheep surgery. *The International Fetal Medicine and Surgery Society*, April 2003, Zermatt, Switzerland. *Journal of Pediatric Surgery* 2005 Feb; 40(2):418-22.

13. Aaronson, OS, Tulipan, NB, Cywes, R Robot-assisted endoscopic intrauterine myelomeningocele repair: a feasibility study. *Pediatric Neurosurgery* 2002; 36:85-9.

In: Robotics in Surgery: History, Current and Future Applications ISBN 1-60021-386-3
Editor: Russell A. Faust, pp. 205-222   © 2007 Nova Science Publishers, Inc.

Chapter 12

ROBOTIC APPLICATIONS IN ADVANCED GYNECOLOGIC SURGERY

Arnold P. Advincula
Department of Obstetrics & Gynecology
University of Michigan Medical Center, Ann Arbor, Michigan USA

Abstract

The use of robot-assisted laparoscopy in gynecology is a promising alternative to conventional laparoscopy for the minimally invasive management of female pelvic pathology.

Keywords: robotics, gynecologic surgery, laparoscopy, myomectomy, hysterectomy

INTRODUCTION

The first known report of an endoscopic procedure dates back to 1807. A physician by the name of Bozzini visualized the urethra with a candle and simple tube-like device. Over a century later, Boesch in 1936 described the first gynecologic use of laparoscopy with tubal sterilization. It was not until the early 1970s that laparoscopy revolutionized gynecology. Since then minimally invasive surgery has become increasingly popular and demanded by both surgeons and patients in the field of gynecologic surgery.

Technical advancements have brought about improvements to modern day laparoscopy. These include high intensity xenon and halogen light sources as well as improved hand instrumentation. As technology surrounding minimally invasive gynecologic surgery continues to grow by leaps and bounds, the days of a surgeon peering through an eyepiece during a diagnostic laparoscopy have long passed. Today three-dimensional imaging is possible for both the surgeon and observers while complex procedures are performed with advanced laparoscopic instrumentation. Studies have clearly shown that laparoscopic surgery allows faster recovery with less postoperative pain. Despite these technological advancements and benefits, more complex procedures such as the management of advanced endometriosis, and procedures that require extensive suturing such as myomectomy, pelvic reconstructive surgery, and tubal reanastomosis are typically still managed by laparotomy. Another example is hysterectomy. In 2002, Farquhar & Steiner reported that approximately 10% of hysterectomies were performed with the assistance of laparoscopy (1).

One major obstacle to the more widespread acceptance and application of minimally invasive surgical techniques to gynecologic surgery has been the limitations encountered with conventional laparoscopy. These include counter-intuitive hand movement, two-dimensional visualization, and limited degrees of instrument motion within the body. Additional challenges are the issues surrounding training and acquisition of advanced skills. In their quest to overcome these obstacles, modern day gynecologic surgeons have begun to apply robot-assisted surgery to their endoscopic armamentarium. The following chapter will review the evolution and current state of robot-assisted laparoscopy in gynecology.

HISTORY

One of the early predecessors and first applications of robotic technology to the field of gynecology was with a voice-activated robotic arm known as Aesop® (Computer Motion Inc.®, Goleta, CA). The primary role of Aesop® was to operate the camera during laparoscopic surgery. One study by Mettler et al. compared the system to a surgical assistant holding the laparoscope during gynecologic surgery (2). The authors found that the time required to perform surgery was faster with the robotic camera holder because it allowed the two surgeons to use both hands for operating thereby improving efficiency.

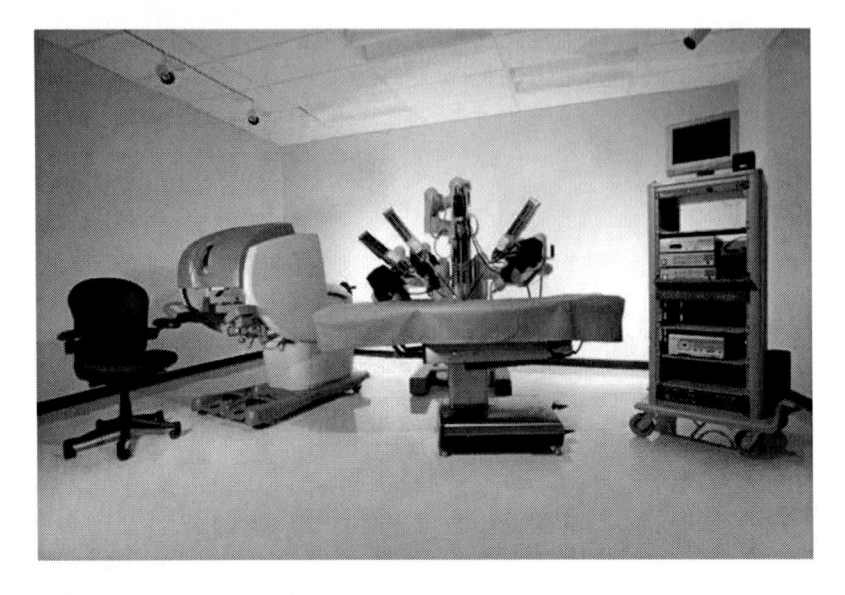

Figure 1. Photograph of the da Vinci® Robotic System. From left to right: surgeon's console, patient-side surgical cart, and InSite® vision tower. Photo courtesy of Intuitive Surgical®, Inc.

Another predecessor to the current platform of surgical robots was Zeus® (Computer Motion Inc.®, Goleta, CA). Early studies reported on its successful application to tubal reanastomosis. In one prospective study, pregnancy rates were evaluated in ten patients with previous tubal ligations who underwent laparoscopic tubal reanastomosis using the identical technique used at laparotomy (3). A post-operative tubal patency rate of 89% was demonstrated in 17 of the 19 tubes anastomosed with a pregnancy rate of 50% at one year. There were no complications or ectopic pregnancies.

The use of robotic technology to facilitate laparoscopic procedures in gynecology has rapidly increased over the past five years, particularly with the introduction of the latest FDA approved platform in surgical robotics, the daVinci® surgical system (Intuitive Surgical®, Sunnyvale, CA). The daVinci® surgical system is comprised of three components (Figure 1). The first component is the surgeon console where the surgeon controls the robotic system remotely. A stereoscopic viewer as well as hand and foot controls is housed in this unit. The second component of the daVinci® surgical system is the InSite® vision system which provides the three dimensional imaging through a 12 mm endoscope. The third component of the daVinci® surgical system is the patient-side cart with telerobotic arms and Endowrist® instruments. Currently this system is available with either three or four robotic arms. One of the arms holds the laparoscope while the other two to three arms hold the various laparoscopic surgical instruments such as a Debakey forceps and round-tip scissors. These Endowrist® instruments are unique in that they possess seven degrees of movement which replicates the full range of motion of the surgeon's hand. The fulcrum effect seen with conventional laparoscopy is eliminated.

In numerous studies across various disciplines, it has been shown to be a safe and effective alternative to conventional laparoscopic surgery, particularly when dealing with complex pathology. In the area of gynecology, there are reports of robot-assisted laparoscopy with the daVinci® surgical system for tubal reanastomosis, ovarian transposition, hysterectomy, myomectomy, and the repair of vaginal vault prolapse (4-7). We have utilized a three-armed daVinci® surgical system in gynecology at the University of Michigan Medical Center since 2001, with an emphasis on myomectomy and hysterectomy.

LEIOMYOMATA

Uterine fibroids (leiomyomata) are benign tumors of fibrous tissue and smooth muscle. They are the most frequent pelvic tumors seen in gynecology and account for approximately 30% of the hysterectomies performed annually in the United States (8). The symptoms are typically pelvic pain and pressure or abnormal uterine bleeding, depending on the location.

Fibroids can be found in the cavity of the uterus (submucosal) or in varying locations in the wall (intramural or subserosal) of the uterus (Figure 2). Occasionally they can grow on a stalk (pedunculated) on the outside of the uterus. The etiology of uterine fibroids is unknown. For women who desire future fertility or uterine conservation, the primary surgical management of symptomatic fibroids is myomectomy. Today many cases of intramural and subserous fibroids are managed with laparoscopic myomectomy as a result of improvements in technology (9). The ability to enucleate leiomyomata and repair the uterus with a multi-layer sutured closure is crucial and technically challenging when done laparoscopically. Despite having a skilled surgeon, the surgical limitations that exist with conventional laparoscopy are thought to affect conversion rates to laparotomy and may play a role in cases of uterine rupture. As a result, the overwhelming majority of cases are still performed through laparotomy. In an attempt to improve the minimally invasive management of leiomyomata, a robotic approach with the daVinci® surgical system is utilized at the University of Michigan Medical Center.

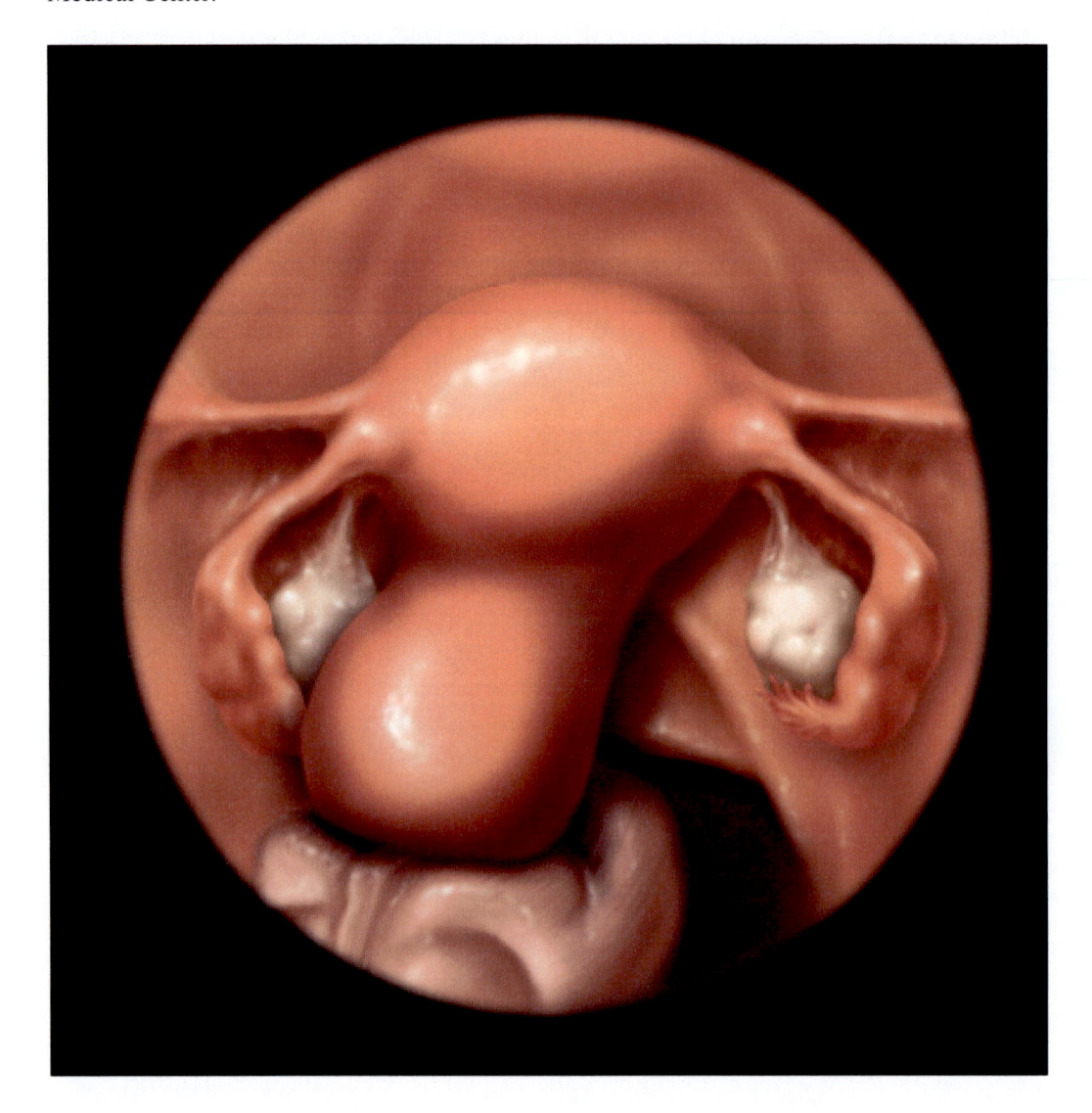

Figure 2. Schematic of large posterior subserosal fibroid compressing rectosigmoid.

ROBOTIC (DAVINCI) MYOMECTOMY - TECHNIQUE

All patients are placed in low dorsal lithotomy position with arms padded and tucked at their sides after general endotracheal anesthesia is administered (Figure 3). The bladder is drained with a Foley catheter and a uterine manipulator is placed. We utilize either a ZUMI®

or RUMI® uterine manipulator (Cooper Surgical®, Trumbull, CT) (Figure 4). Four trocars are typically utilized after pneumoperitoneum is obtained. A 12 mm trocar is placed either at or above the umbilicus depending on the size of the pathology (Figure 5). This trocar accommodates the dual optical channel endoscope. Occasionally a left upper quadrant entry with a 3 mm microlaparoscope is performed in order to help guide operative trocar placement. Indications for this added step would be patients with a markedly enlarged uterus or who are at risk for pelvic adhesions such as prior abdominal surgery. Two-8 mm trocars which mount directly to the surgical carts two operating arms are placed in the left and right lower quadrants respectively. In cases where the uterus sizes to above the pelvic brim, lateral trocar placement is moved cephalad in order to allow adequate working distance between the superior-most border of the tumor and the port site. A fourth trocar which serves as an accessory port is placed between the camera port and the right lower quadrant port. This is typically 12 mm – 15 mm in order to facilitate introduction of suture, a tissue morcellator, and suction/irrigation instruments.

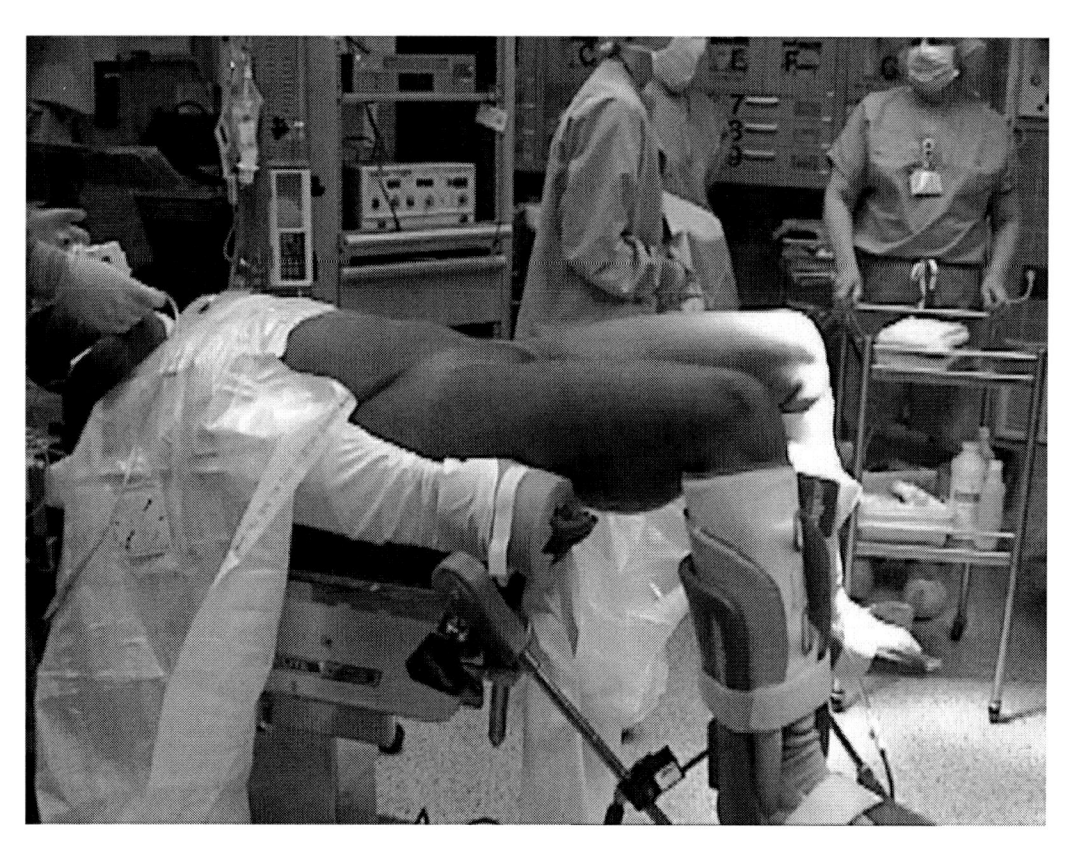

Figure 3. Proper positioning for robotic cases with patient in dorsal lithotomy and arms padded and tucked at sides.

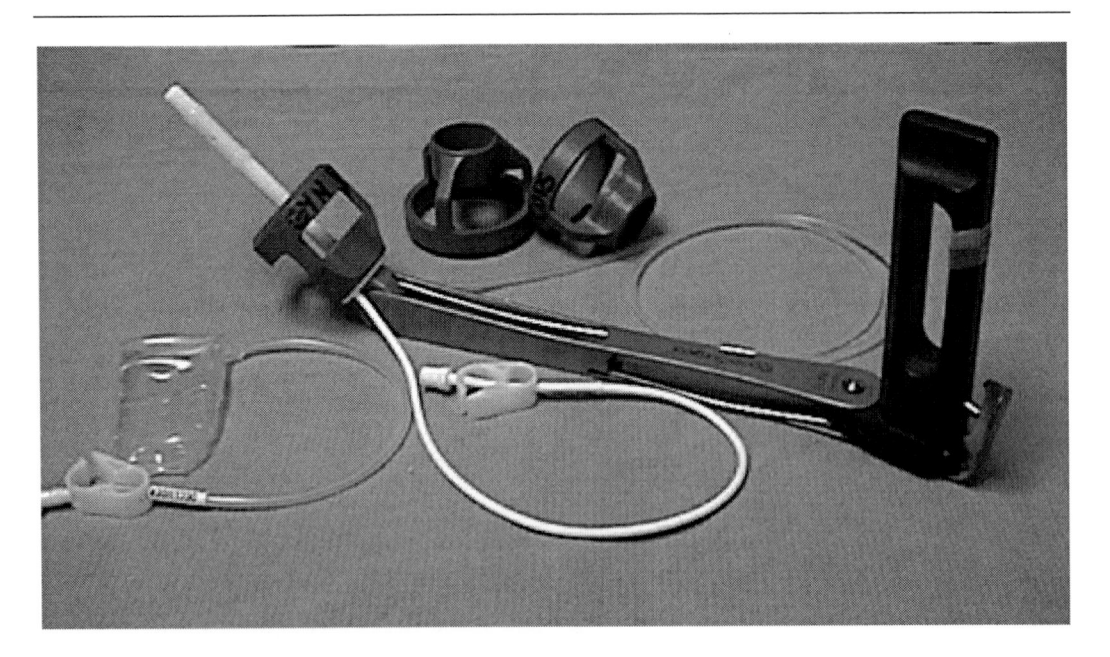

Figure 4. RUMI® uterine manipulator in conjunction with Koh® colpotomy rings and a vaginal pneumo-occluder balloon (all Cooper Surgical®, Trumbull, CT)

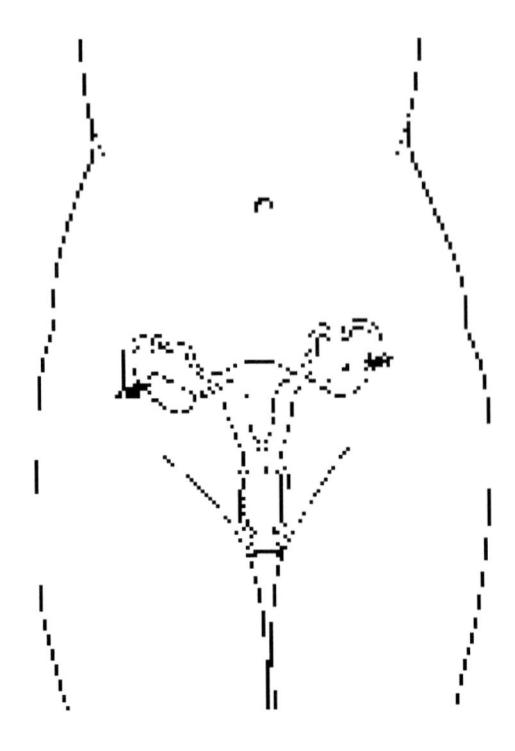

Figure 5. Port Placement. The camera port (A) - 12 mm either at the umbilicus or above depending on the size of the uterus. The lateral ports (B) - 8 mm da Vinci® ports in the right and left lower quadrants of the abdomen. The assist port (12 -15 mm) placed between the camera port and the right lower quadrant port.

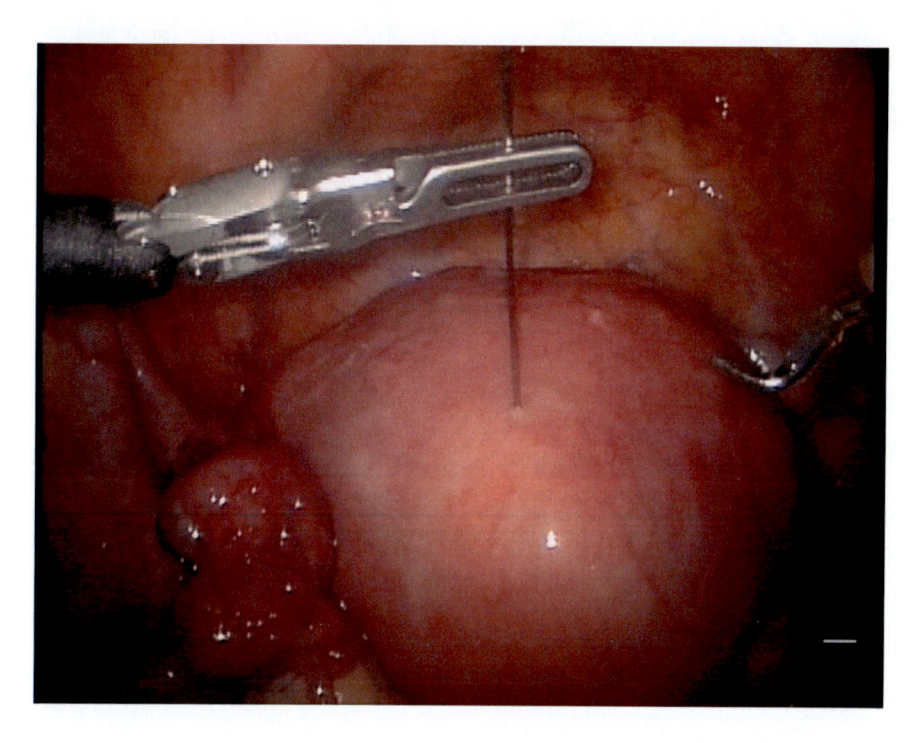

Figure 6. Application of vasoconstrictive agent through 7 inch 22 gauge spinal needle into myometrium as adjunct for hemostasis prior to start of myomectomy.

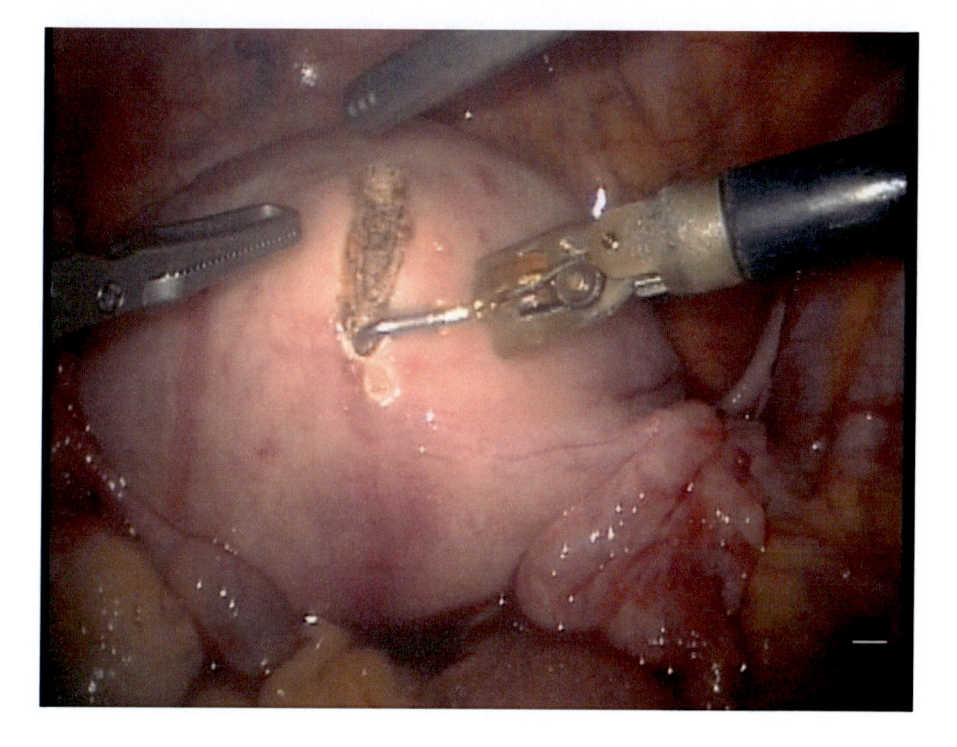

Figure 7. (a) Serosal incision over leiomyoma with Endowrist® permanent cautery hook.

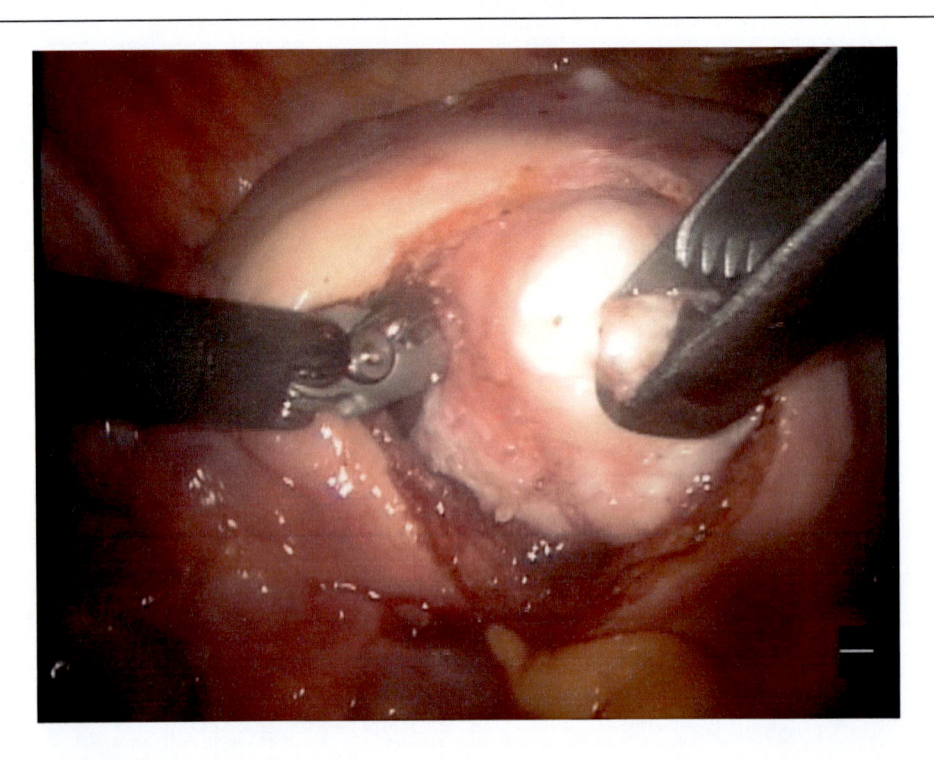

Figure 7. (b) Enucleation of intramural leiomyoma.

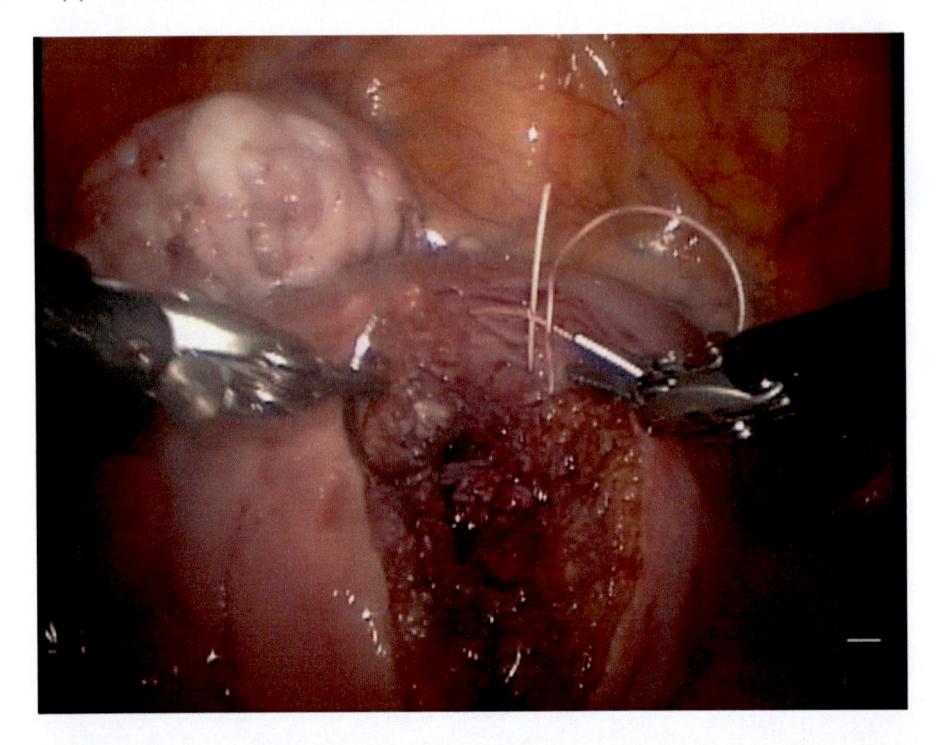

Figure 8. Multilayer-sutured closure of uterine defect with excised leiomyoma in anterior cul de sac.

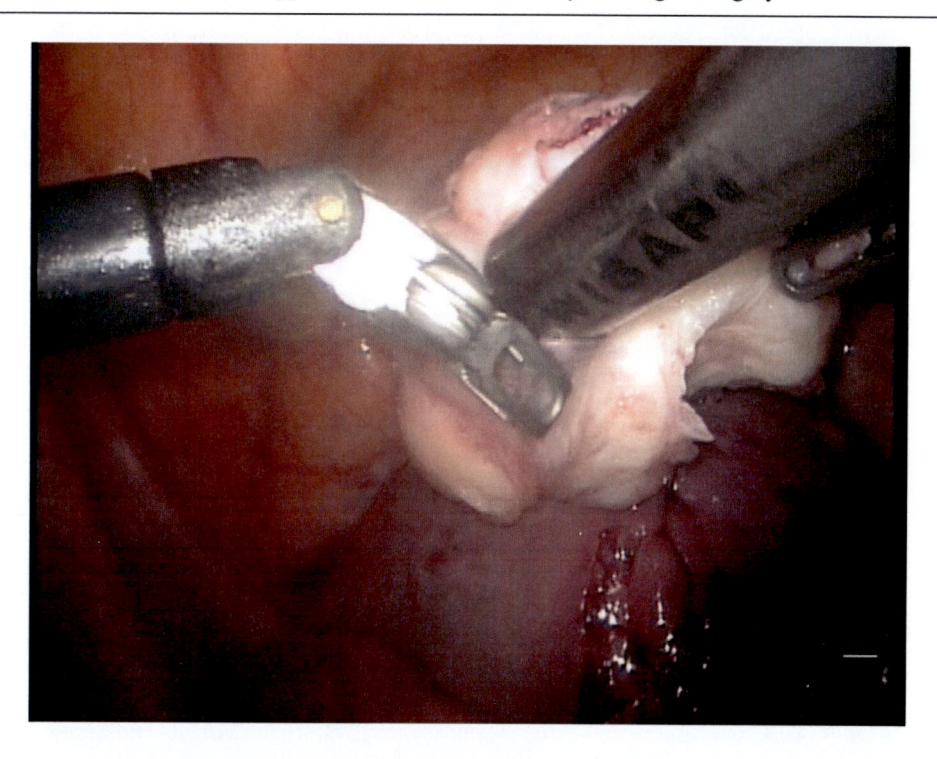

Figure 9. Extraction of leiomyoma with a tissue morcellator

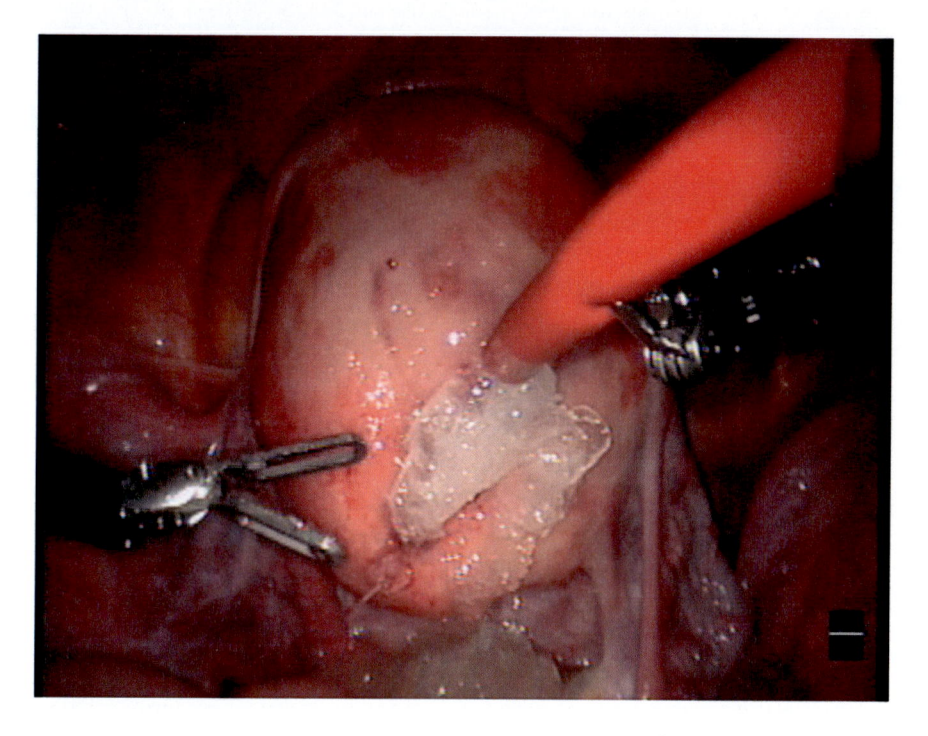

Figure 10. Application of slurry of Seprafilm™ (Genzyme Biosurgery®, Cambridge, MA) as adhesion barrier.

Once all four trocars are in place, the patient is placed in steep Trendelenburg and the patient-side cart with three robotic arms is brought between the patients legs and docked. A survey of the operative field is performed, after which a dilute concentration of vasopressin is infiltrated via a 7 inch 22 gauge spinal needle transabdominally into the myometrium surrounding the fibroid as an adjunct for hemostasis (Figure 6). Heavy grasping instruments such as a Cadiere® (fenestrated forceps) or CobraGrasper® and a permanent cautery hook or spatula, all Endowrist® instruments, are attached to the right and left operating arms and used to incise the serosa as well as enucleate the leiomyomata (Figure 7). Counter-traction is provided by the bedside assistant through the accessory port with a myoma grasper or cork screw. Adequate hemostasis is obtained with the combination of the vasoconstrictive agent administered at the onset of the case, monopolar electrocautery, and bipolar coagulation. Once the myoma(s) are successfully enucleated, attention is directed towards closure of the myomectomy resection bed(s). Endowrist® instruments are changed to a Debakey forcep and needle driver. A three layer closure modeled after traditional open surgical technique is utilized. Interrupted sutures of 0-Vicryl™ on CT-2 needles in addition to 3-0-Vicryl™ on a SH needle are used to complete this portion of the procedure in an intracorporeal fashion (Figure 8). Once the uterine defect(s) are repaired, a Wisap® tissue morcellator is introduced through the accessory port in order to extract the specimen(s) (Figure 9). A low pressure check is performed to ensure hemostasis. Once hemostasis is confirmed, the robot-assist device is undocked. An adhesion barrier such as SurgiWrap™ (MAST Biosurgery®, San Diego, CA) or slurry of Seprafilm™ (Genzyme Biosurgery®, Cambridge, MA) is left in the pelvis as an adhesion prophylaxis measure prior to the conclusion of the case (Figure 10).

ROBOTIC (DAVINCI) MYOMECTOMY – PRELIMINARY RESULTS

We have incorporated robotics in order to complete a myomectomy endoscopically since 2001. In the fall of 2004, our preliminary experience was published in the *Journal of Minimally Invasive Gynecology* (10). Thirty-five robot-assisted laparoscopic myomectomies were attempted in a university hospital setting. All patients desired either future fertility or uterine conservation and possessed leiomyomata thought to be a relative contraindication to removal by conventional laparoscopic techniques. In the thirty-one successfully completed robotic myomectomies, a total of 48 leiomyomas were removed. The mean weight was 223 grams (range 11-1127 grams) with the majority in the range of zero to 250 grams. The mean number of myomas removed was 1.6 (range 1-5). The mean diameter was 7.9 cm (range 3-17 cm) with the majority of myomas falling into the greater than 5 cm range. The locations of the leiomyomata were distributed in all areas of the uterus with the majority being intramural.

The ability to adequately enucleate leiomyomata and suture a uterine defect laparoscopically has always been a subject of debate and cause for concern regarding conversion rates and risk for uterine rupture. In fact, laparoscopically-assisted myomectomy has been suggested in the past with enucleation of myomas performed laparoscopically and uterine closure done through a mini-laparotomy incision (11). In our preliminary experience, we found that the ability of the Endowrist® instruments to replicate the complex motions of the surgeon's hands readily overcame the limitations of conventional laparoscopy despite the size and location of the leiomyomata. These limitations were also overcome despite the absence of tactile or haptic feedback.

Our preliminary experience noted a conversion rate of only 8.6%. In one study involving conventional laparoscopic myomectomy, with an 11.3% conversion rate, four pre-operative factors were found to be independently related to the risk of conversion to laparotomy (12). These factors were myoma size greater than or equal to 5 cm, intramural myoma, anterior location, and the pre-operative use of gonadotrophin-releasing hormone (GnRH) agonists. In comparison to the previously cited study, our conversion rate remained low despite the fact that the majority of leiomyomas were greater than 5 cm and intramural.

In the thirty-one completed cases, the mean estimated blood loss was 169 ml and median was 100 ml (range 50-1000 ml). There were no blood transfusions performed and in our series, estimated blood loss was comparable to or better than published studies. One recent series reported a post-operative blood transfusion rate of 39.2% with a conventional laparoscopic approach (13).

The mean operating time was 230.8 minutes (range 93-384 minutes). Although operative times were much longer than in most published studies of laparoscopic myomectomy, a definite trend of decreasing times in this early series was seen as experience with the robot-assisted approach grew (13-16). Finally, the overall median length of stay for all patients in our series of completed cases was one day (range 0-5 days). Today, this experience remains the only published robotic myomectomy series to date which describes not only technique but also early surgical outcomes.

ROBOTIC (DAVINCI) HYSTERECTOMY FOR BENIGN & MALIGNANT DISEASE

Approximately 600,000 hysterectomies are performed annually in the United States with the majority due to benign conditions (1,8,17). Prior to the introduction of laparoscopic-assisted vaginal hysterectomy in the late 1980s, hysterectomies were approached by either a vaginal or abdominal route (18). Since the 1990s, a definite trend toward laparoscopic hysterectomy has been seen. This trend has also affected the way that gynecologic cancers are treated. As a result, laparoscopic approaches for many gynecologic surgical procedures for cancer have been developed resulting in the reduction of post-operative morbidity and emerging evidence of outcomes that appear to match those of laparotomy (19-21).

Despite the increasing acceptance of laparoscopy for the treatment of both benign and malignant disease, hysterectomy via laparotomy remains the most common route. Two reasons often cited are the technical limitations of conventional laparoscopic instruments and the condition of the surgical field, one example being pelvic adhesions. Additionally, the surgeon's skill level and the lengthy training interval to attain laparoscopic competence have been known to affect the ability to complete a hysterectomy in a minimally invasive fashion (22). Despite these concerns, there are a growing number of investigators applying robotics as a means to complete a hysterectomy in a minimally invasive fashion while treating complex pelvic pathology.

ROBOTIC (DAVINCI) HYSTERECTOMY – TECHNIQUE

The technique at the University of Michigan Medical Center for both benign and malignant disease is very similar. All patients are placed in low dorsal lithotomy position with arms padded and tucked at their sides after general anesthesia is administered. The bladder is drained with a Foley catheter and the stomach is evacuated with a nasogastric tube. For patients with an intact uterus, a ZUMI® or RUMI® uterine manipulator is placed in conjunction with a Koh® colpotomy ring and vaginal pneumo-occluder balloon (all Cooper Surgical®, Trumbull, CT) (Figure 4). For patients with an absent uterus, a sponge stick is placed in the vagina for delineation of the vaginal cuff. Four ports are typically utilized and placed in a fashion similar to that described with a robotic myomectomy after pneumoperitoneum is obtained (Figure 5).

The patient is then placed in steep Trendelenburg and the patient-side cart is brought between the patient's legs and docked. The bedside assistant is responsible for Endowrist® instrument changes and for use of the assist port to aid in traction and exposure or removal of specimens as well as passage of suture. Typical Endowrist® instruments utilized included Cadiere® forceps, DeBakey forceps, round-tip scissors, needle driver, and monopolar electrocautery using a permanent cautery hook.

A survey of the operative field is performed and if altered surgical anatomy is encountered, attention is turned towards normalization of anatomy prior to initiation of the hysterectomy. In cases either concerning or involving a malignancy, pelvic washings are obtained prior to the onset of any operative intervention.

The approach to hysterectomy is carried out in a fashion analogous to open surgical technique. All of the procedures are consistent with either AAGL type IVE or LSH III laparoscopic hysterectomies (23). All vascular pedicles including the infundibulopelvic ligament and the uterine artery pedicles are skeletonized and subsequently suture ligated with either 0-Vicryl™ on CT-2 needles or free ties of 0-Vicryl™ prior to transection. Counter-traction is provided by the bedside assistant through the accessory port. Adequate hemostasis is obtained with the combination of suture ligation and electrocautery. In cases where a total laparoscopic hysterectomy is intended, the monopolar cautery hook is utilized to divide the cardinal and uterosacral ligament complex bilaterally. Completion of both the anterior and posterior culdotomy is facilitated by the Koh colpotomy ring while upward uterine traction is provided by the bedside assistant thereby improving visualization of the colpotomizer and displacing the ureters laterally. Pneumo-peritoneum is maintained by inflation of the vaginal pneumo-occluder balloon. Once the uterus and cervix are completely detached, the specimen with or without adnexae is delivered into the vagina. The uterine fundus is then used to maintain pneumo-peritoneum during the closure of the vaginal cuff. This is accomplished with interrupted sutures of 0-Vicryl™ on CT-2 needles in an intracorporeal fashion (Figure 11). Once the vaginal cuff is closed, the specimen is removed from the vagina and a low pressure check is performed to ensure hemostasis. Finally, the robot-assist device is undocked.

In cases where laparoscopic subtotal hysterectomy is intended, the monopolar cautery hook is used to amputate the uterine corpus below the internal os. The cervical stump is closed with interrupted sutures of 0-Vicryl™ on CT-2 needles. A tissue morcellator is used to extract the specimen through the accessory port.

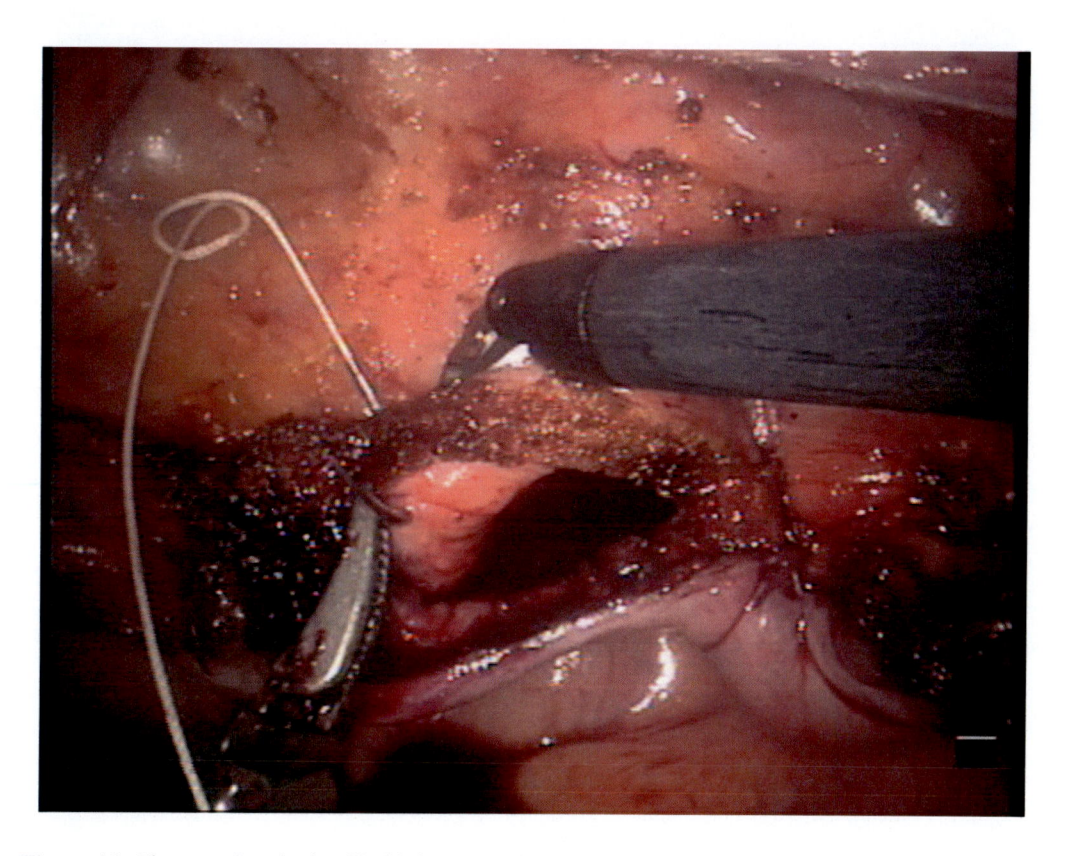

Figure 11. Closure of vaginal cuff with interrupted sutures.

During cases where an oncologic staging is required, the retroperitoneum is opened by incising lateral and parallel to the infundibulopelvic ligament extending from the pelvic brim to the round ligament. Once the pelvic vessels and ureters are identified, lymph nodes are isolated and removed by incising tissues lateral and parallel to the external iliac artery extending from the bifurcation of the common iliac artery to the crossover of the deep circumflex iliac vein over the external iliac artery. During this process, care is taken to identify the obturator nerve, which is stripped free of its attachment to the lymphatic tissues. Common iliac and para-aortic nodes up to the level of the inferior mesenteric artery are also obtained by extending the peritoneal incision above the pelvic brim and reflecting the peritoneum medially to expose the common iliac vessels in addition to incising the peritoneum over the right common iliac artery and extending along the aorta (Figure 12).

Attaining high para-aortic nodes above the inferior mesenteric artery is difficult without re-docking the patient-side cart in an over the patient's head and shoulders orientation. Alternatively, the robot can be undocked in exchange for a conventional laparoscopic approach. In cases where omentectomy is required for staging, the omentum is removed robotically after elevating the transverse colon and dividing the underlying vascular tissues.

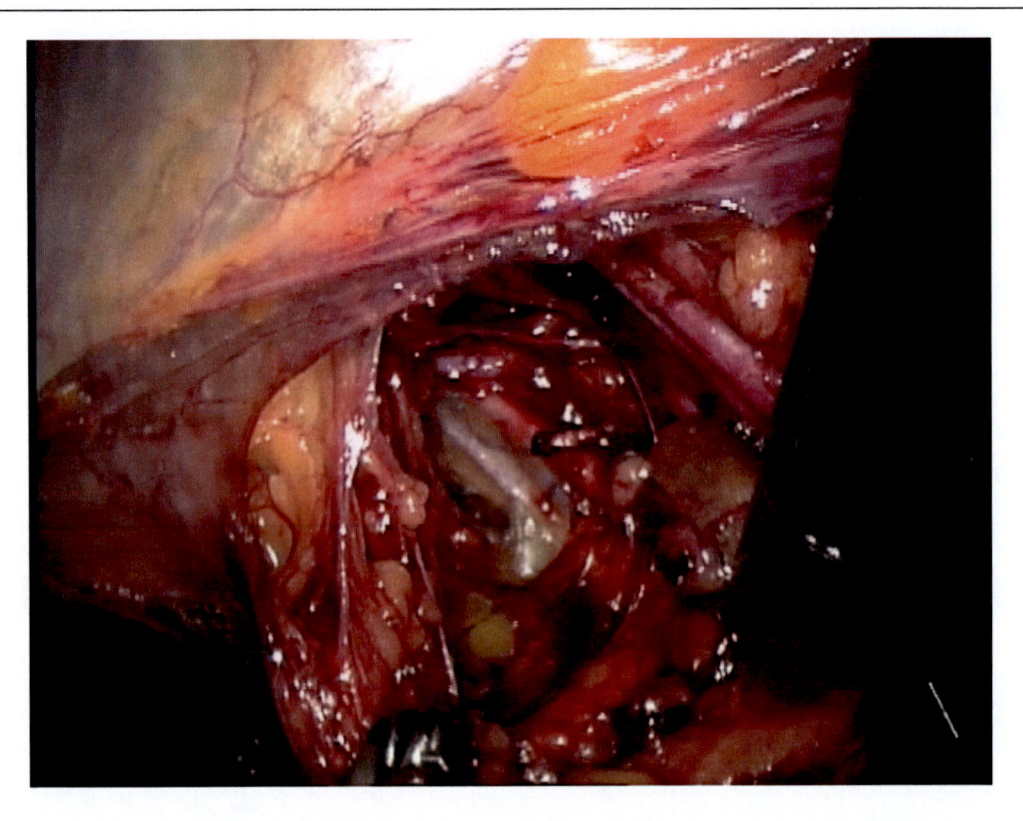

Figure 12. Lymphadenectomy along right pelvic sidewall with obturator nerve in center of photograph.

ROBOTIC HYSTERECTOMY – PRELIMINARY RESULTS

There have been several published series that describe the application of robotic technology to hysterectomy. The earliest reports were by Diaz-Arrastia et al. and Marchal et al., both of whom described the application of the daVinci® surgical system to both benign and malignant disease (24-25). In the series of eleven patients by Diaz-Arrastia et al., hysterectomies were classified as AAGL type IIB and consistent with a laparoscopically-assisted vaginal hysterectomy (23). Operative times in this series ranged from 4 1/2 hours to 10 hours with one conversion to laparotomy. In the series of thirty patients by Marchal et al. out of Europe, 23 hysterectomies were vaginally assisted and 6 were completely performed with the robot with only one conversion to laparotomy. In the 12 patients with malignant disease, a mean follow-up of ten months revealed all patients to be disease free. Operative times ranged from 43 minutes to 315 minutes. Beste et al. recently described their experience with total laparoscopic hysterectomy (AAGL type IVE) in 10 out of 11 successfully completed cases for benign uncomplicated disease (26). Operative times ranged from 148 minutes to 277 minutes.

The experience at the University of Michigan Medical Center in both benign and malignant disease has recently been published (27-28). Advincula and Reynolds looked at the feasibility of applying the robotic approach to six patients with markedly altered anatomy in the form an obliterated anterior cul de sac. They found that the improved dexterity and precision of the Endowrist® instruments readily overcame the technical limitations that typically plagued a conventional laparoscopic approach. There were no conversions to laparotomy however given the significant pelvic adhesive disease that was addressed; the mean operating time was 254 minutes.

We also reported our early experience with robot-assisted laparoscopic staging in seven patients with gynecologic malignancies. Feasibility with an adequate lymph node count (median 15) and disease free follow-up at between 4 months and 25 months was clearly demonstrated. There were no conversions to laparotomy and mean operating time was 257 minutes with an average estimated blood loss of 50 mL.

OTHER ROBOTIC APPLICATIONS IN GYNECOLOGY

Although the majority of the literature surrounding robotics in gynecology is in the area of hysterectomy, there are also reports of its use with tubal reanastomosis and sacrocolpopexy.

Both Degueldre et al. and Dharia et al. performed feasibility studies in the area of tubal reanastomosis (4, 29-30). In the first series, eight patients underwent tubal reanastomosis with the daVinci® surgical system. At four months follow-up, 5/8 patients demonstrated at least unilateral patency and 2/8 achieved a pregnancy. Dharia et al. compared 18 patients undergoing tubal reanastomosis with the daVinci® surgical system with 10 patients undergoing the procedure with traditional open surgical techniques. They found not only comparable patency and pregnancy rates of 100% and 50% respectively, but also comparable costs in a preliminary cost-effective analysis.

DiMarco et al. described the use and benefit of robotic-assisted laparoscopic sacrocolpopexy in the treatment of five patients with post-hysterectomy vaginal vault prolapse (7). The authors utilized the daVinci® surgical system's improved instrument dexterity and precision to suture the mesh to the sacral promontory. Their analysis suggested that the robotic technique may provide the same long-term durability of open sacrocolpopexy with the benefit of a minimally invasive approach. Finally, in a less common procedure, Molpus et al. described the benefits of the daVinci® surgical system in the case of an ovarian transposition in order to preserve ovarian function prior to radiotherapy for a gynecologic malignancy (5).

CONCLUSION

The use of robot-assisted technology such as the daVinci® surgical system is feasible for the treatment of both benign and malignant gynecologic pathology in an endoscopic fashion. The improved instrument precision and dexterity as well as three-dimensional imaging are able to overcome many of the limitations encountered with conventional laparoscopy. This in turn may begin to allow many of the gynecologic procedures performed by laparotomy to be completed in a minimally invasive fashion. These benefits are clearly being realized at the University of Michigan Medical Center as our experience is well over 100 cases.

The technical advantages gained with robotics may also provide a way to improve surgical training and the acquisition of advanced skills. A recent study evaluated this concept. The impact of robotics on surgical skills was assessed by comparing conventional laparoscopy with the daVinci® surgical system in the performance of four training drills. Surgeons completed drills faster with the robotic system. Most importantly, the study found that the playing field between novice and expert surgeons was leveled with use of the robotic system (31).

Although the daVinci surgical system provides advanced instrumentation and imaging, the absence of tactile feedback and longer operative times remain limitations. Costs may also be prohibitive as each daVinci® surgical system retails for over $1,000,000. Additional costs also exist in terms of the Endowrist® instruments and drapes. Currently, the robot-assisted approach may not offer a distinct advantage when it comes to operative time or costs however as with any new technology, cost is likely to decrease over time. Preliminary cost-effective analyses do suggest comparable costs per delivery when the robotic approach is compared to conventional laparoscopic or open surgical techniques (27, 30). This review of the current literature also indicates that with increasing experience, operative time becomes progressively shorter. Overall, evolving robotic technology may further improve patient outcomes while presenting new options for the minimally invasive management of gynecologic pathology in the future. One caution to make is that although technical advancements in surgery have brought us these endoscopic improvements, proper studies must be conducted in order to determine the exact role of robotic technology in the practice of minimally invasive gynecologic surgery.

REFERENCES

1. Farquhar CM, Steiner CA. Hysterectomy rates in the United States 1990-1997. *Obstetrics & Gynecology* 2002; 99:229-234.

2. Mettler L, Ibrahim M, Jonat W. One year of experience working with the aid of a robotic assistant (the voice-controlled optic holder AESOP) in gynecologic endoscopic surgery. *Human Reproduction* 1998; Oct, 13 (10): 2748-2750.

3. Falcone T, Goldberg JM, Margossian H, Stevens L. Robotically assisted laparoscopic microsurgical tubal anastomosis: a human pilot study. *Fertility and Sterility* 2000; 73 (5):1040-1042.

4. Degueldre M, Vandromme J, Huong PT, Cadiere GB. Robotically-assisted laparoscopic microsurgical tubal reanastomosis: a feasibility study. *Fertility and Sterility* 2000; 74 (5): 1020-1023.

5. Molpus KL, Wedergren JS, Carlson MA. Robotically assisted endoscopic ovarian transposition. *Journal of the Society of Laparoendoscopic Surgeons* 2003; 7: 59-62.

6. Diaz-Arrastia C, Jurnalov C, Gomez G, Townsend C Jr. Laparoscopic hysterectomy using a computer-enhanced surgical robot. *Surgical Endoscopy* 2002; 16: 1271-1273.

7. Dimarco DS, Chow GK, Gettman MT, Elliott DS. Robotic-assisted laparoscopic sacrocolpopexy for treatment of vaginal vault prolapse. *Urology* 2004; 63 (2):373-376.

8. Wilcox LS, Koonin LM, Pokras R, Strauss LT, Xia Z, Peterson HB. Hysterectomy in the United States, 1988-1990. *Obstetrics & Gynecology* 1994;83 (4):549-555.

9. Falcone T, Bedaiwy MA. Minimally invasive management of uterine fibroids. *Current Opinion in Obstetrics and Gynecology* 2002;14 (4):401-407.

10. Advincula AP, Song A, Burke W, Reynolds RK. Preliminary experience with robot-assisted laparoscopic myomectomy. *Journal of the American Association Gynecologic Laparoscopists* 2004 Nov;11(4):511-518.

11. Nezhat C, Nezhat F, Bess O, Nezhat, CH, Mashiach R. Laparoscopically assisted myomectomy: a report of a new technique in 57 cases. *International Journal Fertility and Menopausal Studies* 1994 Jan-Feb; 39(1): 39-44.

12. Dubuisson JB, Fauconnier A, Fourchotte V, Babaki-Fard K, Coste J, Chapron C. Laparoscopic myomectomy: predicting the risk of conversion to an open procedure. *Human Reproduction* 2001 Aug; 16(8):1726-1731.

13. Sinha R, Hegde A, Warty N, Patil N. Laparoscopic excision of very large myomas. *Journal American Association Gynecologic Laparoscopists* 2003, 10(4):461-468.

14. Takeuchi H, Kuwatsuru R. The indications, surgical techniques, and limitations of laparoscopic myomectomy. *Journal of the Society of Laparoendoscopic Surgeons* 2003 Apr-Jun; 7(2):89-95.

15. Darai E, Dechaud H, Benifla JL, Renolleau C, Panel P, Madelanat P. Fertility after laparoscopic myomectomy: preliminary results. *Human Reproduction* 1997 Sep 12(9): 1931-1934.

16. Seinera P, Arisio R, Decko A, Farina C, Crana F. Laparoscopic myomectomy: indications, surgical technique and complications. *Human Reproduction* 1997 12(9):1927-1930.

17. Lepine LA, Hillis SD, Marchbanks PA, Koonin LM, Morrow B, Kieke BA, Wilcox LS. Hysterectomy surveillance – United States, 1980-1993. *Morbidity and Morgality Weekly Report. CDC surveillance summaries* 1997 Aug 8; 46(4):1-15.

18. Reich H, Decaprio J, McGlynn F. Laparoscopic hysterectomy. *Journal Gynecological Surgery* 1989; 5: 213-216.

19. Reynolds RK, Burke WM. The evolving role of laparoscopic surgery for treatment of gynecologic masses and cancers. *The Female Patient* 2004; 29 (4): 25-32.

20. Eltabbakh GH, Shamonki MI, Moody JM, Garafano LL. Laparoscopy as the primary modality for the treatment of women with endometrial carcinoma. *Cancer*. 2001 Jan 15;91(2):378-87..

21. Querleu D, Papageorgiou T, Lambaudie E, Sonoda Y, Narducci F, Leblanc E. Laparoscopic restaging of borderline ovarian tumors: Results of 30 cases initially presumed as stage IA borderline ovarian tumor. *BJOG: an international journal of obstetrics and gynecology* 2003 Feb, 110(2): 201-4.

22. Wattiez A, Cohen SB, Selvaggi L. Laparoscopic hysterectomy. *Current Opinion in Obstetrics and Gynecology* 2002 Aug; 14(4): 417-22. Review.

23. Olive DL, Parker WH, Cooper JM, Levine RL. The AAGL classification system for laparoscopic hysterectomy. Classification committee of the American Association of Gynecologic Laparoscopists. *Journal of the American Association of Gynecologic Laparoscopists* 2000 Feb; 7(1): 9-15.

24. Diaz-Arrastia C, Jurnalov C, Gomez G, Townsend C Jr. Laparoscopic hysterectomy using a computer-enhanced surgical robot. *Surgical Endoscopy* 2002 Sep;16(9):1271-3. Epub 2002 Jun 27.

25. Marchal F, Rauch P, Vandromme J, Laurent I, Lobontiu A, Ahcel B, Verhaeghe JL, Meistleman C, Degueldre M, Villemot, Guillemin F. Telerobotic-assisted laparoscopic hysterectomy for benign and oncologic pathologies: initial clinical experience with 30 patients. *Surgical Endoscopy* 2005, May 3 [Epub ahead of print].

26. Beste TM, Nelson KH, Daucher JA. Total laparoscopic hysterectomy utilizing a robotic surgical system. *Journal of the Society of Laparoendoscopic Surgeons/Society of Laparoendoscopic Surgeons* 2005 Jan-Mar; 9(1):13-15.

27. Reynolds RK, Burke WM, Advincula AP. Preliminary experience with robot-assisted laparoscopic staging of gynecologic malignancies. *Journal of the Society of Laparoendoscopic Surgeons/Society of Laparoendoscopic Surgeons* 2005; 9(2):149-158.

28. Advincula AP, Reynolds RK. The Use of robot-assisted laparoscopic hysterectomy in the patient with a scarred or obliterated anterior cul de sac. *Journal of the Society of Laparoendoscopic Surgeons/Society of Laparoendoscopic Surgeons* 2005; 9(3):287-291.

29. Dharia SP, Steinkampf MP, Whitten SJ, Malizia BA. Robotic assisted tubal reanastomosis in a fellowship training program [abstract]. ESHRE Annual Meeting; Berlin, Germany, June 2004.

30. Dharia SP, Steinkampf MP, Whitten SJ, Malizia BA. Robotically assisted tubal sterilization reversal: surgical technique and cost-effectiveness versus conventional surgery [abstract]. American Society for Reproductive Medicine Annual Meeting; Philadelphia, PA, October 2004.

31. Sarle R, Tewari A, Shrivastava A, Peabody J, Menon M. Surgical robotics and laparoscopic training drills. *Journal Endourology* 2004 Feb; 18(1): 63-67.

Chapter 13

APPLICATIONS IN OTOLARYNGOLOGY-HEAD AND NECK SURGERY

David M. Walters and David J. Terris
Department of Otolaryngology-Head and Neck Surgery
Medical College of Georgia, Augusta, GA, USA

Abstract

Beginning with the introduction of the first endoscopic procedures in the 1980's, the field of minimally invasive surgery has progressed beyond the use of endoscopes and laparoscopic instruments to include both passive and active robot-assisted surgery as well as transcontinental telesurgery. The integration of minimally invasive techniques in Otolaryngology-Head and Neck Surgery has advanced steadily despite the anatomic and spatial constraints often encountered within the head and neck. The current and future benefits associated with minimally invasive robotic surgery will be weighed against the substantial costs incurred to provide access to these new frontiers in surgery. Future breakthroughs in otolaryngologic surgery will inevitably include minimally invasive approaches to common pathologic problems in the head and neck. If the recent past is any predictor of the future, robots will assume an increasingly prominent role in the operating theater leading to increased patient safety and satisfaction.

INTRODUCTION

Twenty-first century otolaryngologists continue to embrace and perform historically proven, maximal-access surgical interventions demonstrated to be effective through years of professional collaboration, data collection and analysis. This paradigm is shifting as minimally invasive approaches to the head and neck become increasingly popular and in some cases preferred in appropriately selected patients. Minimally invasive surgery traces its origin back to the development and application of the endoscope. The concept of endoscopic technology dates back as early as 1805 when the "curiosity" of Philip Bozzini motivated him to develop the "Lichtleiter" for which he was sternly criticized by the medical faculty of Vienna (**Figure 1**). His innovation would later be recognized with the publication of work by the father of the cystoscope, Maximilian Nitze, in 1876.[1] The incremental application of endoscopic technology in medicine ultimately produced the nidus for modern minimally invasive surgery on March 17, 1987 when Philippe Mouret performed the first laparoscopic cholecystectomy in Lyon, France.[2]

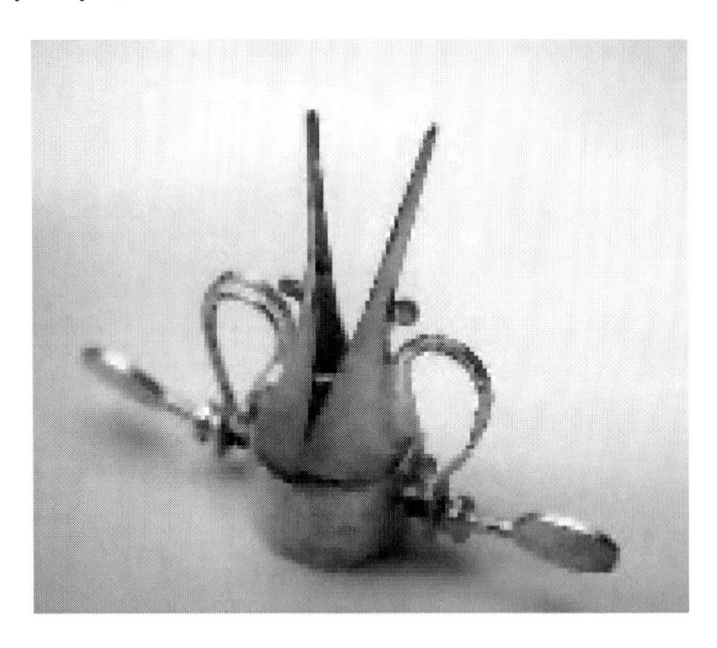

Figure 1. Philip Bozzini's Lichtleiter developed in 1805.

The clinical benefits of minimally invasive procedures include the use of smaller incisions leading to decreased and less visible scarring, diminished blood loss and an overall reduction in postoperative morbidity and mortality. These improvements in patient outcome are achieved without substantially increasing perioperative risk or compromising traditional surgical objectives. The growing popularity of minimally invasive surgical techniques is a catalyst for research into the applications of robotic technology within the surgical profession.

The National Aeronautics and Space Administration (NASA) began investigating the use of surgeon-controlled robotic handpieces as part of their virtual reality technology in the 1980's.[3] SRI International (Menlo Park, CA) using funding from the National Institutes of Health (NIH) developed a prototype system that caught the attention of the Defense Advanced Research Projects Administration (DARPA). DARPA quickly realized the potential of this technology to provide early access to life-saving surgical care for injured soldiers on the battlefield until they could be evacuated to a military hospital. The military surgeons, operating from a distant location utilizing a remote manipulation robot, would have minimal exposure to the dangers present on the frontlines. Ironically, the greatest advances in the application of robotic surgery are a result of commercial growth and development. The medical applications of robots represent a logical progression in the continued evolution of minimally invasive surgery.[4] Throughout this chapter, the history and taxonomy of robotic surgery will be integrated into a discussion of the current applications of robotics in the field of Otolaryngology-Head and Neck Surgery including current advances in endoscopic and minimally invasive surgery involving the head and neck.

TAXONOMY

Classification of function is required to understand the various roles that robots assume within the operating theater. Historically, surgical robots have been classified as active, semiactive or passive based on the actions performed during a procedure. Additional published classifications include technology-based (autonomous vs. teleoperated) and application-based (cardiology vs. urology); however, the role-based classification broadly communicates to both developer and end-user the anticipated level of robot participation. Camarillo et al.[5] define a procedural role-based taxonomy according to the following 3 distinct categories:

1. Passive: robot participation is limited in scope or involvement and is low risk.
2. Restricted: robot responsible for more invasive tasks and assumes higher risk, but remains restricted from certain portions of the procedure.
3. Active: robot intimately involved in the procedure and incurring high risk and responsibility.

The authors compare these classifications to the progression of a surgeon's career through medical school, residency and eventually independent clinical practice.[5] The Food and Drug Administration (FDA) has not yet approved any active-role robots for use in the United States. Passive and restricted-role robots have received FDA approval in minimally invasive cardiac and gastrointestinal surgery.

Telerobotic surgery connotes surgical robotic technology that allows the surgeon to utilize a remote console within the operating theater which projects a virtual 3-dimensional image of the operative field to perform a surgical procedure with robotically-controlled instrumentation. Telepresence surgery implies an expansion of telerobotics that allows a surgeon at remote location to receive virtual images and manipulate a telerobot to perform an operation without ever physically encountering the patient.[6] For example, transatlantic telepresence laparoscopic cholecystectomy was performed successfully in both a porcine model and a human subject by Marescaux, et al.[7] The surgeon was located in New York (USA) and the 68 year old female patient was in Strasbourg, France. Telementoring is a natural extension of telepresence surgery which allows new surgical techniques to be demonstrated by renowned surgeons to nearly any remote location in the world.

The opportunities to apply robotic surgical techniques within Otolaryngology-Head and Neck Surgery are widespread. Clinical and laboratory research experiences utilizing porcine, canine, cadaveric and human models are appearing frequently in the otolaryngology literature. The future of robotic surgery within the head and neck is best understood by examining the previously published experiences within general head and neck surgery as well as the associated subspecialties.

GENERAL OTOLARYNGOLOGY

The greatest potential application of minimally invasive techniques such as endoscopic and robot-assisted surgery probably exists within the practice of general Otolaryngology-Head and Neck Surgery. The spectrum of possible procedures includes excision of benign and malignant lesions of the oral cavity and oropharynx, as well as treatment of thyroid, parathyroid, salivary gland and lymph node pathology within the neck. Both endoscopic and robotic procedures have progressed as a result of the pioneering work in endoscopic neck surgery that has been published since the mid-1990's. Development of endoscopic neck techniques was necessary to facilitate the transition to robot-assisted, minimally invasive procedures.

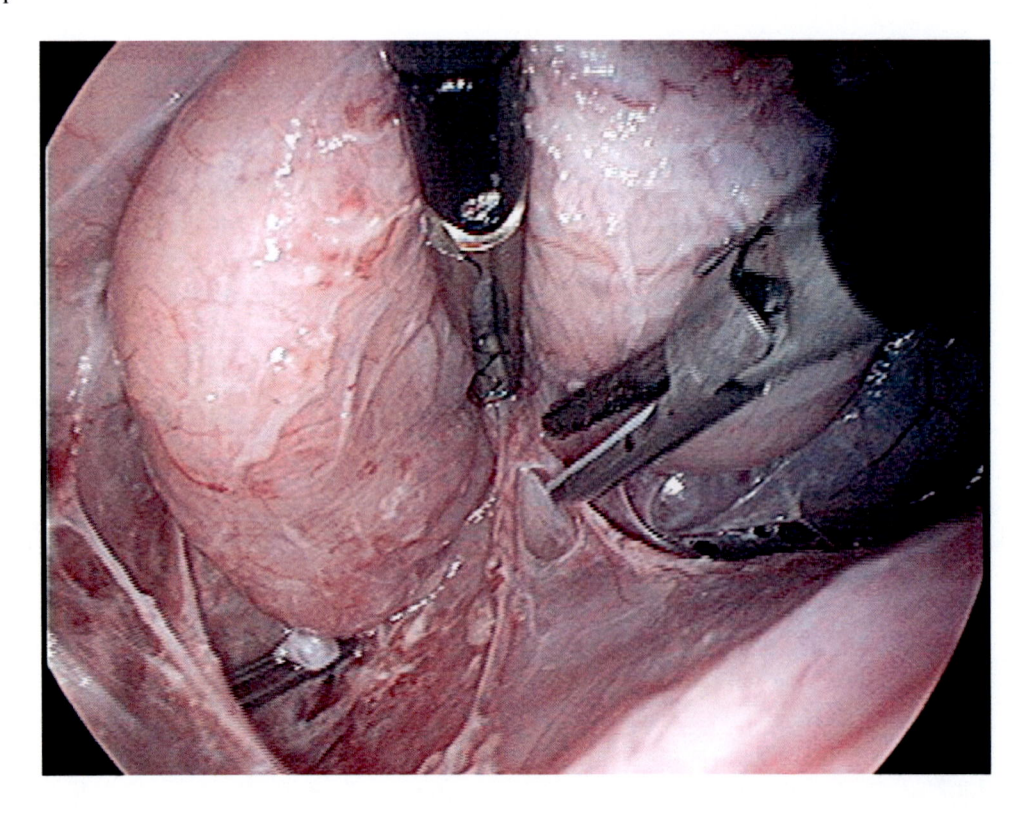

Figure 2: Endoscopic view of porcine submandibular gland (SG) with arrow pointing to the ligated proximal facial artery. (Reprinted with permission from: Monfared A, Saenz Y, Terris DJ. Endoscopic resection of the submandibular gland in a porcine model. *Laryngoscope* 2002, 112:1089-1093).

The first endoscopic neck surgery in humans was a parathyroidectomy reported by Gagner in 1996.[8] Miccoli and colleagues[9] contributed heavily to the development of endoscopic approaches to the parathyroid and published their experience two years later. During the late 1990's, several investigators reported their experience with the logical progression to endoscopic surgery of the thyroid.[10-13] Carreno et al.[14] was the first to attempt upper cervical neck exploration via an endoscopic approach. They experienced a number of major complications including subcutaneous emphysema, carbon dioxide (CO_2) embolism, pneumothorax and a discouraging 40% mortality rate. Dulguerov's group reported improved outcomes in both animal and cadaver models utilizing a combination of CO2 insufflation and hernia balloon dissection.[15-16] In 2000, Ikeda and Takami described an axillary approach to the thyroid and three years later published their experience with 58 patients who underwent axillary or anterior chest approaches for endoscopic thyroidectomy.[17-18] Building on the efforts of their predecessors, Terris et al.[19] published the successful endoscopic resection of 12 submandibular glands in a porcine model with low CO2 insufflation pressures and none of the previously published pitfalls or complications (**Figure 2**). The Terris group subsequently reported 14 successful endoscopic neck dissections in a porcine model.[20] The sternomastoid muscle, thymus, submandibular gland, lymph nodes and fibrofatty tissue were removed with no major complications and no conversions to open neck dissection (**Figure 3**). Application of their endoscopic model was extended to the thyroid compartment, in which they systematically evaluated five distinct anatomic approaches. Precordial, superior, axillary, lateral axillary, and superficial axillary approaches were evaluated to determine if one was superior to the others. After analyzing for estimated blood loss, operative time, and changes in blood pressure and pH the superior approach was found to be the fastest, but the axillary approaches offered improved cosmesis. Of the three axillary approaches evaluated, the superficial axillary approach provided the best overall template for modeling access to the thyroid compartment in humans.[21]

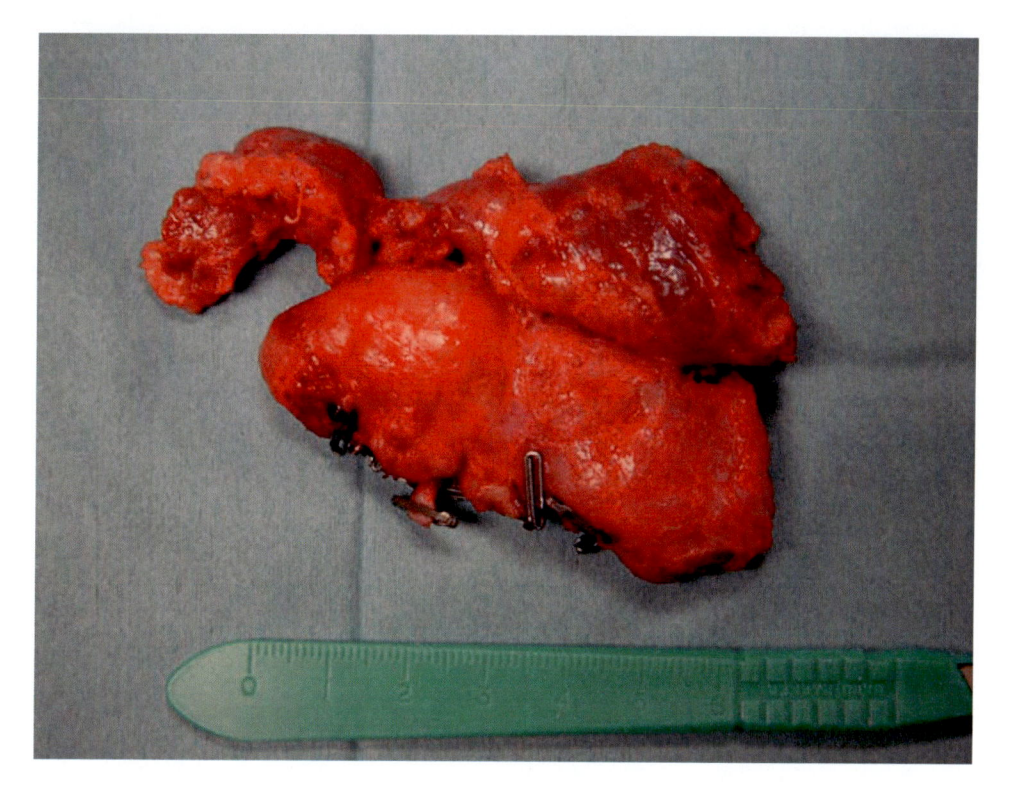

Figure 3. Endoscopic selective neck dissection specimen showing en bloc excision of lymph nodes (LN), submandibular gland (G), sternomastoid muscle (SM) and thymus (T). (Reprinted with permission from: Terris DJ, Monfared A, Thomas A, Kambham N, Saenz Y. Endoscopic selective neck dissection in a porcine model. *Arch Otolaryngol Head Neck Surg* 2003, 129:613-617).

Following the success of endoscopic neck surgery in the porcine model, Terris and colleagues[22] examined the feasibility of totally endoscopic excision of the submandibular gland in a cadaver model. Eight consecutive submandibular excisions were performed endoscopically on 6 cadavers. There were no conversions to an open approach and no postoperative evidence of any neural or vascular injuries. Additionally, histologic examination of the specimens revealed no evidence of excessive trauma or thermal injury. The operative pocket was created and maintained with a hernia balloon and low pressure (only 4 mmHg) CO2 insufflation. Prospective unpublished data collected from ongoing clinical trials currently underway at the Medical College of Georgia further confirms that endoscopic approaches to the neck are both safe and feasible. The complication rate is low and the cosmetic result is superior to conventional open surgical techniques (**Figure 4**). All currently published data suggests that endoscopic neck surgery is a safe and feasible minimally invasive approach in properly selected patients. Further studies remain necessary to define the appropriate scope of practice for endoscopic procedures of the head and neck.

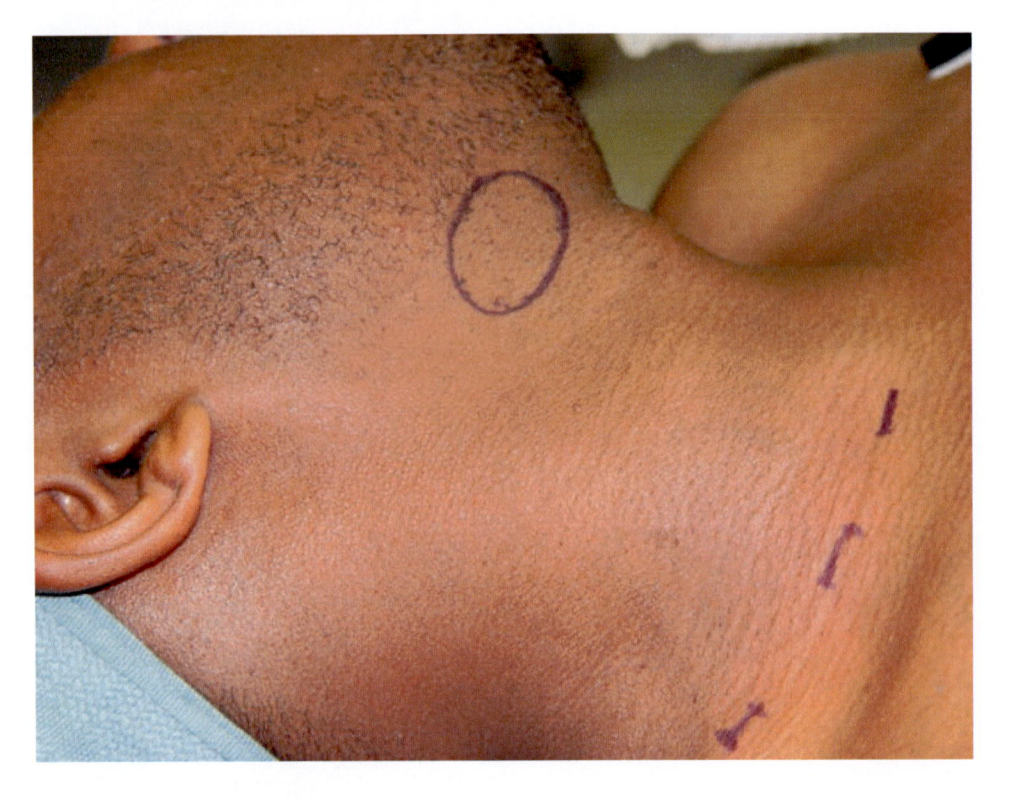

Figure 4: Preoperative photograph marking the location of the submandibular gland to be resected and the planned camera port and trocar incisions.

The application of the master-slave daVinci Robotic System to general otolaryngology procedures was a natural extension of these endoscopic techniques. Terris' group was the first to report the use of the daVinci Robotic System for head and neck procedures.[23] They utilized a porcine model to perform several procedures (partial parotidectomy, thymectomy, submandibular gland resection, selective neck dissection) to demonstrate that endo-robotic neck surgery is a safe and efficient alternative to the previously described endoscopic neck techniques (**Figure 5 a-c**). The advantages over endoscopic surgery include enhanced surgical dexterity and precision, improved ease of surgery, three-dimensional visualization and decreased surgical time (**Figure 6 a-b**). Limitations included occasional instrument interference between surgical arms and decreased haptics or tactile feedback. Their subsequent work in cadaver models[23] confirmed that the approach could be applied in the human (**Figure 7**). A series of submandibular glands were removed with an overall surgical time (including time for robotic assembly) that was shorter than with conventional endoscopic resection (**Figure 8 a-b**). Melder et al. subsequently reported four robot-assisted total thyroidectomies in human patients during their presentation at the American Academy of Otolaryngology- Head and Neck Surgery Annual Meeting in San Diego, California in September 2002. This experience remains unpublished.

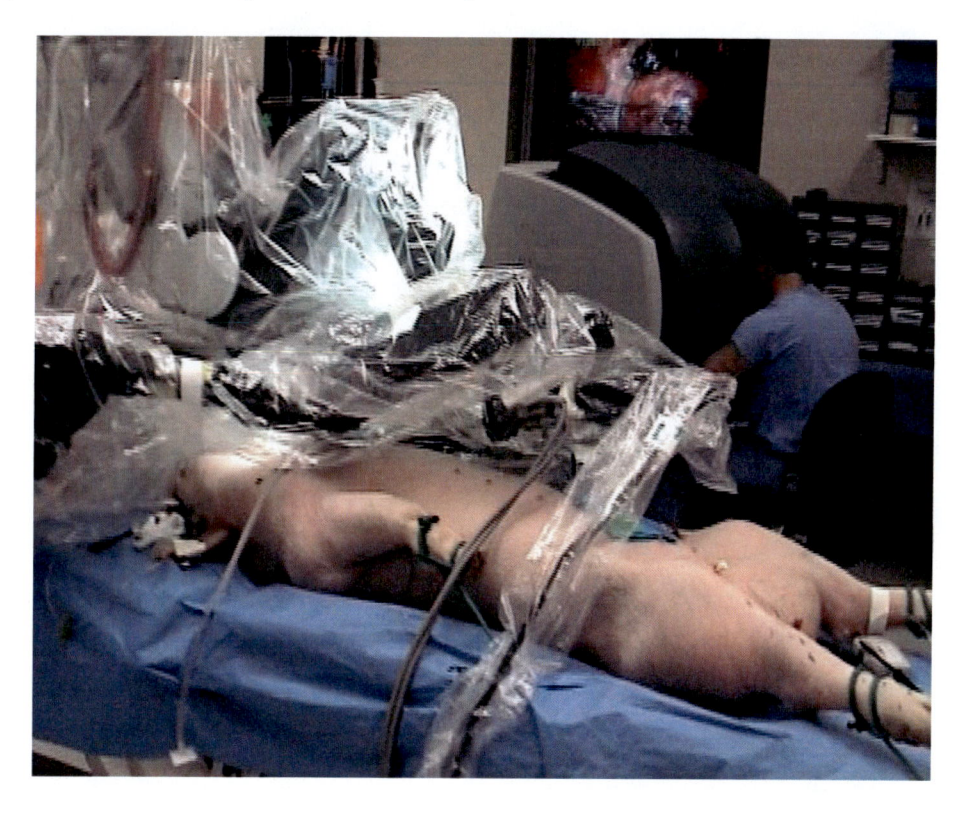

Figure 5a. Setup access for head and neck procedures in the porcine model with the daVinci Robotic System in the foreground and the surgeon console with three-dimensional imaging and operative controls visible in the background.

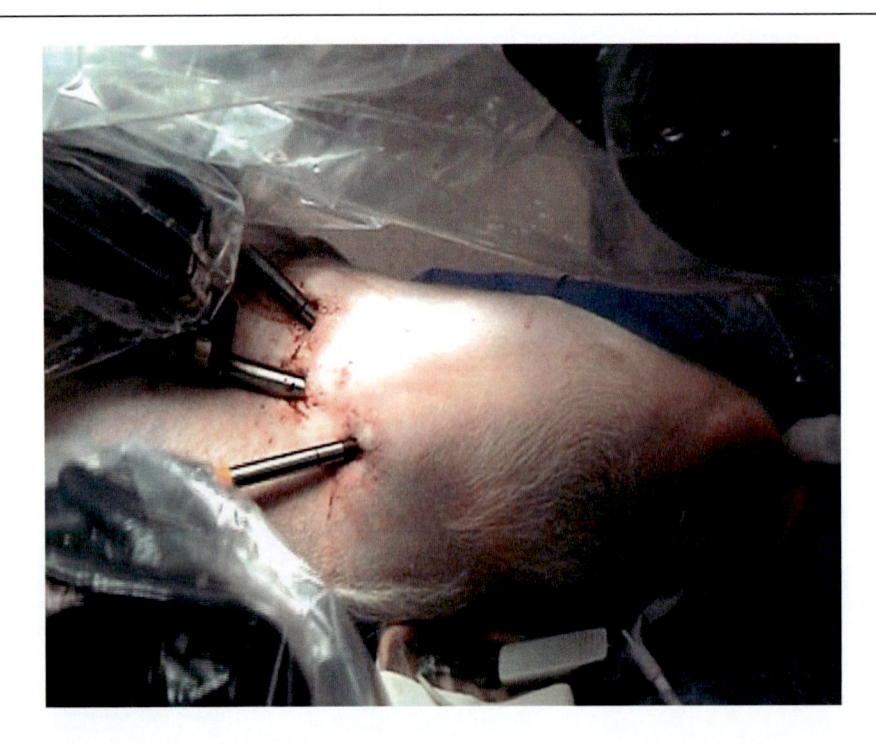

Figure 5 b. External view of the all three trocars in place through cosmetically favorable low anterior neck incisions.

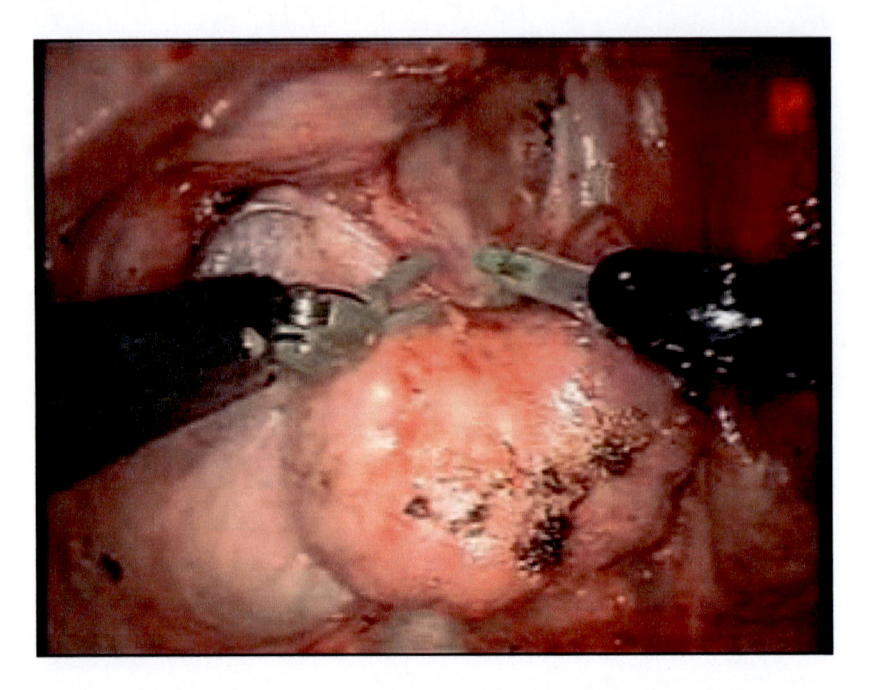

Figure 5c. Endoscopic view of the operative pocket created by inflation of hernia balloon and maintained by low pressure (4 mm Hg) CO_2 insufflation. The submandibular gland is retracted with endoscopic graspers and dissection is accomplished utilizing monopolar electrocautery. (Reprinted with permission from: Haus BM, Kambham N, Le D, Moll FM, Gourin C, Terris DJ. Surgical robotic applications in otolaryngology. *Laryngoscope* 2003, 113:1139-1144).

Applications in Otolaryngology-Head and Neck Surgery 231

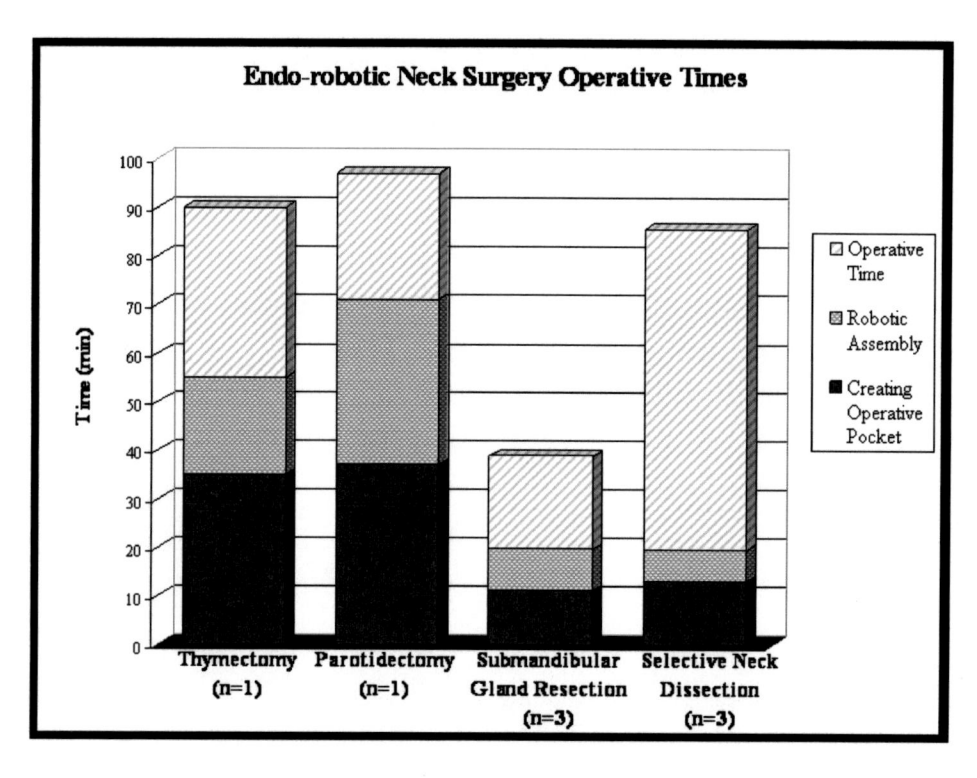

Figure 6a. Bar graph depicting the amount of time required for creation of an operative pocket, robot assembly and actual operative time for each endo-robotic neck procedure.

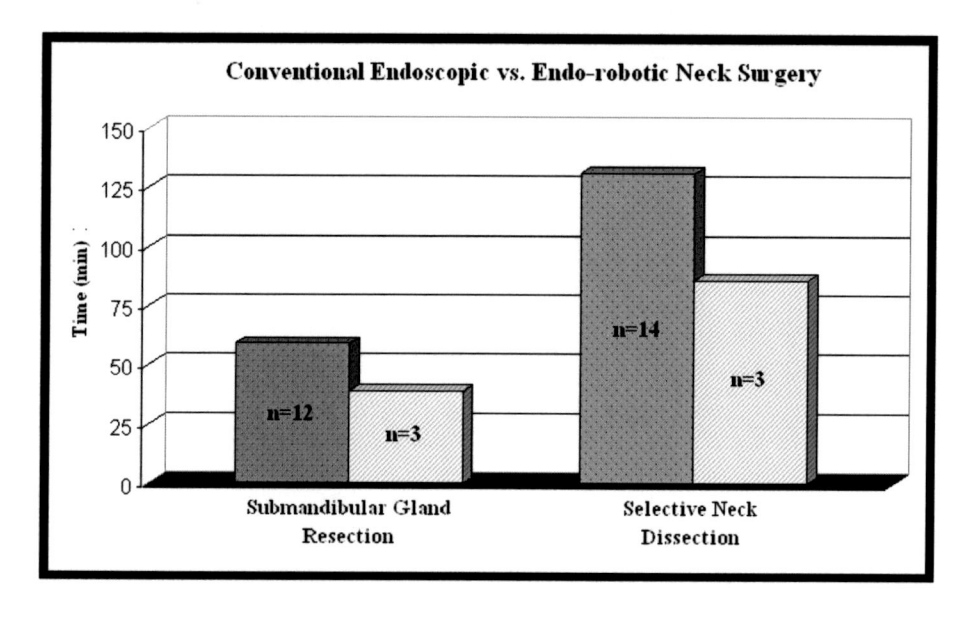

Figure 6b. Bar graph comparing operative times between conventional endoscopic and endo-robotic submandibular gland excision and selective neck dissection. This data suggests that endo-robotic surgery is more efficient than conventional endoscopic techniques. (Reprinted with permission from: Haus BM, Kambham N, Le D, Moll FM, Gourin C, Terris DJ. Surgical robotic applications in otolaryngology. *Laryngoscope* 2003, 113:1139-1144).

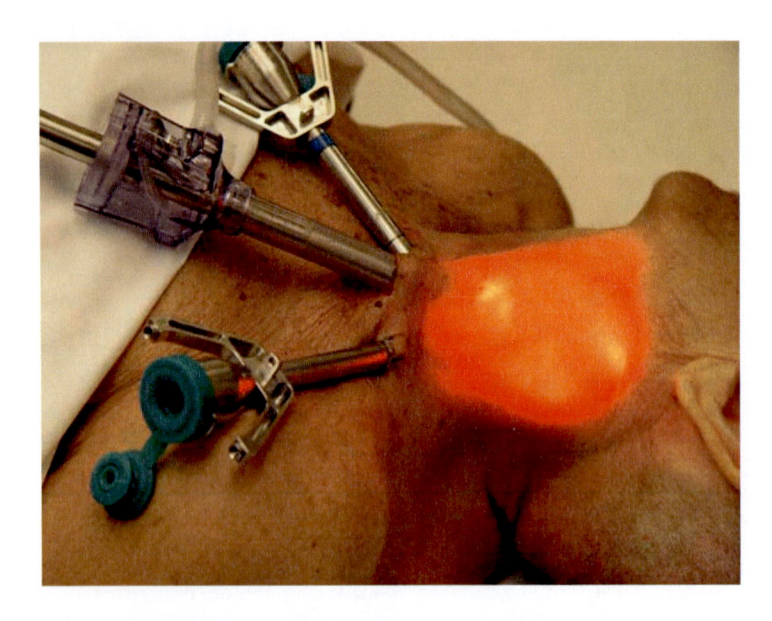

Figure 7: External view of the ideal placement of all three robotic trocars. Operative instruments are inserted through 7-mm trocars while the laparoscope passes through the 12-mm trocar. The optimal placement of the central trocar is over the clavicular head of the sternocleidomastoid muscle. [Reprinted with permission from: Terris DJ, Haus BM, Gourin CG, Lilagan PE. Endo-robotic resection of the submandibular gland in a cadaver model. *Head Neck* (In press)].

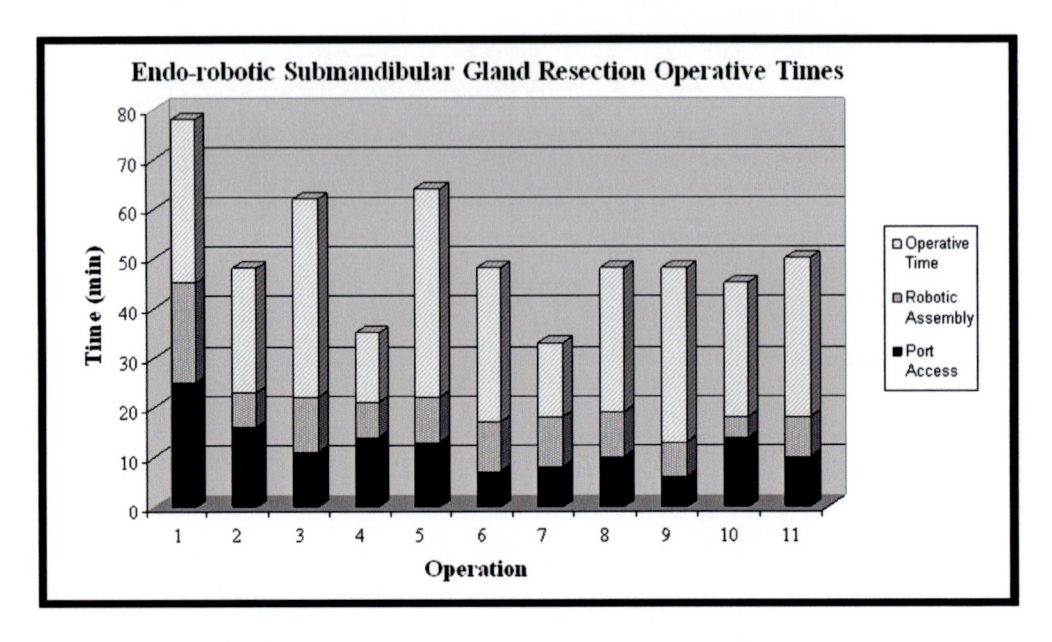

Figure 8a. Bar graph depicting the operative times of a series of endo-robotic submandibular gland excisions in a cadaveric model. Times are separated into port access, robotic assembly and operative time.

Applications in Otolaryngology-Head and Neck Surgery 233

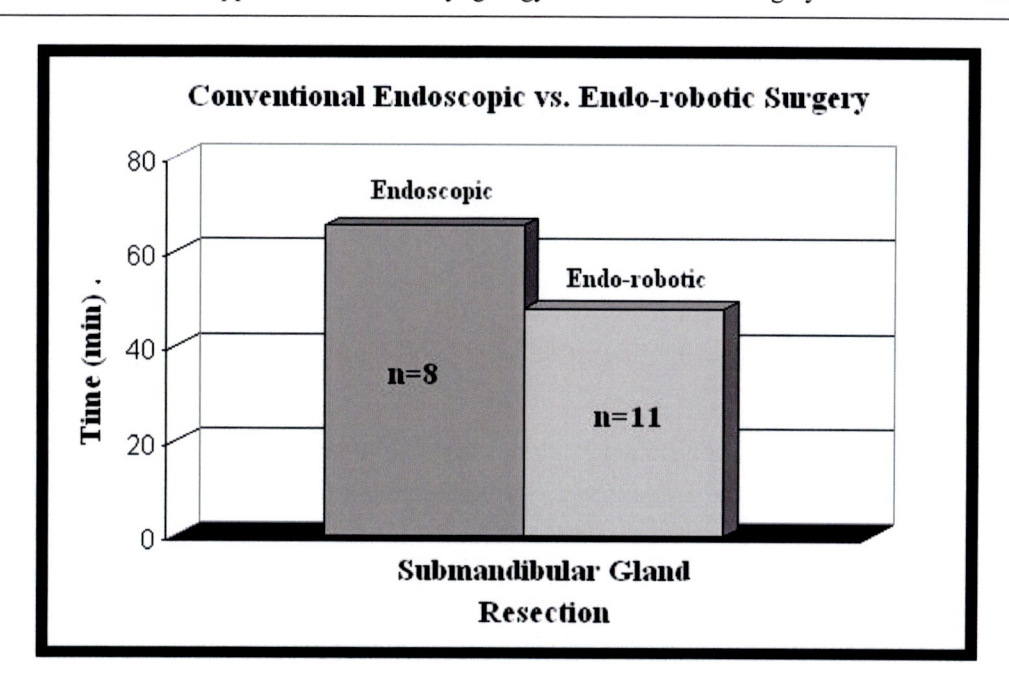

Figure 8b. Bar graph comparing operative times for conventional endoscopic versus endo-robotic submandibular gland excision indicating decreased time required for the end-robotic approach. [Reprinted with permission from: Terris DJ, Haus BM, Gourin CG, Lilagan PE. Endo-robotic resection of the submandibular gland in a cadaver model. *Head Neck* (In press)].

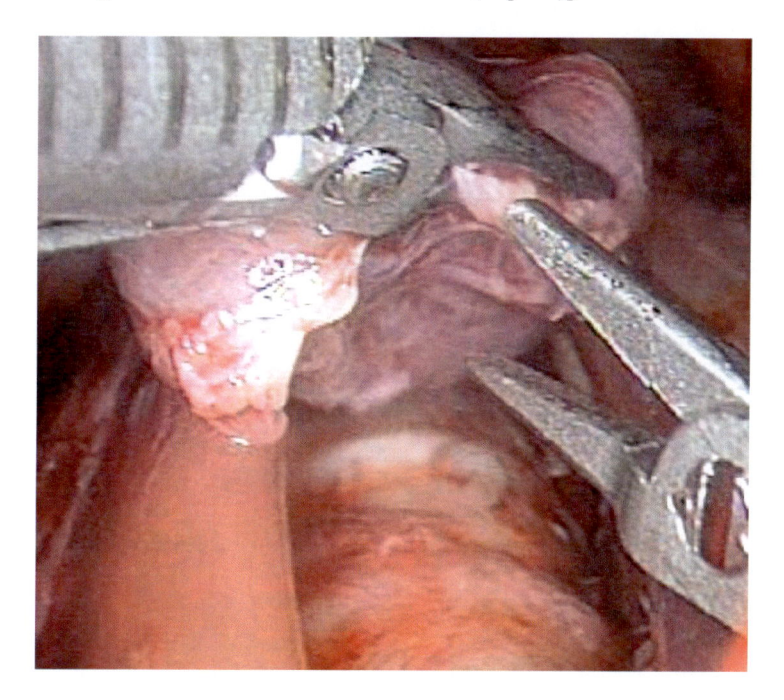

Figure 9. Endoscopic view of operative pocket in 4.2 kg piglet with thyroid specimen dissected free and ready for removal. (Printed with permission from Russell Faust).

Faust et al. combined the principles from the endoscopic thyroidectomy[21] with the previously described implementation of robotic technology[23-24] to accomplish robot-assisted thyroidectomy in an infant porcine neck model, which represents the approximate size of a human infant neck. Faust's group reports an effective surgical workspace between 2 to 4 cubic centimeters which necessitates the use of smaller dissection balloons and 3 to 5 mm instrumentation. (**Figure 9**) This experience is not yet published and was obtained through personal correspondence with permission to be included in this text. McLeod and Melder[25] published the successful excision of a vallecula cyst utilizing the daVinci Robotic System. The limited space within the oral cavity required a human surgical assistant to provide suction and tissue counter-traction. While total reported operative time was 109 minutes, approximately 75 minutes was dedicated to setting up the daVinci system. The procedure was completed without complication and the patient was discharged home the same day.

Although the volume of publications detailing robot-assisted head and neck surgery is limited, the data that has been published offers promising results. A critical determinant of the successes in robot-assisted surgery to date is appropriate patient selection. As surgeons' experience increases, the opportunity to "push the envelope" with more challenging cases will undoubtedly stretch the limits of robot-assisted surgery to new frontiers.

OTOLOGY

Otologic procedures were among the earliest applications of robotic surgery within Otolaryngology-Head and Neck Surgery. The experimental designs within otology focus primarily on improving the performance of delicate, drill-oriented procedures by overcoming limitations of human dexterity and tactile responsiveness. These goals are achieved by utilizing computer sampling and robotic systems to mitigate human inconsistency resulting from tremor, jerking and drifting or overshooting.[26] Rothbaum et al.[27] designed a surgical model to evaluate the accuracy of stapedotomy fenestration performed with the Steady Hand (SH) robotic system on an artificial foam stapes footplate. The SH robot is co-manipulated by the surgeon to assist with the performance of a stapedotomy fenestration. The force applied to the stapes footplate was reduced nearly 58% with robot assistance in force feedback mode and 30% in force scaling mode with no significant differences occurring between junior and senior surgeons. Interestingly, SH robot assistance helped junior surgeons with fenestration targeting while senior surgeons experienced an 80% increase in fenestration displacement with robot assistance. While this study suggests that robot assistance may improve the accuracy of stapes fenestration by less experienced surgeons and reduce the amount of force applied to the stapes bone by all surgeons, the clinical application of this procedure remains limited by ergonomic challenges such as line-of-sight obstruction and modified angle of approach to the stapes footplate.

Federspil et al.[28] describe the first force-controlled milling of the temporal bone to create cavities for implantable hearing aids. The RX-130 robot with serial kinematics and 6 degrees of freedom was computer controlled and programmed to mill an implant bed within cadaveric temporal bones with instructions to abort its action if forces greater than 40 Newton were encountered. During the milling process, the cutting burr was observed moving along the dura without inducing any damage. The successful force-based control almost mimics the adjustments that are made when this type of procedure is performed by human hands. The high degree of precision achieved by the robot during this experiment is encouraging for the future of robot-assisted otologic surgery. Future applications may include ultrasound-based sensors to guide local anatomic navigation and ultimately robot-assisted mastoidectomy.

RHINOLOGY

A strong case can be made that no subspecialty within Otolaryngology-Head and Neck Surgery has benefited more from the advent and proliferation of endoscopy than the field of rhinology. In addition to traditional handheld physician-directed endoscopy, robotic technology has been adapted to control endoscopes intraoperatively potentially replacing the need for a surgical assistant. As early as 1990, May et al.[29] published on the use of a "surgical assistant" to stabilize the endoscope during endoscopic sinus surgery thereby allowing the surgeon to use both hands to operate. In 1994, the automated endoscopic system for optimal positioning (AESOP; Computer Motion, Inc., Goleta, CA, USA) became the first robotic system to receive FDA approval for clinical use in humans. AESOP consists of a robotic arm designed to stabilize and control the movement of a surgical endoscope. Movement of AESOP is controlled by hand, foot or voice–activated controls allowing the operating surgeon to operate without restriction utilizing both hands.[6] In 2000, Obando et al.[30] reported the use of AESOP with voice recognition and a pediatric Foley catheter to create a closed circuit for optimal visualization during five cases of endoscopic sinus surgery. Continuing the use of AESOP with voice recognition Obando's group reported on the use of this robotic arm in performing 7 transnasal endoscopic hypophysectomies with their neurosurgical colleagues.[31]

Based on these operative experiences, the proposed benefits of AESOP include precise, steady scope movement, tremor reduction, advantages of a "third hand", decreased risk of aspiration, maintenance of clean endoscope lens, reduced need for nasal packing post operatively and reduced time and money expenditure by alleviating the need for a surgical assistant.[30] The recently enacted resident work hour restrictions may prompt increased use of AESOP and other robot-assisted surgery especially at smaller institutions, both academic and private, where human resources may be limited.[4] While anatomic constraints may limit the role of active robot-assisted rhinologic surgery, Steinhart et al.[32] have reported the performance of 5 sphenoidectomies in a cadaveric model utilizing a robot with combined automated (active role) and telemanipulation roles performed in association with CT guidance. The Neuroptic T-30 (Polydiagnost Inc., Pfaffenhofen, Germany) and RV-1a articulating arms robot with controller CR1-571 (Mitsubishi Electric, Tokyo, Japan) was utilized to perform pre-programmed drilling through the anterior sphenoid wall. Following entry into the sphenoid sinus, the operating surgeon took over via telemanipulation to complete the dissection of the anterior sphenoid to achieve the desired size and exposure.

While the anatomy of the nose and paranasal sinuses may not allow the optimal exposure necessary for pursuing robotic surgery, the use of AESOP and the favorable results achieved involving the sphenoid sinus in cadavers are encouraging signs that robot-assisted surgery has a role in the future of rhinologic surgery.

LARYNGOLOGY

The greatest challenges in robot-assisted surgery of the pharynx and larynx are related to the limited anatomic workspace, need for airway management and the available methods for suspending instruments to allow adequate exposure and access to the structures of interest. In 2002, Melder and Mair reported early evaluation of endolaryngeal manipulation utilizing the daVinci Surgical Robot at Walter Reed Army Medical Center in porcine and cadaveric models (presented but not published). Suspension laryngoscopy was performed with atraumatic manipulation of supraglottic tissues. A significant early challenge identified in the lab was limited freedom of motion from instrument interference both externally and at the operative site. Access and maneuverability was improved with the use of the Pointsetter pneumatic endoscopic arm (Karl Storz, Culver City, CA, USA) to hold the endoscope. Subsequent adjustments in the size and number of instruments available for use with the daVinci Surgical Robot have also reduced the impact of these issues. Among the proposed new instruments is a robotic laser tip that is ideally designed for endolaryngeal procedures. **(Figure 10)**

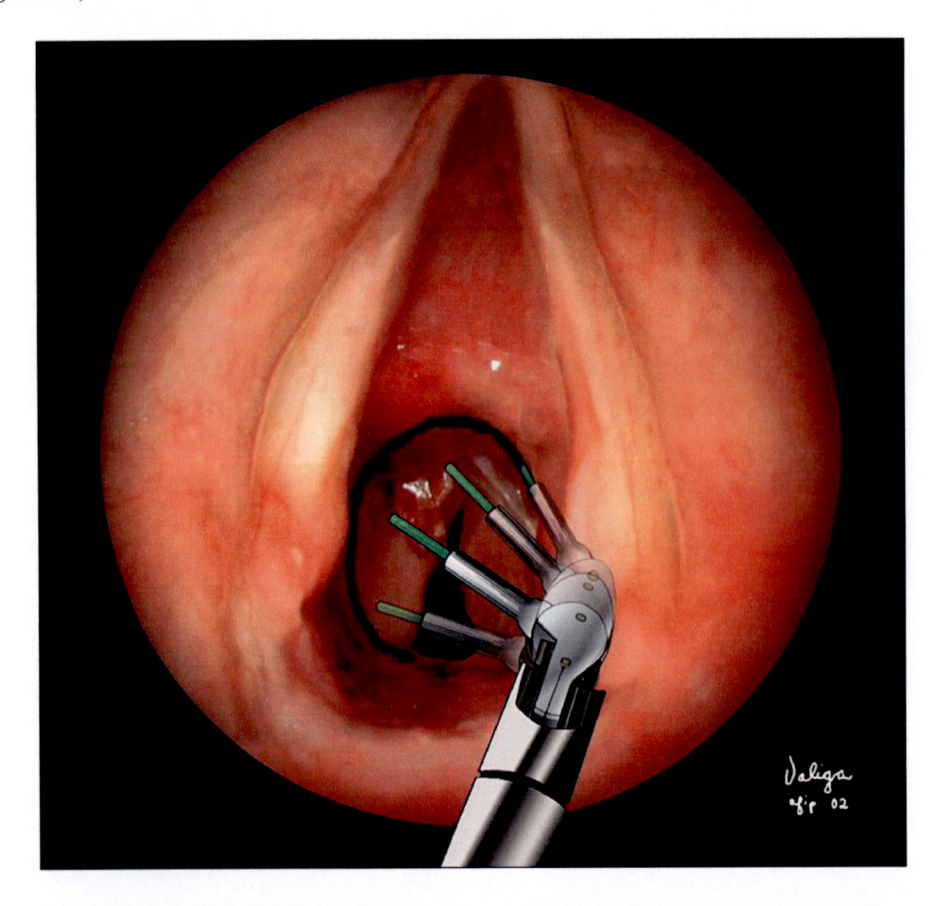

Figure 10: Artist rendering of EndoWrist Laser Tip Instrument for daVinci Robotic System.

Hockstein et al.[33] have built on Melder's work with a technical feasibility study to examine the use of the daVinci Surgical Robot for microlaryngeal procedures. An airway mannequin (Laerdal Airway Management Trainer 250000, Wappingers Falls, NY, USA) was enlisted to determine the optimal setup to perform robot-assisted microlaryngeal surgery with the greatest possible surgical field exposure and range of motion for the robotic arms. Their findings suggest that the optimal combination includes the McIvor mouthgag, 30-degree three-dimensional endoscope, 5mm instruments at the glottic level and 5mm or 8mm instruments at the hypopharynx and supraglottic levels (**Figure 11**).[32]

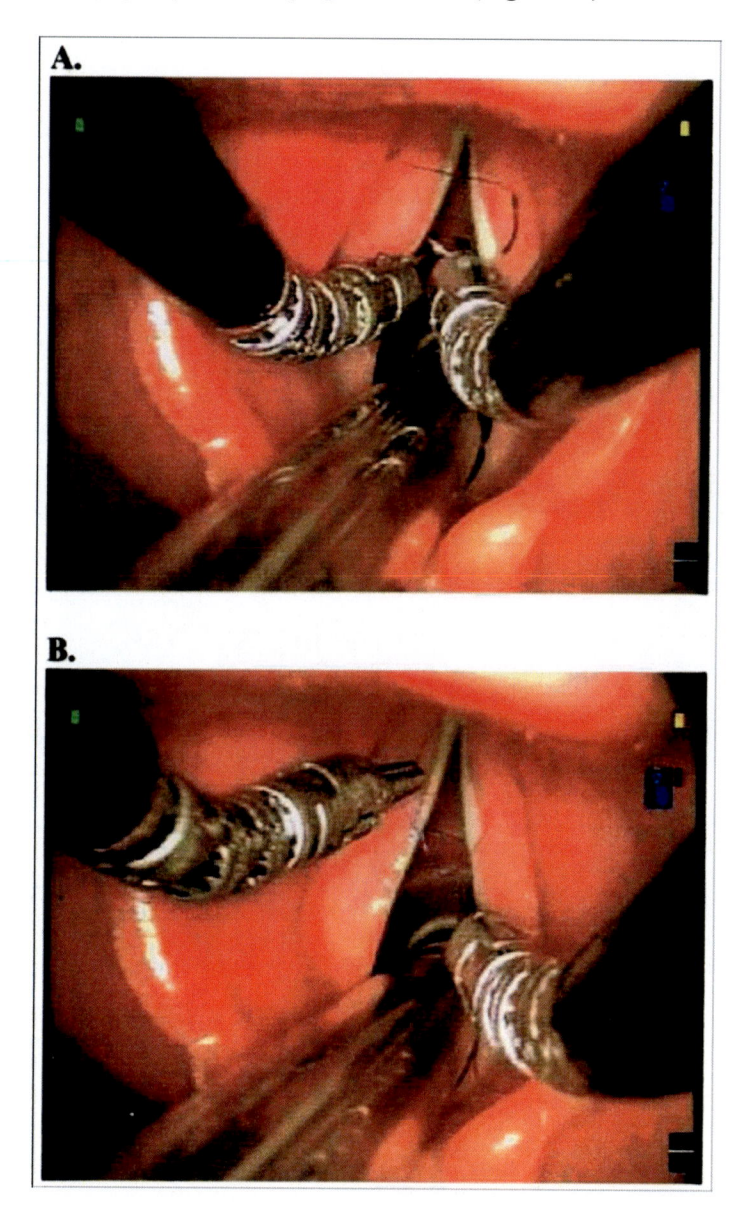

Figure 11. (A,B) Endolaryngeal view of an intubated mannequin showing suturing and knot tying technique utilizing 5 mm instrumentation. Note that the needle is removed prior to the tying of the knot. (Reprinted with permission from: Hockstein NG, Nolan JP, O'Malley BW Jr., Woo YJ. Robotic microlaryngeal surgery: A technical feasibility study using the daVinci surgical robot and an airway mannequin. *Laryngoscope* 2005, 115:780-785).

A subsequent study by Hockstein and colleagues[34] evaluated six procedures within the larynx and pharynx in a cadaver model again utilizing the daVinci Surgical Robot. The procedures include bilateral true vocal cord stripping, rotation of mucosal flap from epiglottis to anterior commissure, partial vocal cordectomy, arytenoidectomy, partial epiglottectomy with thyrohyoid dissection and partial base of tongue resection. The optimal setup configuration as determined in their previous study was utilized with substitution of a Dingman mouth gag with integrated cheek retractors for the McIvor mouth gag. All robotic dissections were performed safely and effectively in times that were felt to be comparable to other modalities. The setup time to get the robot in position and ready to operate was 30 minutes and procedure times ranged from 6 minutes for both left vocal cord stripping and partial vocal cordectomy to 28 minutes to rotate the mucosal flap from the epiglottis to the anterior commissure. All other procedures fell within these timeframes and endotracheal intubation did not adversely affect the ability to carry out the partial epiglottectomy and thyrohyoid dissection, arytenoidectomy or base of tongue excision.

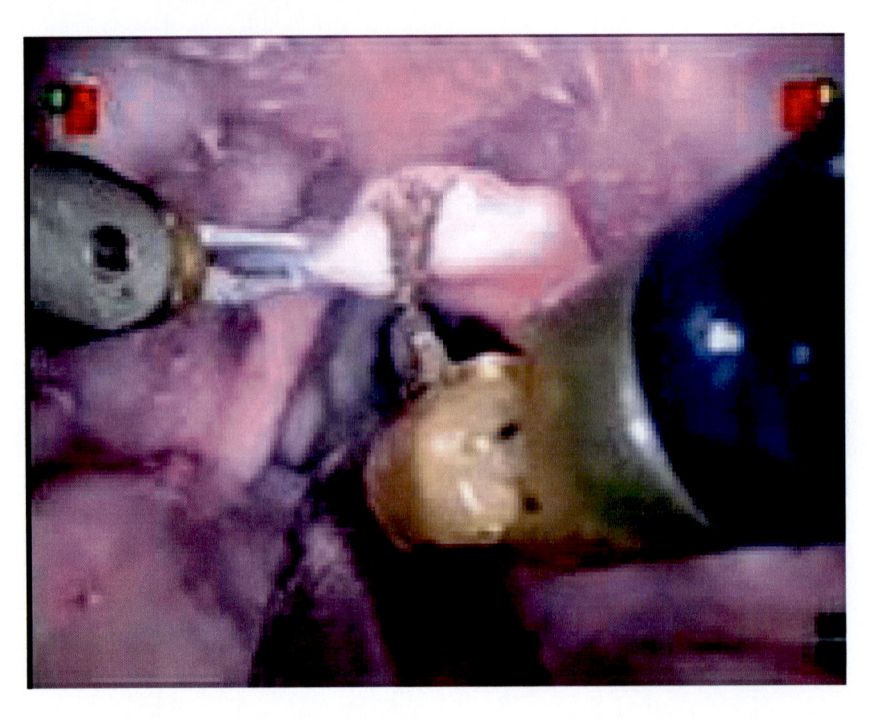

Figure 12a. Endoscopic view of vertical division of epiglottis utilizing monopolar spatula cautery visible in the right of the surgical field.

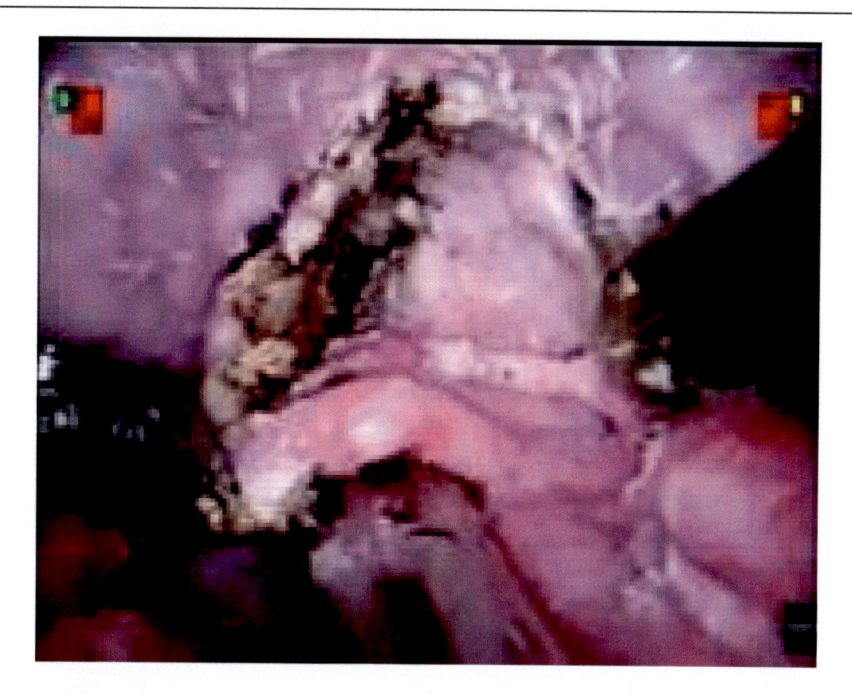

Figure 12b. Continued dissection of specimen along thyrohyoid membrane to identify the superior aspect of the thyroid cartilage.

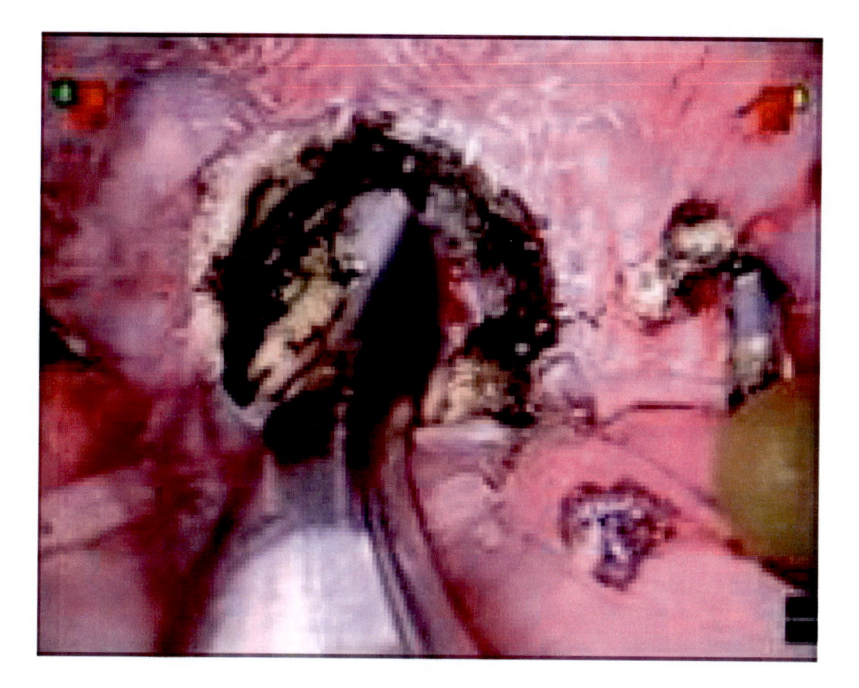

Figure 12c. Operative field following transoral robotic supraglottic partial laryngectomy in canine model. (Reprinted with permission from: Weinstein GS, O'Malley, BW Jr., Hockstein NG. Transoral robotic surgery: supraglottic laryngectomy in a canine model. *Laryngoscope* 2005, 115:1315-1319).

The Hockstein group reported an additional canine study in which they pursued transoral robotic supraglottic partial laryngectomy.[35] One mongrel dog underwent the procedure utilizing the daVinci Robotic System and 8mm instrumentation including a bipolar triangular forceps and monopolar spatula cautery as well as the 30 degree, three-dimensional endoscope. There was no difficulty maintaining the correct dissection planes and the bisected surgical specimen was excised leaving the true vocal cords, arytenoids and pyriform sinuses completely intact (**Figure 12 a-b**). The authors comment on the paucity of published data regarding the use of monopolar cautery in supraglottic procedures.

Based on the findings of these recent efforts, it seems likely that the daVinci Surgical Robot will be used in a clinical setting for surgery of the pharynx and larynx. Given the advanced articulating technology of these instruments, the potential exists for revolutionary breakthroughs in the treatment of laryngeal and pharyngeal pathology previously accessible only through external open approaches.

CONCLUSIONS

As one of the oldest surgical subspecialties, Otolaryngology-Head and Neck Surgery has a long history of adopting innovative surgical techniques to improve the efficiency and efficacy of the many diverse procedures utilized to treat pathology of the head and neck. The paradigm shift toward minimally invasive surgery continues to gain momentum, and even those surgeons who are reluctant to embrace these techniques acknowledge that patient demand will likely ensure its survival. Likewise, the integration of robots into the surgical theater seems inevitable. Multiple feasibility studies using porcine, cadaver, canine and mannequin models demonstrate that robot-assisted surgery in the head and neck can be performed safely and efficiently. The spectrum of passive to active robot assistance offers great diversity when selecting the degree of robot involvement and responsibility desired for a given procedure. While the integration of telesurgery utilizing master-slave robotic systems is well-established in specialties such as urology, cardiothoracic and pediatric surgery, the opportunities within Otolaryngology-Head and Neck Surgery are still being identified. As robotic technology continues to improve, each otolaryngologic subspecialty will realize increased opportunities to utilize robot-assisted surgical techniques in clinical models. Seemingly inconceivable or impossible clinical applications of today may become a reality for tomorrow's head and neck surgeons.

REFERENCES

1. Cuschieri A, Dubois F, Mouiel J, Mouret P, Becker H, Buess G, Trede M, Troidl H. The European experience with laparoscopic cholecystectomy. *Am J Surg* 1991, 161:385-387.

2. Mouret P. How I developed laparoscopic cholecystectomy. *Ann Acad Med Singapore* 1996, 25:744-747.

3. Satava RM. Surgical robotics: the early chronicles. *Surg Laparosc Endosc Percutan Tech* 2003, 12:6-16.

4. Gourin CG, Terris DJ. Surgical robotics in otolaryngology: expanding the technology envelope. *Curr Opin Otolaryngol Head Neck Surg* 2004, 12:204-208.

5. Camarillo DB, Krummel TM, Salisbury JK Jr. Robotic technology in surgery: past, present and future. *Am J Surg* 2004 Oct, 188(4A Suppl): 2s-15S.

6. Ballantyne GH. Robotic surgery, telerobotic surgery, telepresence, and telementoring. *Surg Endosc* 2002, 16:1389-1402.

7. Marescaux J, Leroy J, Gagner M, Rubino F, Mutter D, Vix M, Butner SE, Smith MK. Transatlantic robot-assisted telesurgery. *Nature* 2001, 413:379-380.

8. Gagner, M. Endoscopic subtotal parathyroidectomy in patients with primary hyperparathyroidism. *Br J Surg* 1996, 83:875.

9. Miccoli P, Bendinelli C, Vignali E, Mazzeo S, Cecchini GM, Pinchera A, Marcocci C. Endoscopic parathyroidectomy: Report of an initial experience. *Surgery* 1998, 124:1077-1079.

10. Huscher CS, Chiodini S, Napolitano C, Recher A. Endoscopic right thyroid lobectomy. *Surg Endosc* 1997, 11:877.

11. Yeung GHC. Endoscopic surgery of the neck. *Surg Laparosc Endosc* 1998, 8:227-232.

12. Bellantone R, Lombardi CP, Raffaelli M, Rubino F, Boscherini M, Perilli W. Minimally invasive, totally gasless video-assisted thyroid lobectomy. *Am J Surg* 1999, 177:342-343.

13. Shimizu K, Akira S, Jasmi AY, Kitamura Y, Kitagawa W, Akasu H, Tanaka S. Video-assisted neck surgery: Endoscopic resection of thyroid tumors with a very minimal neck wound. *J Am Coll Surg* 1999, 188:697-703.

14. Carreno OJ, Wilson WR, Nootheti PK. Exploring endoscopic neck surgery in a porcine model. *Laryngoscope* 1999, 109: 236-240.

15. Dulguerov P, Vaezi AE, Belenger J, Wang D, Kurt AM, Allal AS, Lehmann W. Endoscopic neck dissection in an animal model: comparison of nodal yield with open-neck dissection. *Arch Otolaryngol Head Neck Surg* 2000, 126:417-420.

16. Dulguerov P, Leuchter I, Szalay-Quinodoz I, Allal AS, Marchal F, Lehmann W, Fasel JH. Endoscopic neck dissection in human cadavers. Laryngoscope 2001, 111:2135-2139.

17. Takami H, Ikeda Y. Endoscopic thyroidectomy via an axillary or anterior chest approach. In: Gagner M, Inabnet WB 3rd, eds. *Minimally Invasive Endocrine Surgery*. Philadelphia: Lippincott Williams & Wilkens, 2002:56-63.

18. Takami H, Ikeda Y. Total Endoscopic Thyroidectomy. *Asian J Surg* 2003 Apr, 26(2):82-85.

19. Monfared A, Saenz Y, Terris DJ. Endoscopic resection of the submandibular gland in a porcine model. *Laryngoscope* 2002, 112:1089-1093.

20. Terris DJ, Monfared A, Thomas A, Kambham N, Saenz Y. Endoscopic selective neck dissection in a porcine model. *Arch Otolaryngol Head Neck Surg* 2003, 129:613-617.

21. Terris DJ, Haus BM, Nettar K, Ciecko S, Gourin CG. Prospective evaluation of endoscopic approaches to the thyroid compartment. *Laryngoscope* 2004, 114:1377-1382.

22. Terris DJ, Haus BM, Gourin CG. Endoscopic neck surgery: Resection of the submandibular gland in a cadaver model. *Laryngoscope* 2004, 114:407-410.

23. Haus BM, Kambham N, Le D, Moll FM, Gourin C, Terris DJ. Surgical robotic applications in otolaryngology. *Laryngoscope* 2003, 113:1139-1144.

24. Terris DJ, Haus BM, Gourin CG, Lilagan PE. Endo-robotic resection of the submandibular gland in a cadaver model. *Head Neck* (In press)

25. McLeod IK, Melder PC. Da Vinci robot-assisted excision of a vallecular cyst: a case report. Ear Nose Throat J 2005 Mar, 84(3):170-172.

26. Charles S. Dexterity enhancement for surgery. In: Taylor RH, Lavellee S, Burdea GC, Mosges R. *Computer Integrated Surgery: Technology and Clinical Applications*. Cambridge, Massachussetts: MIT Press; 1996. p. 467-471.

27. Rothbaum DL, Roy J, Stoianovici D, Berkelman P, Hager GD, Taylor RH, Whitcomb LL, Francis HW, Niparko JK. Robot-assisted stapedotomy: Micropick fenestration of the stapes footplate. *Otolaryngol Head Neck Surg* 2002, 127: 417-426.

28. Federspil PA, Geisthoff UW, Henrich D, Plinkert PK. Development of the first force-controlled robot for otoneurosurgery. *Laryngoscope* 2003, 113:465-471.

29. May M, Hoffman DF, Sobol SM. Video endoscopic sinus surgery: a two handed technique. *Laryngoscope* 1990, 100:430-432.

30. Obando MA, Payne JH. The future application of the robotic arm (automatic endoscopic system for optimal positioning or AESOP) with voice recognition in sinus endoscopic surgery. *Op Tech Otolaryngol Head Neck Surg* 2003, 14:55-57.

31. Obando M, Liem L, Madauss W, Morita M, Robinson B. Robotic surgery in pituitary tumors. *Op Tech Otolaryngol Head Neck Surg* 2004, 15:147-149.

32. Steinhart H, Bumm K, Wurm J, Vogele M, Iro H. Surgical applications of a new robotic system for paranasal sinus surgery. *Ann Otol Rhinol Laryngol* 2004, 113:303-309.

33. Hockstein NG, Nolan JP, O'Malley BW Jr., Woo YJ. Robotic microlaryngeal surgery: A technical feasibility study using the daVinci surgical robot and an airway mannequin. *Laryngoscope* 2005, 115:780-785.

34. Hockstein NG, Nolan JP, O'Malley BW Jr., Woo YJ. Robot-assisted pharyngeal and laryngeal microsurgery: Results of robotic cadaver dissections. *Laryngoscope* 2005, 115:1003-1008.

35. Weinstein GS, O'Malley, BW Jr., Hockstein NG. Transoral robotic surgery: supraglottic laryngectomy in a canine model. *Laryngoscope* 2005, 115:1315-1319.

In: Robotics in Surgery: History, Current and Future Applications ISBN 1-60021-386-3
Editor: Russell A. Faust, pp. 243-258 © 2007 Nova Science Publishers, Inc.

Chapter 14

TRANSORAL ROBOTIC SURGERY (TORS)

Neil G. Hockstein[1], Gregory S. Weinstein[2] and Bert W. O'Malley, Jr.[2]

[1]Family Ear, Nose and Throat, Wilmington, DE, USA
[2]Department of Otorhinolaryngology, Hospitals of University of Pennsylvania
Philadelphia, PA, USA

Abstract

Robotic technology has rapidly become integrated into endoscopic abdominal and thoracic surgery. Advantages of robotic surgery include: excellent optics, wristed instrumentation, scaled movements, and tremor filtration. These attributes lend themselves well to pharyngeal and laryngeal microsurgery. Obstacles to the safe performance of robotic pharyngeal and laryngeal microsurgery include: patient and instrument positioning and exposure, means of suctioning, and maintenance of hemostasis. These obstacles are manageable and early experience has demonstrated the technical feasibility of transoral robotic surgery (TORS) using the daVinci Surgical System.

The earliest experiments into TORS involved an airway mannequin model, a cadaver model, and a canine model. These experiments helped to identify methods to expose the laryngopharynx, achieve hemostasis, and control secretions. A variety of retractors and laryngoscopes have been tested and different devices have been identified to be useful at different levels in the pharynx and larynx. Additionally, the potential for patient harm secondary to robotic malfunction or robotic misuse has been assessed.

This early experience indicates that there will likely be value for this technology in the management of neoplastic disorders of the oral cavity, pharynx, and larynx. Additionally, treatments for neurologic voice disorders, functional voice disorders refractory to conservative therapy, obstructive sleep apnea, and transoral approaches to the skull base may be managed with TORS.

INTRODUCTION

The attributes of robotic technology including excellent optics, tremor filtration, motion scaling and wristed instrumentation are exceptionally well suited to treatment of pharyngeal and laryngeal disorders. Potential advantages include both improvements in treatment of diseases currently managed transorally with the operating microscope (with and without carbon dioxide [CO2] laser) and transoral management of diseases currently treated with open surgical approaches.

Conventional microsurgery with the operating microscope has several inherent disadvantages, especially to the less experienced surgeon. First, the long instruments required to perform transoral laryngeal microsurgery create a fulcrum effect. With the fulcrum effect, small movements of the surgeon's hand translate into larger movement by the distal tip of the endoscopic instrument and movements are counterintuitive with movement of the hand in one direction resulting in a movement of the distal tip of the instrument in the other direction. Additionally any movements, including tremor, are further magnified by the power of the operating microscope. The non-wristed instruments also make precise handling of tissues and suturing more challenging. Robotic technology, with wristed microinstruments and tremor filtration eliminate these issues.

Certain disease processes, not amenable to non-robotic transoral management, are potentially treated transorally with robotic technology. Certain areas of the pharynx are difficult to reach with the CO2 laser as line-of-site cannot be achieved. With robotic technology, wristed electrocautery instrumentation and angled endoscopes obviate the need for line-of-site. Parapharyngeal lesions are not managed with conventional transoral procedures, as the great vessels cannot be controlled. With robotic assistance, the great vessels can potentially be dissected and controlled transorally. Robotic technology may decrease the need to perform certain open surgical approaches, including the lateral pharyngotomy approach and the mandibulotomy approach for access to the oropharynx and hypopharynx. In this chapter we discuss our early experience with TORS.

OPERATING ROOM SETUP

In traditional abdominopelvic and thoracic applications of the daVinci Surgical System the patient is placed in the supine position on the operating room table with the head toward the anesthesiologist. The robotic unit is positioned either perpendicular to the patient (adjacent to the chest and abdomen) or between the patient's legs. The arms (in the three armed unit) enter the patient's body cavities from above, through three widely placed ports, perpendicular to the surface of the operating room table.[1,2]

In TORS, this traditional positioning is not technically feasible. Several factors require an alternative strategy for positioning. First, the structures potentially treated with TORS lie in a plane nearly parallel to the surface of the operating room table and, therefore, transoral instrument placement necessitates a nearly parallel trajectory of the robotic arms. Second, to obtain near parallel placement of the robotic arms (which only flex toward the robotic unit and do not sufficiently extend away from the robotic unit, the patient optimally would be placed in line with the robotic unit with the head distal and the legs in stirrups straddling the robot's base. Placement of patients in the lithotomy position is impractical for transoral surgery, and rotating the operating room table to approximately 30-degrees provides for adequate arm positioning. **[Figure 1]** Finally, the funnel created by the mouth, pharynx, and larynx requires the arms to be placed very close to one another with more acute angles for work deeper in the pharynx and larynx.[3,4]

As in non-robotic microlaryngeal surgery, when the operating room table is rotated placing the head (and consequently the airway) remote from the anesthesiologist with cumbersome instrumentation situated in close proximity or inside the patients oral cavity, the airway must be very secure. Means to secure the airway can include use of reinforced endotracheal tubes, which resist kinking, suturing of endotracheal tubes, and providing appropriate slack to the ventilatory circuit.

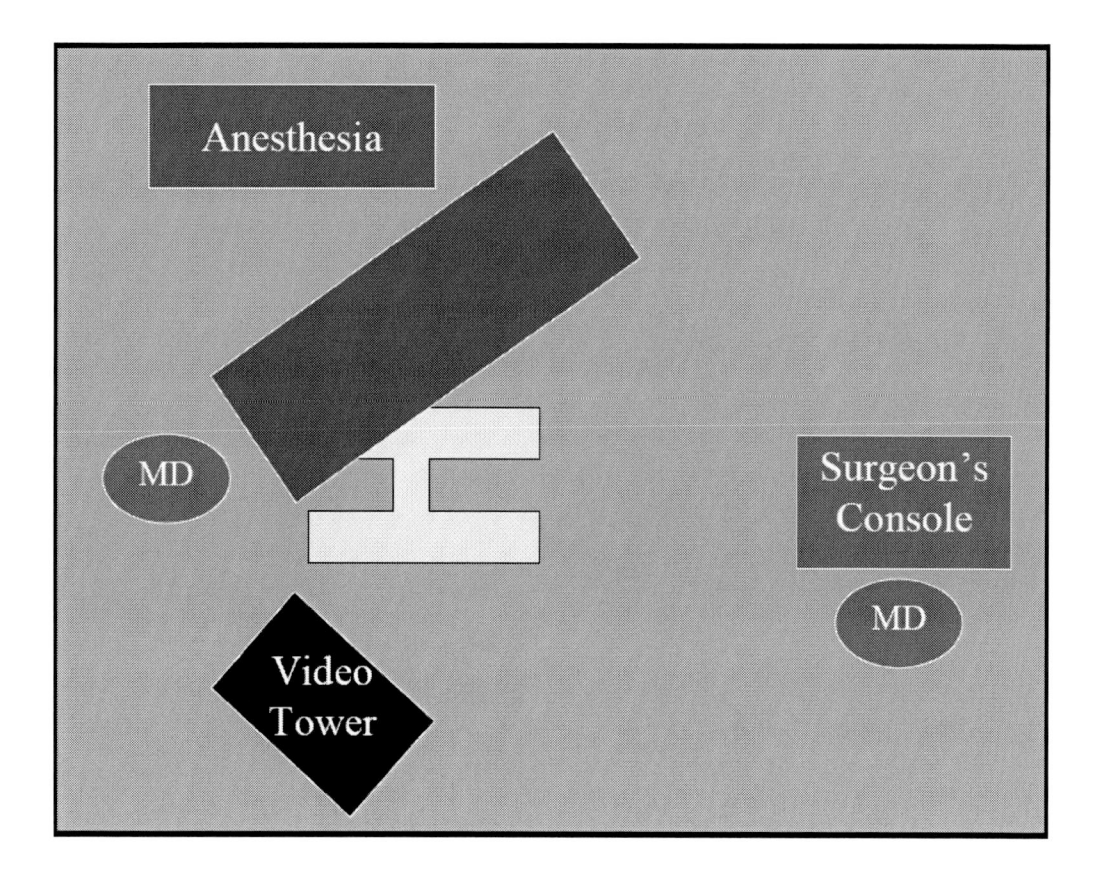

Fig. 1. Schematic of the operating room setup with the operating table rotated to 30-degrees relative to the robot unit and the surgeon sitting at a remote console. An assistant surgeon also sits at the head of the bed as an added measure of safety.

EXPOSURE AND INSTRUMENTATION

Conventional laryngoscopy and microlaryngoscopy rely on the multitude of closed tube laryngoscopes that have been developed and modified over the last century. An enormous variety of laryngoscopes have been developed to optimize visualization of different areas in the pharynx and larynx and an equally large array of sizes exist for use in patients of different body habitus.[5,6,7] Additionally, specialty laryngoscope have been designed for particular procedures including bivalve scopes for endoscopic Zenker's diverticulotomy, slotted laryngoscopes for phonomicrosurgery, and specially coated scopes for use with the CO2 laser.[8,9] Innovation in endoscopic pharyngeal and laryngeal microsurgery reveals the inherent disadvantage of the reliance on closed tube laryngoscopes, in that many surgical innovations require modification of existing laryngoscopes. Further, no individual surgeon or surgical facility can feasibly obtain and maintain the variety of laryngoscopes that are available and mastery of the use of different laryngoscopes is equally challenging for the surgeon.[10]

Attempts at the use of closed tube laryngoscopes in transoral robotic surgery achieved limited success. McLeod and Melder reported a case of a robotic-assisted marsupialization of a vallecular cyst using the daVinci Surgical System and a slotted, closed tube laryngoscope. Using the closed tube laryngoscope, an assistant surgeon was required to manually retract the cyst as space constraints limited the ability to introduce the third robotic arm.[11]

Additional research in the laboratory demonstrated that use of closed tube laryngoscopes was inferior to mouth-gag systems. The use of closed tube laryngoscopes interferes with endoscope excursion and with the daVinci System's wide-angle and high-magnification cameras, the three-dimensional endoscope can be positioned several centimeters proximally from the surgical site and adequate magnification with a wide field-of-view is obtained. A variety of mouth gags provide adequate exposure for work in the proximal pharynx and supraglottis including: the McIvor Mouth-gag, the Dingman Mouth-gag, and the Crow-Davis Mouthgag.[3,4] **[Figure 2]** Like working with closed tube laryngoscopes, different patients and different anatomic locales may require different mouth-gags, but the variety is significantly more limited. Once placed, the mouth-gag does not need repositioning for work in different areas, rather the endoscope can be repositioned more proximally or distally and at different angles to better view different areas.

Once pharyngeal exposure is achieved, either the 0-degree or 30-degree endoscope can be used, depending on the particular operative site. While rotation of the 30-degree endoscope away from the horizon does skew three-dimensional perspective, a limited amount of rotation does allow for better visualization of lateral structures. Although, at extremes of rotation, the viewing-mode can be changed to two-dimensional, the authors' personal preferences are to use the three-dimensional mode even beyond 45-degrees of rotation.

HEMOSTASIS AND SECRETIONS

Maintenance of hemostasis is essential for the safe performance of TORS both to limit intra-operative blood loss and to prevent aspiration. Maintenance of hemostasis requires: the prevention of bleeding, the control of active bleeding, and adequate suction. Hemostasis has not been problematic in robotic laparoscopic and thoracoscopic surgery; in fact, robotic surgeons report decreased blood loss and need for blood transfusion.[1,12,13] Several strategies employed in cardiac and urologic procedures can be applied to TORS. Discontinuation of anticoagulants and antiplatelet agents (aspirin) is recommended prior to surgery, if medically acceptable.[1] Intraoperative techniques for to control bleeding include the use of monopolar

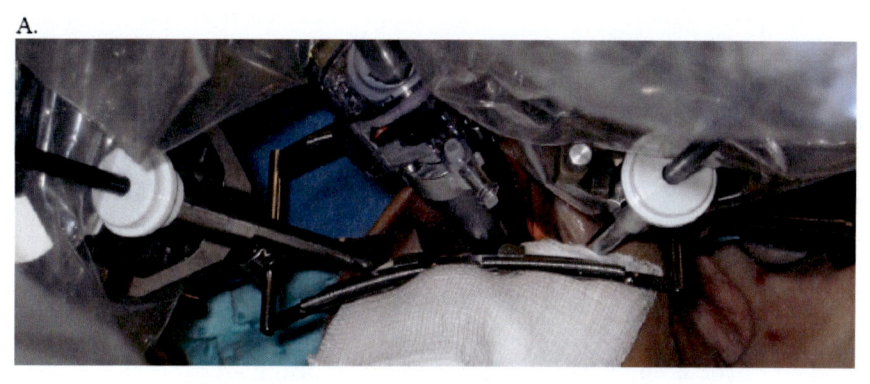

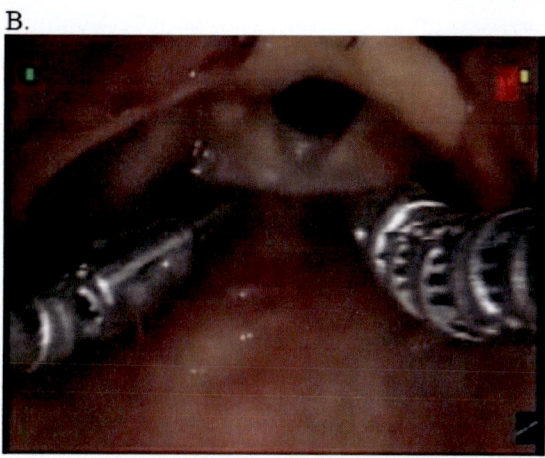

Fig. 2. Use of the Dingman mouthgag in a human cadaver provides a wide oral aperture (A) and excellent laryngeal exposure (B).

and bipolar cautery and robotically and non-robotically controlled hemoclips.[1] Although endoscopic suturing can be performed in TORS, it is seldom necessary for control of bleeding.[3,4,14]

Incision or excision of pharyngeal and laryngeal muscle, cartilage, glandular, and mucosal tissues is commonly performed using monopolar and bipolar electrocautery in conventional open surgical procedures. Although further studies are indicated, robotic control of cautery probably does not alter the thermal properties of the cautery and previous reports have demonstrated that electrocautery produces tissue injury similar to that of the CO2 laser, which is commonly employed in endoscopic laryngeal surgery.[15,16,17] In TORS, large caliber vessels can be ligated with both robotic and non-robotically controlled hemoclips. **[Figure 3]** Large caliber vessels can be managed in TORS in a manner similar to endoscopic laser resections performed in the pharynx and larynx.[18,19,20] In the superficial tissues of the larynx and hypopharynx, there are no large caliber vessels. Oropharynx resections, which involve transection of branches of the lingual arteries, require the use of surgical hemoclips, both robotically driven and hand operated by an assistant surgeon. Both robotically driven and hand operated hemoclip appliers are frequently employed in robotic radical prostatectomy and both are similarly effective in early experience with TORS.[14] Risk of aspiration of surgical hemoclips placed in the oropharynx is similar in TORS and in endoscopic laryngeal and pharyngeal laser surgery and hemoclips are routinely used for ligation of vessels greater than 0.5 to 1 mm in diameter without report of aspiration.[20]

Experience in both the animal laboratory and early experience with patients has demonstrated the limited need for suctioning of secretions or blood.[14] When suction is required, several options exist. In our early experience, we have had a surgical assistant observe the procedure transorally to ensure that the backs of the robotic arms do not injure the patient's cheeks, lips, teeth, and gums. The surgical assistant can also use a rigid suction catheter, either viewing on a video monitor or under direct vision, when needed to clear secretions, however, this is seldom necessary. Additionally, a flexible suction catheter can be placed in the surgical field and grasped and directed with a robotic forceps.[3,21] **[Figure 4]** While suction is not integrated into the robotic instruments currently commercially available, this method of using a flexible suction catheter is effective and obviates the need for integrated suction.

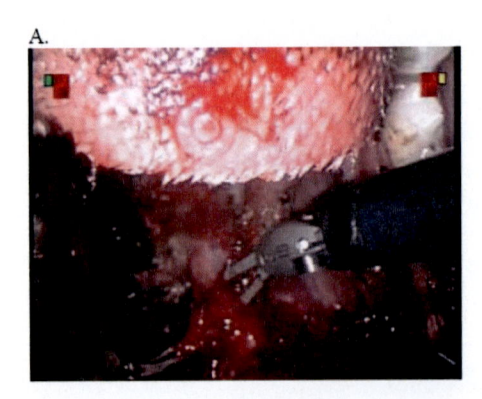

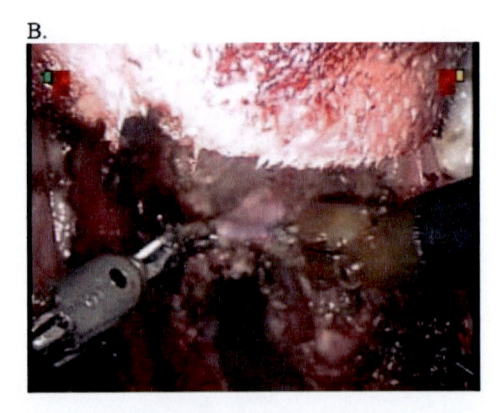

Fig. 3. A. The transected canine lingual artery is grasped with a forceps in the left-handed instrument while a robotically controlled clip is applied with the right instrument. B. The clipped vessel is dissected free of surrounding tissues.

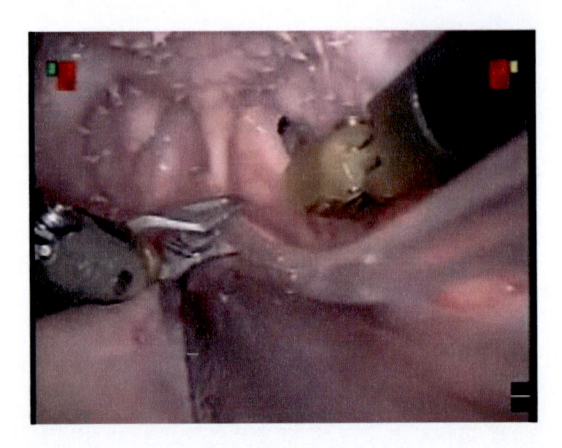

Fig. 4. A flexible respiratory suction catheter is grasped and manipulated with the robotically controlled forceps.

POTENTIAL SURGICAL PROCEDURES

The potential applications for TORS include selected lesions, which are presently approached transorally either with conventional laryngoscopy, microlaryngoscopy, or endoscopic laser microlaryngeal surgery. Additionally, certain lesions not amenable to non-robotic, transoral surgery are potentially treatable with TORS. For these lesions, the benefits of TORS may be related to exposure and the potential to work around corners without the limitations of line-of-site required for CO2 laser surgery. In other areas, the potential for increased precision associated with tremor filtration, motion scaling, and excellent optics will be the principle advantages. Other advantages may include the potentially increased speed of robotic electrocautery over carbon dioxide laser surgery and more facile endoscopic suturing. Finally, the potential for telementoring and telepresence offers advantages to patients without access to surgical subspecialists.

Oral Cavity Lesions

Lesions of the oral cavity are easily reached with conventional instrumentation and seldom require high magnification, therefore there is limited value incorporating robotics into oral cavity surgery. There may be some potential advantages for posteriorly based oral cavity lesions.

Oropharyngeal and Hypopharyngeal Lesions

TORS is well suited to the management of both oropharyngeal and hypopharyngeal tumors, including tumors of the tongue base, tonsil, and pharyngeal walls. **[Figure 5]** Large specimens may be removed en bloc and issues of line of site and exposure associated with the use of an operating microscope and laser are eliminated with the use of the angled endoscope and wristed instruments. Early experience in cadavers and animals has demonstrated the technical feasibility of applying TORS to the management of these lesions.[25] Further study of large patient series with both functional and oncologic outcome measures is warranted.

Malignant Laryngeal Lesions

The endoscopic laser supraglottic partial laryngectomy has been shown to have advantages over the open supraglottic partial laryngectomy for selected patients with oncologically appropriate tumors electing surgical treatment in whom exposure can be achieved.[18] The application of TORS to the management of these tumors is a natural next step. Rather than using the laser to transect tissues, the monopolar and bipolar cautery are used offering potential speed advantages. TORS allows for multiplanar transection of tissues with the ability to cut toward and away from the surgeon which may provide an additional degree of safety when transecting the tissues above the laryngeal ventricle.[14] **[Figure 6]**

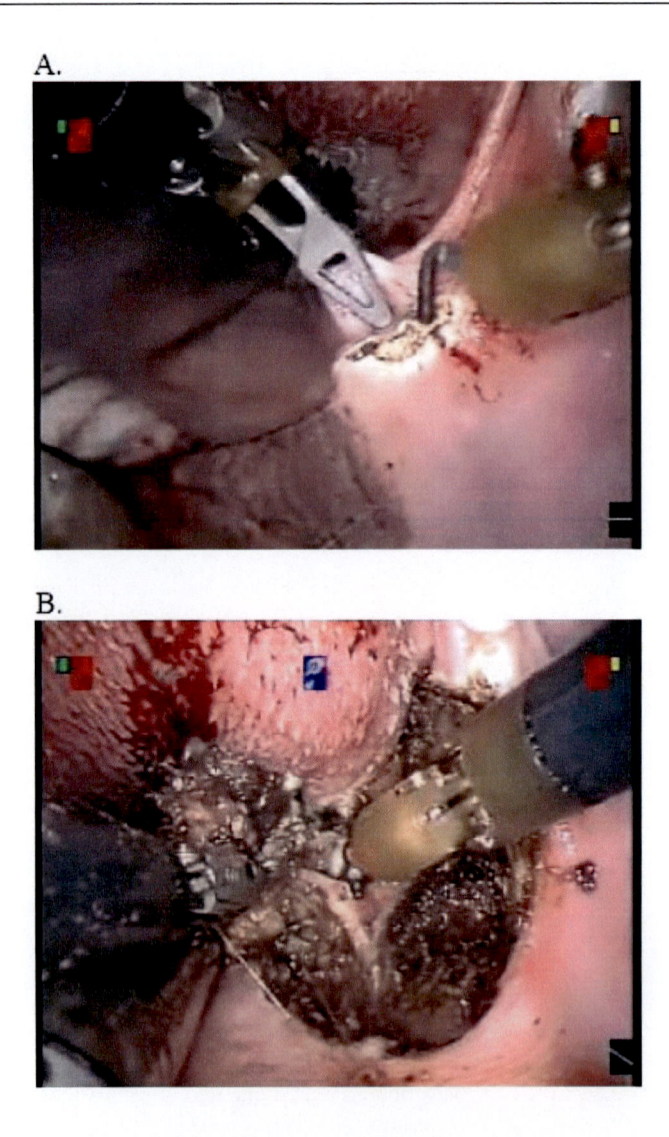

Fig. 5. A. The canine right lateral pharyngeal wall is grasped just superior to the tonsil with a forceps and a cautery hook is used to incise the mucosa. B. The radical tonsillectomy is completed including excision of the constrictor muscles leaving only a thin fascial layer over the carotid artery.

Additionally, the learning curve of the robotic partial supraglottic laryngectomy seems to be more favorable than the laser supraglottic partial laryngectomy, but further study is warranted.

Endoscopic management of T1 glottic cancers provides excellent local control, even in some tumors involving the anterior commissure.[22] Using a hydrodissection technique, superficial tumors can be dissected from Reinke's Space and voice quality can be preserved without compromising margins.[23] The same technique can be employed under robotic control and the advantages of tremor filtration and improved optics may improve dexterity and surgical precision.[10] **[Figure 7]**

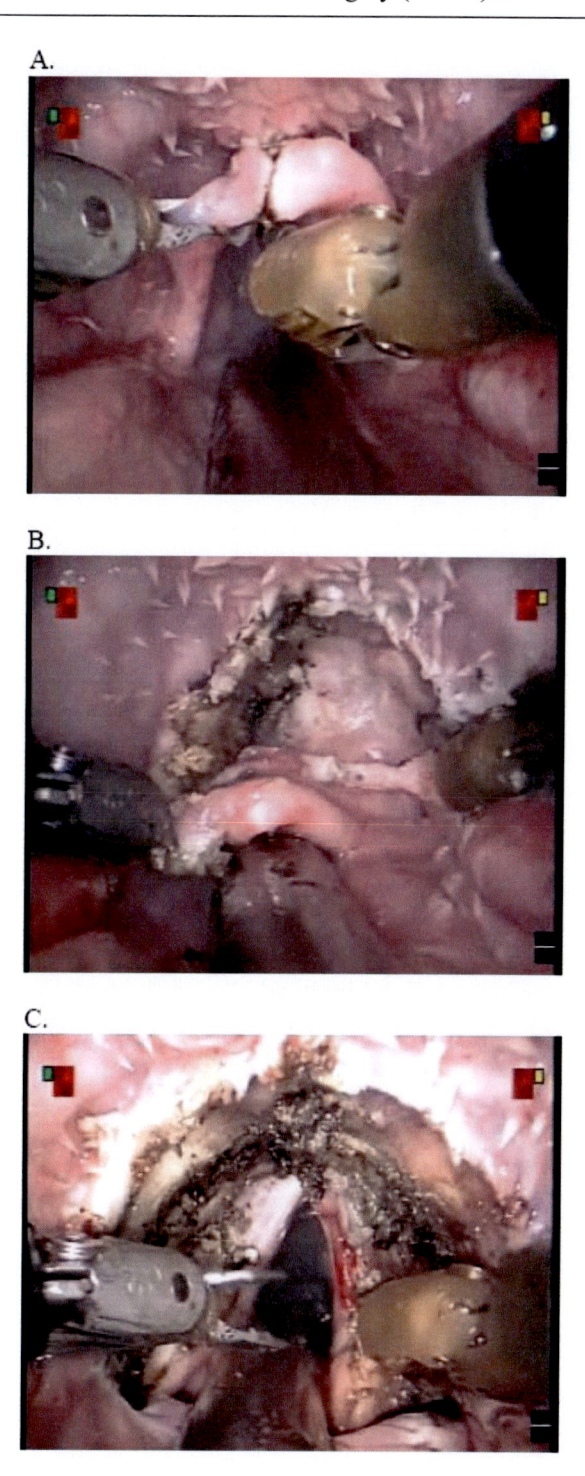

Fig. 6. A. The canine epiglottis is bisected as the initial step in the endoscopic supraglottic partial laryngectomy. B. The dissection continues along the thyrohyoid membrane. C. The completed endoscopic supraglottic partial laryngectomy.

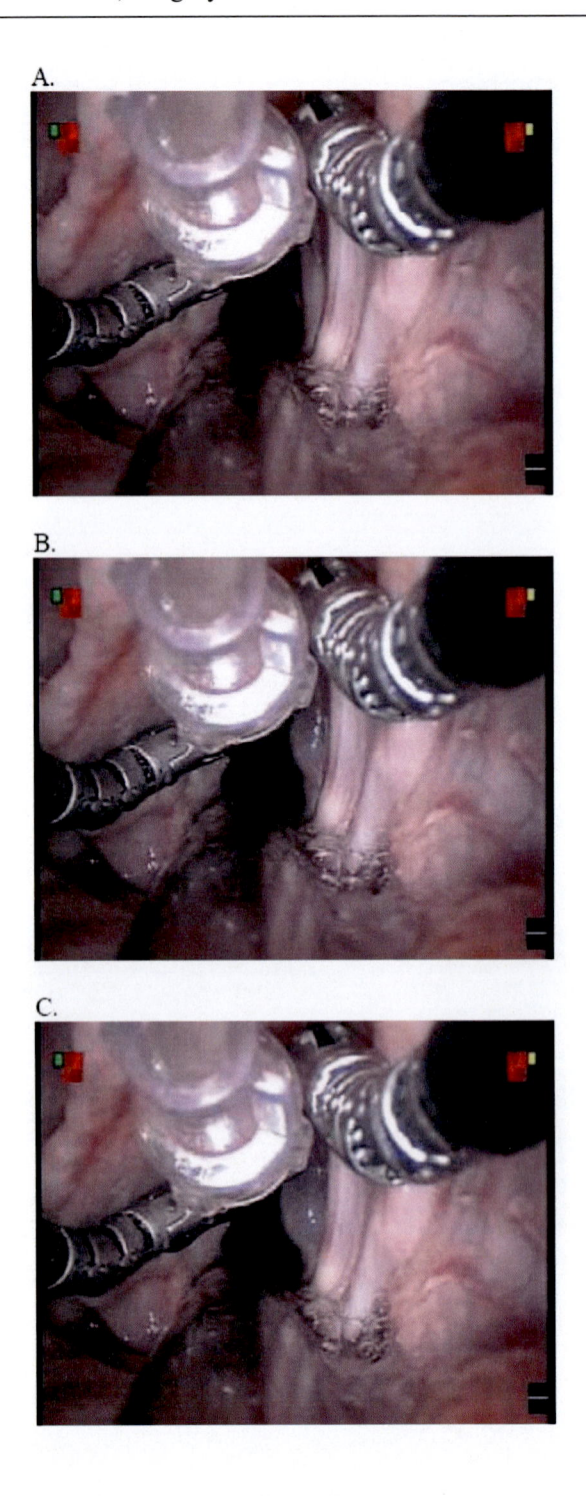

Fig. 7. A., B., C. A 25-gauge needle is used to raise a bleb in the mucosa of the canine true vocal fold under robotic control. This is analogous to the hydrodissection used is excision of superficial vocal fold lesions.

Benign Laryngeal Lesions and Phonomicrosurgery

The inherent advantages that robotics confers upon the treatment of malignant laryngeal lesions can be applied to benign laryngeal disorders as well. The absence of tremor and improved optics offers surgeons the potential to operate with greater precision and to attempt more technically challenging maneuvers. The elevation of microflaps, precise submucosal dissections, and endolaryngeal suturing are all technically feasible with TORS and the learning curve is very advantageous.[4,10] The anatomic confines at the level of the glottis provide the greatest challenge during TORS. **[Figure 8]** Two 5 mm instruments may either obstruct the surgeons view or by nature of their sheer space occupying effect limit surgical access.

Skull Base and Cervical Spine Surgery

Transoral approaches to the skull base and cervical spine with or without mobilization of the palate provide direct access to otherwise difficult to reach surgical sites. These procedures commonly require the transection or resection of bone with both manual and powered instrumentation including drills, rongeurs, and osteotomes. At present, these instruments have not been coupled to surgical robotics, thus limiting the application of robotics to skull base surgery. Potentially, non-robotic instruments can be used to gain access to the skull base and the robot can be used for more delicate handling of tissues and vessels deep within the skull base, but application of this concept has been met with only limited success in the laboratory. Further instrument development is necessary to fully integrate surgical robotics into transoral skull base and spine surgery.

SAFETY ISSUES

The application of robotic technology to transoral surgery potentially exposes patients to new risks, some of which are predictable, others unknown. Ensuring patient safety is of primary importance and while TORS is in its infancy, several issues related to acute surgical risk have been evaluated.

The safety record of the daVinci system in its application to thoracoscopic and laparoscopic surgery establish a solid background of overall device safety.[1,2] Specific issues related to transoral placement of the robotic arms include potential lip and tooth injuries, facial and ocular injuries, mucosal injuries, and neck or spine injuries. While these risks are also associated with conventional transoral surgery, it is unknown if the addition of a robotic device alters the complication rate.

Several studies evaluating the potential for direct patient injury by device misuse have yielded promising results. Attempts to intentionally fracture or extract stable, intact teeth in a cadaver with a variety of robotic instruments were unsuccessful resulting in either instrument failure (breakage) or alarming of the robot. **[Figure 9]** Forcefully impaling the skin and mucosa with the robotic arms and endoscope (either manually or under robotic control) failed to cause significant injury resulting in only superficial lacerations. Attempts to intentionally

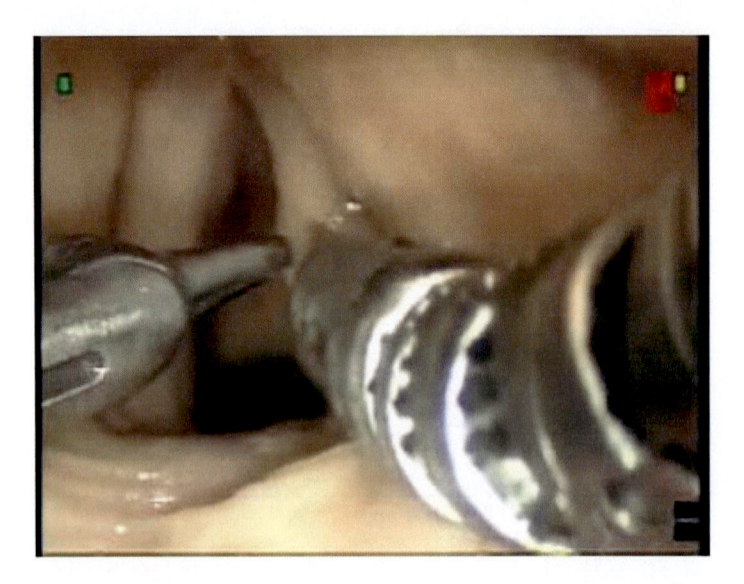

Fig. 8. Glottic resection in a human cadaver with 5mm instruments demonstrates the space constraints working at this level.

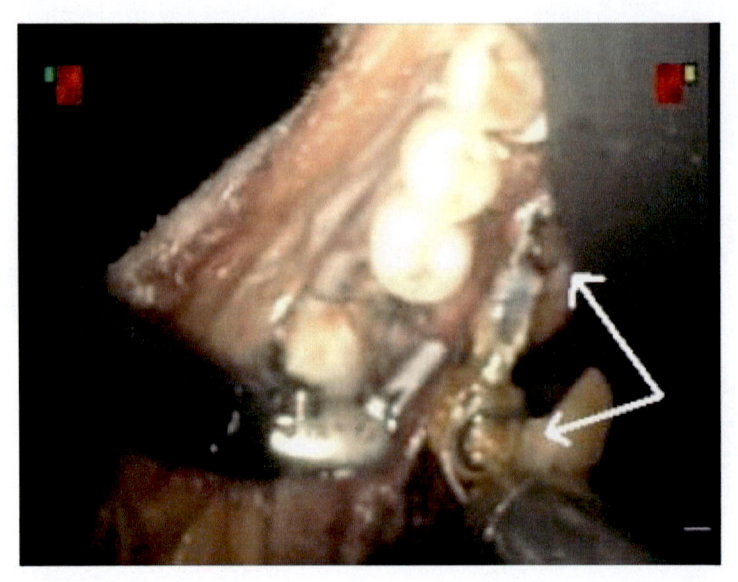

Fig. 9. Robotic instruments were intentionally driven into the cadaver's teeth to attempt to cause dental injury. Instrument breakage occurred prior to tooth injury. Arrows point toward broken distal tip of an 8mm spatula bovie.

fracture the mandible or cervical spine in a cadaver by gross misuse of the robotic arms were also unsuccessful; again, the robot alarmed and entered a safe mode precluding further movement of the robotic arms against resistance.[24] Reckless placement of the robotic arms or endoscope may result in ocular injury or impalement of the orbit, but this risk is similar to any other surgical procedure in which the eyes are in close proximity to the surgical field.

During robotic positioning, the surgeon must be careful to avoid injury to the eyes, however, once the instruments are in the mouth, risk to the orbits is essentially eliminated. For additional safety, protective eyeshields offer at least a theoretical advantage.

FUTURE DIRECTIONS

The excellent optics and wristed movements inherent in TORS provide the surgeon with the potential to obtain transoral vascular control, not possible with conventional techniques.[21] These attributes have already proven useful in surgical management of soft tissues in the oral cavity, pharynx, and larynx. The potential to extend beyond the aerodigestive tract into the soft tissue spaces of the neck has yet to be fully explored. The ability to obtain control of the great vessels will open the door to transoral resection of retropharyngeal and parapharyngeal neoplasms.

The degree to which TORS will become integrated into the surgeon's armamentarium is unknown, currently the field is in its infancy and its true potential has yet to be realized. As technology advances with smaller instrumentation, integrated suction and drills, and haptic technology, the opportunities to apply TORS will only increase. Both intra-operative and long-term safety warrant further assessment as does cost-benefit analysis. Additionally, telementoring and telesurgery offer the potential to provide improved access to specialty healthcare. Perhaps, the greatest excitement in TORS will be the performance of procedures not currently even conceived.

REFERENCES

1. Menon M, Tewari A, Peabody JO, Shrivastava A, Kaul S, Bhandari A, Hemal AK. Vattikuti institute prostatectomy, a technique of robotic radical prostatectomy for management of localized carcinoma of the prostate: experience of over 1100 cases. *Urologic Clinics of North America* 2004; 31(4): 701-17.

2. Tatooles AJ, Pappas PS, Gordon PJ, Slaughter MS. Minimally invasive mitral valve repair using the daVinci robotic system. *Annals of Thoracic Surgery* 2004; 77(6): 1978-82.

3. Hockstein NG, Nolan P, O'Malley BW Jr, Woo YJ. Robotic microlaryngeal surgery: A technical feasibility study using the daVinci® surgical robot and an airway mannequin. *Laryngoscope* 2005; 115(5): 780-5.

4. Hockstein NG, Nolan P, O'Malley BW Jr, Woo YJ. Robot-assisted pharyngeal and laryngeal microsurgery: Results of robotic cadaver dissections. *Laryngoscope* 2005; 115(6): 1003-8.

5. Weed DT, Courey MS, Ossoff RH. Microlaryngoscopy in the difficult surgical exposure: a new microlaryngoscope. *Otolaryngology Head and Neck Surgery;* 1994; 110(2):247-52.

6. Jako GJ. Laryngoscope for microscopic observation, surgery, and photography. The development of an instrument. *Archives of Otolaryngology – Head and Neck Surgery* 1970; 91(2):196-9.

7. Benninger MS. Laryngeal microinstrumentation: a novel design to reduce movement. *Otolaryngology-Head and Neck Surgery* 2003; 129(3):280-3.

8. Thaler ER, Weber RS, Goldberg AN, Weinstein GS. Feasibility and outcome of endoscopic staple-assisted esophagodiverticulostomy for Zenker's diverticulum. *Laryngoscope* 2001; 111(9): 1506-8.

9. Kucharczuk JC, Kaiser LR, Marshall MB. Weerda diverticuloscope: a novel use to remove embedded esophageal foreign bodies. *Annals of Thoracic Surgery* 2003; 76(4): 1276-8.

10. O'Malley BW Jr, Weinstein GS, Hockstein NG. Transoral robotic surgery (TORS): Glottic microsurgery in a canine model. Submitted for publication.

11. McLeod IK, Melder PC. DaVinci robot-assisted excision of a vallecular cyst: A case report. *Ear Nose and Throat Journal* 2005; 84(3): 170-2.

12. Ahlering TE, Woo D, Eichel L, Lee DI, Edwards R, Skarecky DW. Robot-assisted versus open radical prostatectomy: a comparison of one surgeon's outcomes. *Urology* 2004; 63(5): 819-22.

13. Ruurda JP, van Dongen KW, Dries J, Borel Rinkes IH, Broeders IA. Robotic-assisted laparoscopic choledochojejunostomy. *Surgical Endoscopy* 2003; 17(12): 1937-42.

14. Weinstein GS, O'Malley BW Jr, Hockstein NG. Transoral robotic surgery (TORS): Supraglottic laryngectomy in a canine model. *Laryngoscope* 2005; 115(7):1315-9.

15. Oluwasanmi AF, Mal RK. Diathermy epiglottectomy: endoscopic technique. *Journal of Laryngology and Otology* 2001; 115(4):289-92. Review.

16. Carew JF, Ward RF, LaBruna A, Torzilli PA, Schley WS. Effects of scalpel, electrocautery, and CO2 and KTP lasers on wound healing in rat tongues. *Laryngoscope* 1998; 108(3):373-80.

17. Liboon J, Funkhouser W, Terris DJ. A comparison of mucosal incisions made by scalpel, CO2 laser, electrocautery, and constant-voltage electrocautery. *Otolaryngology-Head and Neck Surgery* 1997; 116(3):379-85.

18. Rudert HH, Werner JA, Hoft S. Transoral carbon dioxide laser resection of supraglottic carcinoma. *Annals of Otolaryngology Rhinology and Laryngology* 1999; 108:819-27.

19. Steiner W, Ambrosch P. *Endoscopic Laser Surgery of the Upper Aerodigestive Tract: With Special Emphasis on Cancer Surgery.* 1st edition. Stuttgart, Germany: Georg Thieme Verlag; 2000.

20. Puxeddu R, Pirri S, Bacchi PC, Salis G, Ledda GP. Endoscopic CO2 laser treatment of supraglottic carcinoma. *Acta Otorhinolaryngologica Italica* 2003; 23:459-466.

21. Hockstein NG, Weinstein GS, O'Malley BW Jr. Maintenance of hemostasis in transoral robotic surgery (TORS). *ORL; Journal for Oto-Rhino-Laryngology and its Related Specialties* 2005; 67(4):220-4. Epub 2005; Sep 5.

22. Steiner W, Ambrosch P, Rodel RM, Kron M. Impact of anterior commissure involvement on local control of early glottic carcinoma treated by laser microresection. *Laryngoscope* 2004; 114(8):1485-91.

23. Mirza N, Perloff JR. Submucosal dissection technique for the treatment of benign and premalignant lesions of the vocal folds. *Operative Techniques in Otolaryngology-Head and Neck Surgery* 2003; 14(1): 18-21.

24. Hockstein NG, O'Malley BW Jr, Weinstein GS. Assessment of intra-operative safety in transoral robotic surgery (TORS). *Laryngoscope* 2006; 116: 165-168.

SECTION III

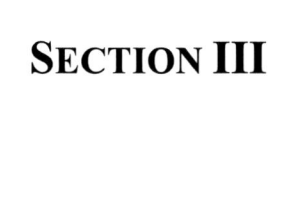

Chapter 15

ROBOTIC SURGERY OF THE UPPER AIRWAYS: ADDRESSING THE CHALLENGES OF DEXTERITY ENHANCEMENT IN CONFINED SPACES

Nabil Simaan[1], Russell H. Taylor[2], Alecxander Hillel[3] and Paul Flint[3]

[1]Department of Mechanical Engineering,
Columbia University, New York, NY USA
[2]Mechanical Engineering, Radiology, Surgery,
Johns Hopkins University, Baltimore, MD USA
[3]Department of Otolaryngology – Head and Neck Surgery,
Johns Hopkins School of Medicine, Baltimore, MD 21287 USA

Abstract

This paper provides an overview of minimally invasive surgery of the throat. After outlining the surgical setup and the currently available instruments, it focuses on the current limitations of throat MIS. The paper addresses the main hurdles impeding surgeons from performing complex surgical MIS procedures inside the throat. These hurdles stem from the strict space limitation coupled with dexterity restrictions as surgeons manipulate multiple (two to three) instruments through a pre-determined single access port, i.e. the laryngoscope. The paper then lists surgical procedures that can benefit from improved dexterity in performing fine suturing, complex tissue manipulation, or fine tissue reconstruction inside the throat. The paper reviews the previous works on dexterity enhancement in MIS. Then it presents a new tele-robotic system designed to aid surgeons in performing complex operations currently very difficult (or impossible) to perform in a MIS of the throat and upper airways. This tele-robotic system uses a novel slave manipulator to operate two to three robotic arms through the laryngoscope. Each robotic arm is equipped with a novel Distal Dexterity Unit (DDU) that supports downsize scalability while providing the required dexterity and forces for surgical tool manipulation. The Distal Dexterity Units (DDU's) are also designed to support multiple functionalities ranging from tissue manipulation and suturing, laser ablation, improving visualization, and delivery of fluids or aspiration. Each distal dexterity unit is composed from a Snake-Like Unit

(SLU) and a Parallel Manipulation Unit (PMU) that provide the necessary dexterity, accuracy, and tool detachment capability. Experiments and simulations on both large scale and small scale SLU present the capabilities of this unit in performing suturing in small confined spaces by using rotation mode about their central backbone. The paper then reviews the current challenges we are facing while developing this robotic system and presents an updated design of the slave robot to answer some of these challenges. Then the paper presents our outline of the planned system.

INTRODUCTION

Minimally Invasive Surgery (MIS) benefits patients with reduced trauma and healing time. For this reason, MIS has gained increasing importance and popularity since its first successful application during the 1980's. The MIS approach allows surgeons to access internal organs of the patient through a limited number of ports through which surgical tasks are performed. *These access ports typically provide access for a single instrument per a port.* While MIS is beneficial to the patient, it presents surgeons with increased difficulties; hence it is often called *minimal access surgery*. Since the surgical tools are constrained to an incision point fixed in space, they possess only 4 Degrees-of-Freedom (DoF) and limited distal dexterity. Added to the limited dexterity, tactile and force sensing are limited or non-existent in most available surgical tools.

To help surgeons in overcoming these difficulties, a large number of robotic devices and systems have been developed [1-4]. An updated comprehensive review of these systems, and others, was given in [5] and an outline of the challenges of MIS and the potential applications of robotics for MIS in [6]. The early stages of robotic-assisted surgery focused on well defined problems of orthopedic surgery where the integration of pre-operative imaging, registration and tracking of surgical devices, and surgical robotic devices was used to improve orthopedic surgical procedures [3, 7-10]. Robotic and computer-assisted MIS mainly focused on laparoscopy [1, 2, 11-19]. All these works formed substantial advances in applications of MIS beneficial to surgeons. Despite these developments, current robotic instruments are still too large and/or have insufficient dexterity for many surgical domains. Minimally invasive surgery of the throat and the upper airways is an example of such a surgical domain. In all surgical procedures exceeding the capabilities of current MIS tools/robots, surgeons must resort to open surgery, exposing the patient to otherwise an avoidable trauma and prolonged post-operative pain had they had the adequate tools. The following section reviews the clinical setup of MIS of the throat and lists the challenges hindering the implementation of current hand-held and robotic devices for operations on the throat and the upper airways.

MINIMALLY INVASIVE SURGERY OF THE THROAT AND UPPER AIRWAYS: HISTORY, CURRENT SETUP AND CHALLENGES

The upper airway is a long, narrow, and irregularly shaped organ that includes the pharynx (throat), hypopharynx, and larynx, commonly referred to as the voice box. These areas are subject to a variety of benign and malignant growths, paralysis, and scar tissue formation requiring surgical interventions for excision and/or reconstruction. These procedures (e.g. partial or total laryngectomy, vocal fold repositioning, and laryngotracheal reconstruction) are routinely performed using open surgical techniques on the expense of damaging the integrity of the framework supporting the laryngeal cartilage, muscle, and the connective tissue vital to normal function. Minimally invasive endoscopic procedures are generally preferred over open procedures, thereby, preserving laryngeal framework integrity, promoting faster recovery and frequently overcoming the need for tracheostomy. Open surgery of the larynx provides good exposure and dexterity of instrumentation; however, healthy tissue, especially the delicate framework of the larynx, is often damaged on the approach. In contrast, endoscopic laryngeal surgery utilizes natural body openings and therefore minimizes resultant damage.

The history of endoscopic laryngeal surgery spans almost a century. In 1915 Lynch first reported the use of a laryngoscope for excision of glottic cancer [20]. Lynch's use of suspension laryngoscopy enhanced the endoscopic approach by allowing for bimanual operation of instruments. Four decades later Rosemarie Albrecht described using a microscope to examine the larynx [21]. Laryngeal microsurgery was introduced in the early 1960's by Jako and Kleinsasser [22-24], which advanced laryngeal surgery by magnifying and illuminating the operator's view as well as providing depth perception with binocular vision. Microlaryngeal scissors, graspers, grippers, mirrors, elevators and suction devices evolved to accompany this new operative approach. A decade later Strong and Jako merged the carbon dioxide laser with the operating microscope to add a new tool to the endoscopic laryngologist's armamentarium [25, 26]. Since that time, lasers have been refined with the microspot laser and microlaryngeal instruments have been miniaturized. Recently a powered microdebrider has been introduced in an attempt to lessen the operative time of and thermal damage caused by the laser [27, 28].

Other than these few advancements endoscopic laryngeal surgery has evolved little in the past thirty years. Laryngologists remain restricted by the operator's distance from the surgical field, the laryngoscope's relatively small exposure, and reduced depth perception with binocular vision. These combine to restrict the surgeon's ability to manipulate instruments across the long distance from the oral cavity to the larynx resulting in poor sensory feedback (both visual and tactile) and magnification of the operator tremor. While microsurgical instruments have been miniaturized they otherwise remain unchanged. They still have long handles and lack maneuverability at the distal end of the instrument. The lack of distal freedom often results in damage to surrounding healthy tissue and limits healing from surgical trauma in endoscopic laryngeal surgery. Though Woo and Buess established distinct laryngeal endosuture techniques, suture repair of vocal fold wounds remains challenging and has yet to be accepted due to technical complexities and increase in operative time [29, 30]. The inability to suture such wounds results in larger scar formation. A recent study by

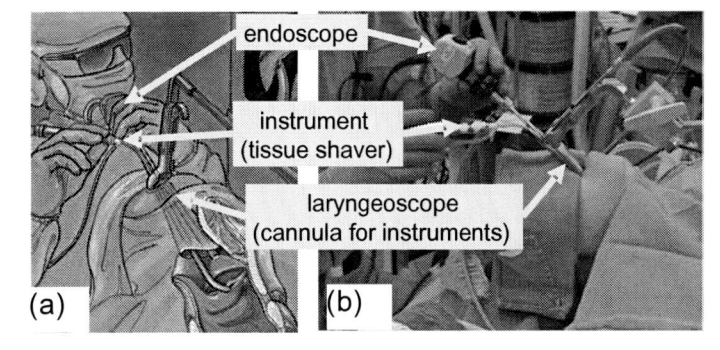

Figure 1. A typical surgical setup for MIS of the throat (a) artist rendering (b) actual surgical setup

Fleming et al. demonstrated a 75% larger scar area when laryngeal defects healed with secondary intention vs. primary intention [31]. A larger scar, likely due to unhindered collagen deposition results in worse voice outcomes. At this time endoscopic laryngeal surgery has reached an impasse as the lack of distal instrument mobility, complexity of suture technique and poor three-dimensional (3D) viewing field limit surgical techniques that are routine in other surgical subspecialties.

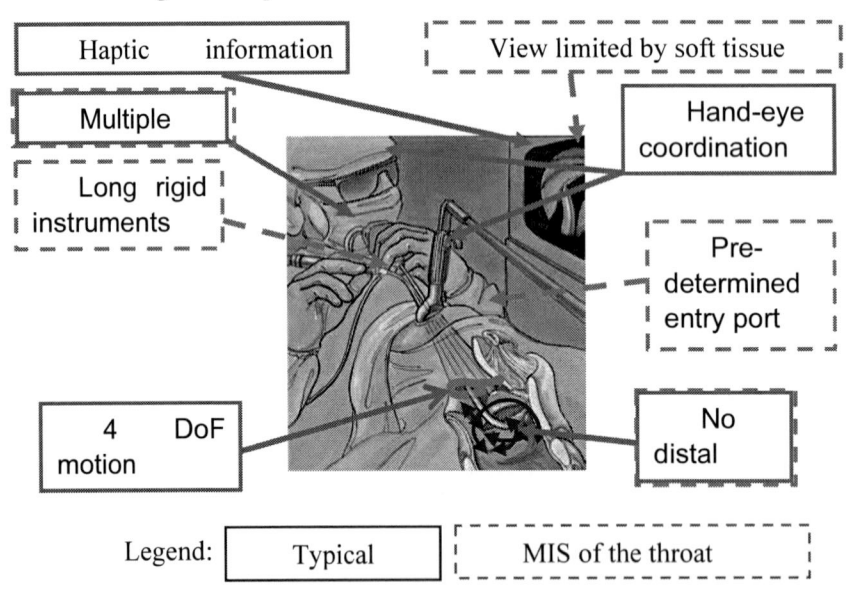

Figure 2. Limitations of MIS of the throat compared to typical MIS

Figure 1 shows a typical MIS setup for endoscopic laryngeal surgery. The internal regions of the airway are accessed by using an array of long instruments (usually ranging between 240 to 350 mm long) through a laryngoscope that is inserted into the patient's mouth and serves as a visualization tool and a guide for surgical instrumentation. The laryngoscope is typically 180 mm long with an oval cross-section usually ranging between 16-20 mm in width at its smallest cross section. This surgical setup requires the surgeon to manipulate several long tools (for example one tool for suction and another for tissue manipulation) that are constrained to 4 DoF motions and lacking tool-tip dexterity. *For these limitations, laryngeal MIS is currently* **limited to simple operations** *such as microflap elevation, excisional biopsies, and removal of pappiloma using laser or powered microdebrider.* Functional reconstructive procedures (e.g. tissue flap rotation or suturing), are not performed in throat MIS; although, reconstruction of the vocal fold structures as accurately as possible is crucial for maintaining the voice characteristics. Suture closure of surgical defects has been shown to reduce scar tissue, shorten healing time, and result in improved laryngeal function and sound production [29, 31]. This seemingly simple operation is very difficult, if not impossible, to perform in laryngeal MIS. *Our current work addresses these needs by developing a tele-robotic system to allow surgeons to perform complex functional reconstruction tasks and suturing in MIS of the upper airway.*

Figure 2 summarizes the additional limitations that MIS of the throat and the upper airways compared to typical laparoscopy. *The main challenging aspect of MIS of the throat is the requirement to manipulate multiple tools through a pre-determined narrow single access port, i.e. the laryngoscope.* This limits both the space available for the surgical tools, their workspace, and their dexterity. In order to enable surgeons to perform complex surgical operations and tissue reconstructive procedures, a significant improvement in distal dexterity of the surgical tools is necessary. This requires a new generation of dexterous, yet small, surgical instrument carriers that are capable of performing the most important operation for tissue reconstruction, i.e. suturing.

DEXTERITY ENHANCEMENT IN MINIMALLY INVASIVE SURGERY

Since distal dexterity of surgical tools is a necessary enabler for complex operations in MIS [32] (e.g. suturing), it received considerable attention from the research community [1, 19, 33-56]. The works dealing with distal dexterity enhancement in MIS included planar and spatial linkages [38, 42], parallel wrists [39-41], serial articulated wrists [1, 19, 36, 37], and more recently snake-like devices [34, 35, 37, 42-46, 48, 49] to allow surgeons to control the orientation of surgical tools. Distal dexterity improvement was investigated in robotic systems for laparoscopy [1, 18, 19, 33, 38, 49], arthroscopy [43], gastro-intestinal surgery [44-46], neurosurgery [35, 36], fetal surgery [34], Microsurgery [47], and is currently being developed by us [50-54] and by Ikuta et al. [35] for ENT surgery. Recently, Weinstein et al. [57] demonstrated the use of the 8mm da-Vinci instruments on a canine model for partial laryngectomy. The actuation methods for these devices included wire actuation [1, 19, 33-37, 49], hydraulic actuation [40], shape memory alloy actuation [43], mechanical actuation through linkages [38, 55], gear transmission [42], embedded miniature electromechanical motors [56], and recently we used push-pull actuation using flexible super-elastic members [50-52]. Despite this large number of works dealing with dexterity enhancement in MIS, a small number of commercial tele-robotic systems uses distal dexterity wrists. The da-Vinci system by Intuitive-Surgical has a wide array of distal dexterity wrists used for MIS with designs based on wire actuated devices stemming from [1]. Distal dexterity enhancement had also many other applications in active bending catheters and endoscopes that are not included here since our focus is on distal dexterity enhancement for surgical tool manipulation.

Wrists for dexterity enhancement offered a solution to the distal dexterity problem and proved to be successful in supporting suturing in laparoscopy [19, 58]. However, it was shown in [33] that certain wrist designs are optimal for shallow suturing approach angles (as in thoracoscopy) while other wrist designs are suitable for steep approach angles (as in laparoscopy) and in [59] that snake-like devices offer better dexterity than articulated wrists. It is was also shown that it is beneficial to optimize the location of the access ports in MIS to ensure optimal performance [60-62]. In MIS of the throat, the entry port is pre-determined (the laryngoscope), hence the requirement for distal dexterity enhancement and size reduction of tools were the main guiding principle in the design of our robotic slave for throat MIS. *For these reasons we focused on developing highly dexterous, down-scalable, distal dexterity units that use a combination of a snake-like unit a micro-parallel wrist at its tip.*

PREVIOUS WORKS AND APPLICATIONS OF DEXTERITY ENHANCEMENT IN MINIMALLY INVASIVE LARENGEAL SURGERY

Minimally invasive robotic surgery has the potential to significantly advance laryngeal surgery. As early as 1997, Plinkert recognized the need for steerable modular instruments with increased degrees of freedom and 3D viewing [30] to improve distal dexterity and facilitate laryngeal suturing. Independently steerable arms and 3D imaging were incorporated in the da Vinci Surgical Robot (Intuitive Surgical, Sunnyvale, CA). In 2005 the first accounts in the literature describe testing the technical feasibility of the da Vinci surgical robot on a mannequin and cadavers [63, 64]. Hockstein et al. reported an increase in freedom of instrument mobility, improved depth perception with the 3D imaging, scaling of movement (from the large movement of operators hand to the small movement of instrument), and removal of tremor. McLeod and Melder reported the first robotic-assisted surgery with the da Vinci system to remove a vallecular cyst [65]. During operation with the robot, both groups reported limited access through the laryngoscope/mouth gag resulting in instrument crowding and a lack of suction device included in the robot. Hockstein et al. reported increased instrument access through the mouth gag – a device that retracts the mouth and controls the tongue with a blade [63]. However, it appears that the procedure is performed with a wide angle between instruments causing a technically complex and awkward operation. These concerns have been remedied in the new generation of the da Vinci robot and should result in an integrated suction device, increased distal dexterity and instrument maneuverability.

A robot with the ability to maneuver in a tight space with multiple instruments would have wide utility in laryngeal surgery and other surgical fields. This system would facilitate resection of small lesions, such as papillomas or carcinomas, and suture repair of the wound. An efficient and accurate suturing method would additionally improve the repair of laryngeal microflaps and glottic web flaps. Further utility would be seen in repair of tracheo-esophageal fistulas and laryngeal clefts, endoscopic positioning of arytenoids, medialization and lateralization procedures, and refine endoscopic cricoid split procedures for airway expansion [66]. Outside of laryngology, a multi-armed robotic system would have utility in

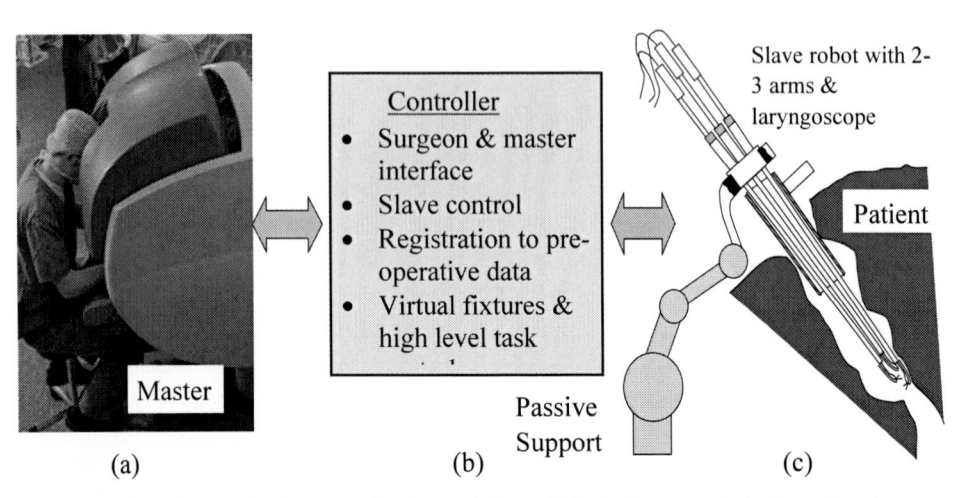

Figure 3. The tele-surgical system for throat MIS will include a novel design of a slave robot equipped with 2-3 arms and small distal dexterity units.

microsurgical procedures at the base of the skull, sinus surgery, single port gastrointestinal and thoracic access surgery, and microvascular anatamoses.

OUTLINE OF OUR SYSTEM FOR MIS OF THE THROAT

Figure 3 presents the system we are currently developing for throat MIS. This system has the same master-slave architecture as the da-Vinci® [1] or any other tele-surgical robot. The specialized component in this system is the slave robot, which is custom-designed for throat surgery. Figure 3-(c) presents the initial concept for this slave robot presented in [50]. It is a three-armed robot working through a laryngeoscope equipped with a standard endoscope. The detailed concept for this slave robot is shown in figure 4. Our concept includes a standard laryngoscope, a base link, two similar Distal Dexterity Units (DDU's) for tool/tissue manipulation, and another DDU for suction. Each DDU is a 5 DoF hybrid robot mounted on a corresponding DDU holder, which is manipulated by a corresponding 4 DoF tool manipulation unit (TMU) that controls the angle of approach, the rotation about, and the position along the axis of the DDU holder. The TMU's are mounted on a rotating base unit (RBU) permitting the system to be oriented within the throat so as to minimize collisions between DDU holders. The DDU holders are thin tubes (about 4.2 mm in outside diameter) providing an actuation pathway for the DDU and possibly a light-source or a suction channel. Each TMU is equipped with a fast clamping device for adjusting the axial location of the DDU. The actuation unit of each DDU is located at its upper extremity and the actuation is by super-elastic tubes operated in push-pull mode [51, 52]. Overall, our system is designed to have 34 actuated DoF for the robotic slave since each DDU has 7 actuated joints and each TMU has 4 actuated DoF.

The actuation unit of each DDU is 74 mm in diameter and 150 mm in height, Fig. 5. It is equipped with standard encoders for control purposes and with an additional set of absolute position high-accuracy potentiometers. This allows easy "homing" ("home configuration" is a

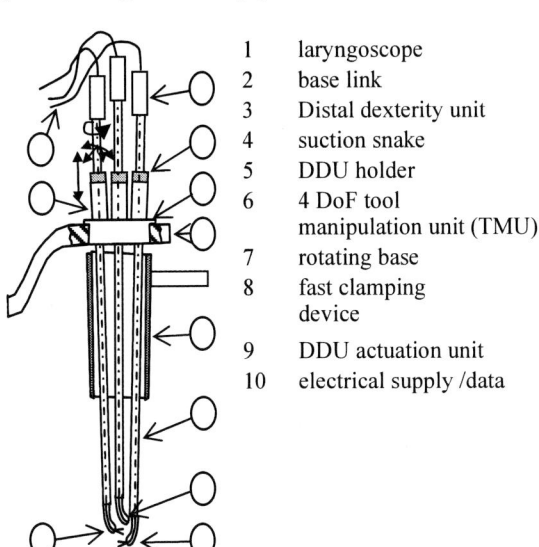

1	laryngoscope
2	base link
3	Distal dexterity unit
4	suction snake
5	DDU holder
6	4 DoF tool manipulation unit (TMU)
7	rotating base
8	fast clamping device
9	DDU actuation unit
10	electrical supply /data

Figure 4. The initial concept for a three-armed slave robot for throat surgery.

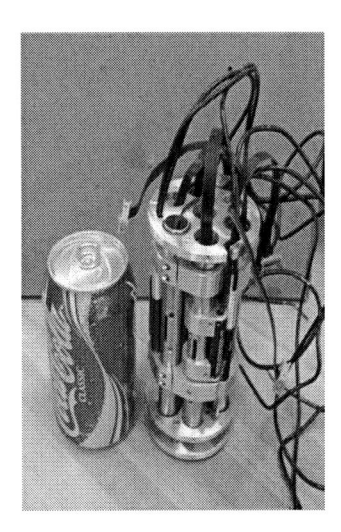

Figure 5. The actuation unit for the DDU has 7 actuated joints and provides actuation redundancy for the 5 DoF DDU.

pre-determined calibrated configuration used as a reference position for control) of the DDU's and provides fail-safe features to our system. The system also uses custom-designed low power DC motor control cards that provide both velocity control, current control and monitoring, [53]. This allows us to measure the joint actuation forces and provides intrinsic force sensing capabilities that will provide the force applied by the DDU on its environment without adding force external sensors to our system.

The size of the actuation unit of Fig. 5, the space limitations imposed by the laryngoscope, and the undesirable flexibility of the long and thin DDU holders led us to change the initial design in Fig. 4 to another design alternative that allows collision avoidance between the two robotic arms operating through a laryngoscope, Fig. 6-(a) (although our eventual goal is 3 arms to be used in surgery, we will conduct the initial validation experiments using 2 arms only). Simulations of two robotic arms operating through a laryngoscope showed that it is better to use a staggered arrangement of the actuation units as shown in figure 6-(a). The design shown in Fig. 6 is one design alternative that is being compared to other design alternatives in terms of feasibility, simplicity, compactness, dexterity, and collision minimization between the robotic arms. Each robotic arm in Fig. 6-(a) is manipulated by a planar 5-bar mechanism with two actuated prismatic actuators. The planar 5-bar mechanisms carry a 2 DoF z-θ stage that rotates/translates the robotic arms about/along the axis of the DDU holder. The z-θ stages are connected to the five-bar mechanism through a passive universal-joint that allows tilting the axis of the DDU holder in any direction. The robotic arms are attached to the z-θ stages through fast locking mechanism. To provide support to the long and thing DDU holders, we will equip the laryngoscope with an internal rubber disk that serves as a fulcrum point for the DDU holders, Fig. 6-(b). By using this rubber disk and the passive universal joint a *passive RCM* (Remote Center of Motion) similar to the one used in AESOP robot [2] is achieved.

The planned surgical setup is illustrated in Fig. 7-(a). The slave robot will be positioned with respect to the patient in the same way the surgeon positions himself with respect to the patient, Fig. 7-(b). Visualization will initially be provided through standard endoscopes that will be fixed to the laryngoscope. The surgeon will be able to intervene and retract the robotic arms outside of the laryngoscope by using the fast clamping device on the z-θ stage. The manipulation of the snake-like units and the parallel manipulation units will be achieved through a smart haptic interface that receives the motion commands to move the surgical tool and resolves the required joint motions for the system to optimize dexterity and avoid joint limits and collisions among instruments and between the instruments and anatomy. Virtual fixtures will be implemented based on the linearized optimization framework presented in [54, 67].

In the authors' opinion the Lindholm laryngoscope[Karl Storz; Tuttlingen, Germany] provides the slave robot the best access to the supraglottis and glottis. The Lindholm's large opening allows space for instrument placement and excellent workspace within the glottis. For operating at the level of the glottis or below the Bouchayer laryngoscope [Micro-France; Bourbon L'Archambault, France] provides better lateral dimension of scope for superior instrument access and maneuverability.

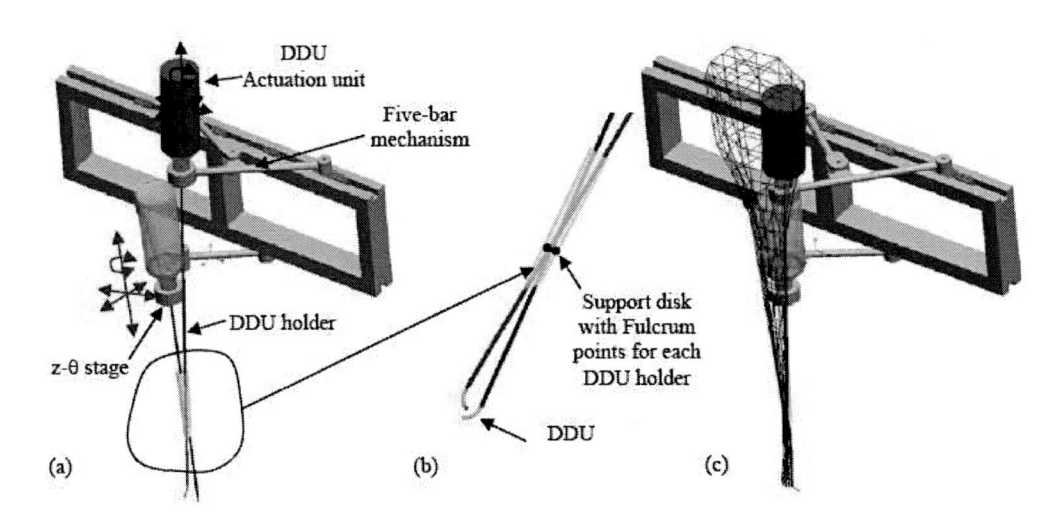

Figure 6. A design alternative for a slave robot with two robotic arms in a staggered configuration (a) the design uses passive RCM design with the center of motion fixed along the axis of the laryngoscope (b) the 4 DoF TMU is an optimized five bar with a workspace corresponding to the limitations of the laryngoscope (c).

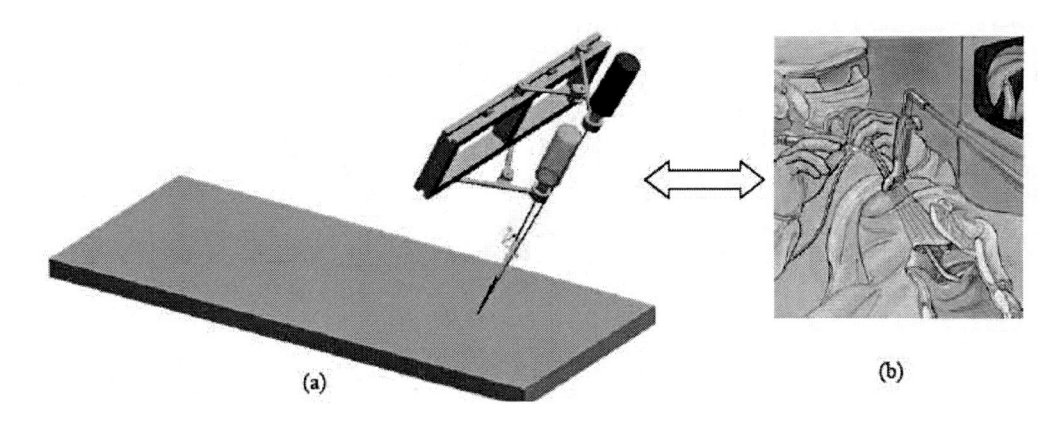

Figure 7. The robotic slave will be assembled above the patient bed in an orientation identical to the current manual surgical setup.

THE DISTAL DEXTERITY UNITS

The main enabling component in out system is the Distal Dexterity Units (DDU's), Fig 8. The DDU is composed from a 2 DoF Snake-Like Unit (SLU) and a 3 DoF detachable Parallel Manipulation Unit (PMU) attached at its tip, Fig. 8. It is designed to bypass obstacles (such as the vocal folds) and to perform suturing by transforming the rotation of the DDU holder about its axis into rotation about the axis of its central backbone. The DDU provides global dexterity by using the bending SNU and local dexterity by using the 3DoF PMU unit which

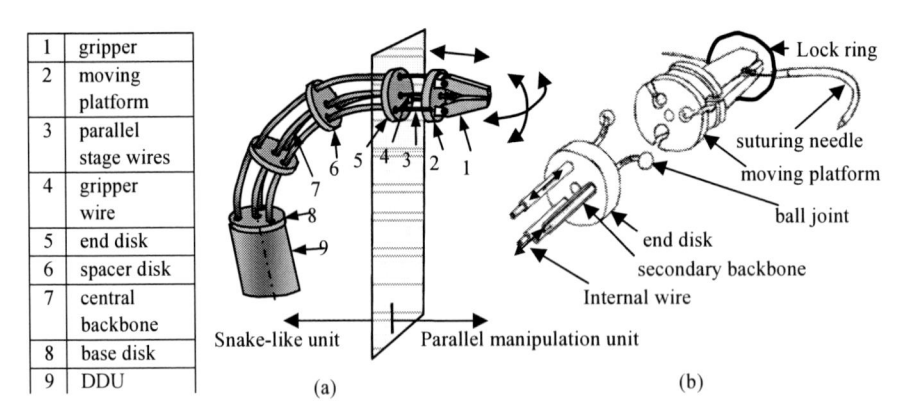

1	gripper
2	moving platform
3	parallel stage wires
4	gripper wire
5	end disk
6	spacer disk
7	central backbone
8	base disk
9	DDU

Figure 8. (a) The DDU (Distal Dexterity Unit) is composed from a snake-like unit and a detachable parallel manipulation unit (b) detachable parallel manipulation unit for precise wrist-like and axial motions; and surgical tool interchangeability.

acts as a high precision wrist at the tip of the SNU. This arrangement provides the gripper with nine DoF since the DDU has 5 DoF and it is mounted on a DDU holder manipulated by a 4 DoF PMU. This kinematic redundancy will be used to provide the required dexterity inside the throat while performing obstacle avoidance among the robotic arms.

The design of the SNU relies on a novel, yet simple concept that uses multiple flexible backbones for actuation and for structural rigidity required from a device for surgical tool manipulation, Fig. 8-(a). This 2 DoF robot is composed from a base disk, an end disk, several spacer disks, and four super-elastic NiTi tubes. These tubes are called the *backbones* of this SLU. The central tube is the *primary backbone* while the remaining three tubes are called the *secondary backbones*. The secondary backbones are equidistant from the central backbone and from one another. The central backbone is attached to both the base and end disks and to all spacer disks while the secondary backbones are attached only to the end disk and are free to slide and bend through properly dimensioned holes in the base and spacer disks. These secondary backbones are used for actuating this snake-like device and they pass through guiding channels in the DDU holder to allow their actuation in both push and pull modes. The spacer disks prevent buckling of the central and secondary backbones and keep an equal distance between them.

The snake-like unit is designed to support multiple secondary functions beside its main function as a distal dexterity enhancement device. Its design has several advantages over other designs (e.g. [1, 19, 33-39, 41-56] that use discrete backbones (articulated serial chains). By using flexible backbones, the dependency on small universal joints and wires is removed. This reduces production costs and enhances downsize scalability. The use of tubes for the backbones provides a secondary application for them as suction channels, actuation channels for the tool mounted on the SLU distal end or as a source of light for imaging. By using three push-pull secondary backbones for actuation, it is possible to implement redundancy resolutions that satisfy the static balance of the structure while preventing buckling of the backbones as was proposed in [51, 52]. This further enhances the downsize scalability while maintaining the force application capability of these SLU's on a level large enough for tool manipulation for delicate tasks (1-2 Newton). This actuation redundancy also provides the option of "stiffness modulation", [68-70], of the DDU's.

The SLU is designed to bend sideways ±90° in any direction to provide 2 DoF for distal dexterity. By controlling 2 out of the three secondary backbones, we have demonstrated a bending capability of more than 70° in any direction [50], Fig. 9. To enhance it with surgical tool interchangeability and additional precise wrist action and axial motion, we are currently designing and constructing the detachable parallel unit of Fig. 8-(b). The parallel mechanical architecture has been chosen for providing precise and high-accuracy motions in a small workspace while utilizing its inherent rigidity and high payload to-weight ratio [15, 71, 72]. The detachable milli-parallel unit is constructed from super-elastic links passing through the secondary backbones, spherical joints, and a moving platform to which a gripper is affixed, Fig. 8-(b). The moving platform is machined with matching groves such that the balls affixed to the end of the actuation wires match its diameter and a fast locking mechanism is used to secure them to the moving platform. We are currently constructing one possible embodiment of this parallel manipulation unit as shown in Fig. 10. The size of this gripper is 5.4×4.4×9.3 mm. The gripper geometry was optimized to provide 40 N of needle gripping force while using a 0.4 mm NiTi wire for actuation. The parallel manipulation unit is currently being designed to supply *local dexterity* at the tip of the snake. Our goal is to provide ±20° tilting in any direction using this parallel manipulation tip.

There are two possible operation modes using the detachable milli-parallel unit. In the first operation mode, the actuation wires are used only to extend axially in order to attach a new moving platform equipped

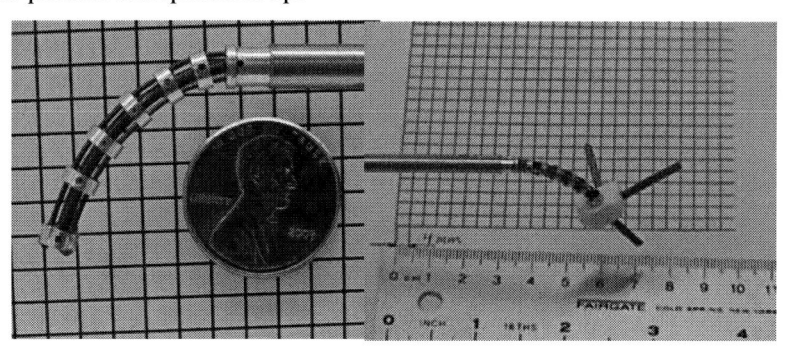

Figure 9. The SNU demonstrating it bending capabilities using two out of three available secondary backbones.

with another tool. Once the tool is attached, then the actuation wires are retracted to secure the moving platform to the end disk of the SLU. In the other mode, for operations requiring small workspace and fine motions, the actuation wires are used to actuate the moving platform of the parallel manipulation unit as a three DoF parallel platform with flexible extensible links. We are also considering another alternative design for this parallel manipulation unit for small-diameter DDU's. This design sacrifices detachability for downsize scalability by eliminating the spherical joints in Fig. 10 and relying completely on the flexibility of the super-elastic links for manipulating the moving platform. A first prototype showing the actuation unit assembled to the snake-like units is shown in Fig. 11. This prototype is currently being used for verification of force application capabilities and redundancy resolution algorithms aiming at optimizing the loads on the backbones of the snake-like unit [51, 52]. Figure 12 demonstrates controlled rotation about the axis of the DDU. When this rotation is coupled with a reverse rotation of the DDU holder (Fig. 4), the tip of the snake-like unit remains stationary in space while the rotation of the DDU holder is translated into rotation about the axis normal to the end disk of the snake-like unit. This rotation about the central backbone is important for suturing in confined spaces. Figure 13 demonstrates this operation mode for suturing on a large-scale snake-like unit [51, 54].

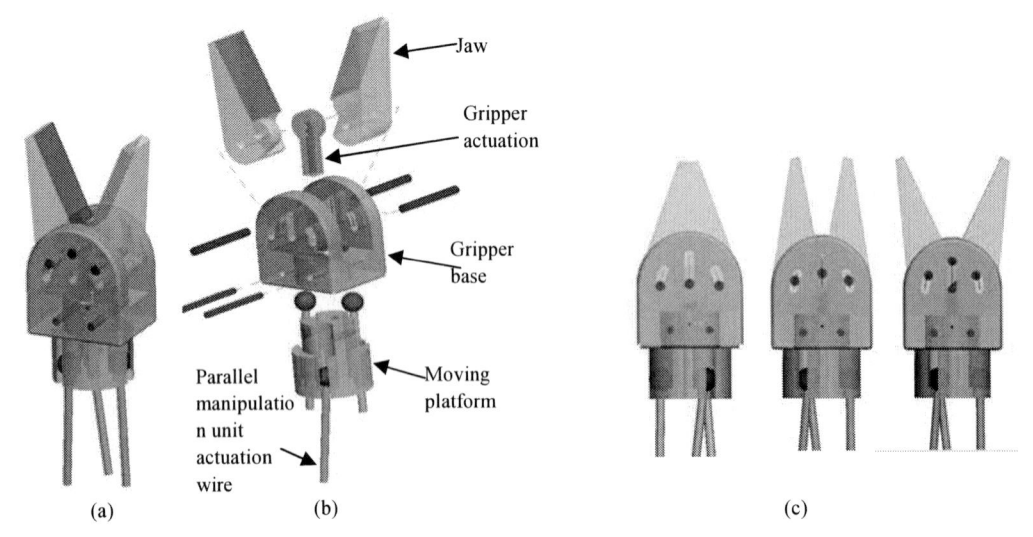

Figure 10. Detachable gripper with the moving platform of the Parallel Manipulation Unit (PMU) (a), exploded view (b), this design minimizes the required gripper actuation force (c).

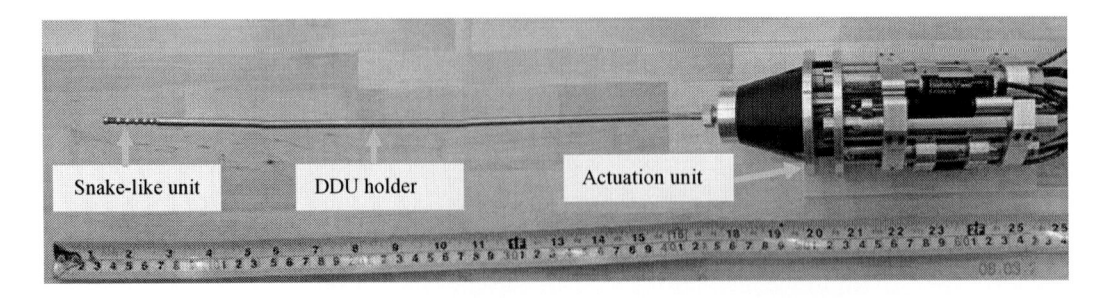

Figure 11. A first prototype of the snake-like unit attached to the actuation unit of the DDU.

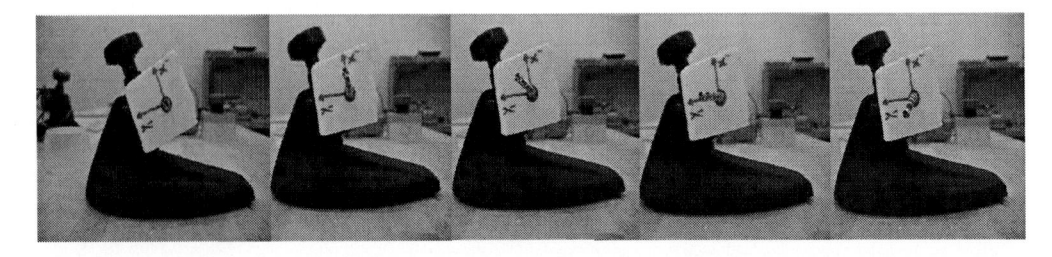

Figure 12. Movie screen shots of the 4 mm SLU demonstrating controlled rotations about the axis of the DDU holder.

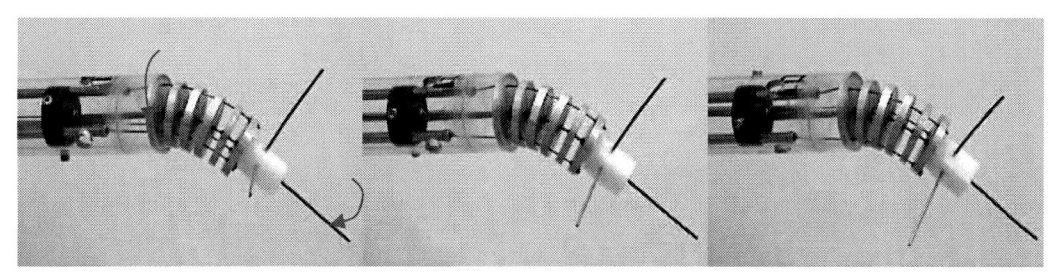

Figure 13. A large-scale snake-like unit performing rotation about its central backbone. This mode of operation is useful for suturing in confined spaces.

CONCLUSION

This paper presented our up-to-date work on designing a high dexterity, high accuracy slave for tele-operated minimally invasive surgery of the throat. The slave robot is capable of simultaneously manipulating up to three surgical tools through a laryngoscope. This system is designed to allow tissue reconstruction of the vocal folds and suturing tasks - currently extremely difficult to perform in a minimally invasive approach.

The main unit of this slave is an eleven DoF DDU (Distal Dexterity Unit) composed from a snake-like unit and a detachable parallel wrist that provides surgical tool exchangeability. The design of the snake-like unit was presented. This unit uses multiple super-elastic tubes as flexible backbones actuated in push-pull modes. This design provides future downsize scalability and manufacturing simplicity that allow constructing surgical tool manipulators with diameters smaller than 5 mm. The DDU is composed from a snake-like unit and a parallel manipulation unit. It provides global dexterity using the snake-like unit and localized dexterity using the parallel manipulation unit, which serves as a wrist at the tip of the snake. The DDU is designed to be simple, down-scalable, and disposable to save repetitive sterilization cost and time.

We expect this system to provide surgeons with suturing capabilities, accurate tissue reconstruction, and to open new possibilities for surgeries that are currently performed in an open surgical approach. The surgical procedures in throat MIS that will benefit from this system include any procedure benefiting from the provided tool-tip dexterity (e.g. partial or total laryngectomy, vocal fold repositioning, resection of small lesions (such as papillomas or carcinomas), and suture repair and laryngotracheal reconstruction. Our future plans include integrating this slave robot with a standard master interface such as the da-Vinci master to evaluate the performance of this system. The benchmark procedure to be initially used for performance evaluation is suturing inside a phantom model of a human larynx.

ACKNOWLEDGEMENTS

This work was partially funded by the National Science Foundation (NSF) under Engineering Research Center grant #EEC9731478, NSF grant #IIS9801684, and by the

National Institutes of Health (NIH) under grant #R21 EB004457-01 and by the Johns Hopkins University internal funds.

REFERENCES

1. Guthart, G. and K. Salisbury, "The Intuitive™ Telesurgery System: Overview and Application," presented at IEEE International Conference on Robotics and Automation, pp. 618-621, 2000.

2. Sackier, J. M. and Y. Wang, "Robotically assisted laparoscopic surgery from concept to development," *Surgical Endoscopy*, vol. 8, pp. 63-66, 1994.

3. Taylor, R., H. A. Paul, P. Kazanzides, B. D. Mittestadt, W. Hanson, J. F. Zuhars, B. Williamson, B. L. Mustits, E. Glassman, and W. L. Bargar, "An image-directed robotic system for precise orthopedic surgery," *IEEE Transactions on Robotics and Automation*, vol. 10, pp. 261-275, 1994.

4. Ghodoussi, M., S. E. Bunter, and Y. Wang, "Robotic Surgery - the Trans-Atlantic Case," presented at IEEE International Conference on Robotics and Automation, pp. 1882-1888, 2002.

5. Taylor, R. and D. Stianovici, "Medical Robotics in Computer-Integrated Surgery," *IEEE Transactions on Robotics and Automation*, vol. 19, pp. 765-781, 2003.

6. Tendick, F., S. Sastry, R. Fearing, and M. Cohn, "Applications of Microelectromechanics in Minimally Invasive Surgery," *IEEE/ASME Transactions on Mechatronics*, vol. 3, pp. 34-42, 1998.

7. Fadda, M., D. Bertelli, S. Martelli, M. Marcacci, P. Dario, C. Pagetti, D. Caramella, and D. Trippi, "Computer Assisted Planning for Total Knee Arthoplasty," in *Lecture Notes in Computer Science (LNCS)*, vol. 1205, J. Troccaz, E. Grimson, and R. Mosges, Eds.: Springer, pp. 619-628. 1997.

8. Leitner, F., F. Picard, R. Minefelde, H.-J. Schultz, P. Cinquin, and D. Saragaglia, "Computer-Assisted Knee Surgical Total Replacement," in *Lecture Notes in Computer Science (LNCS)*, vol. 1205, J. Troccaz, E. Grimson, and R. Mosges, Eds.: Springer, pp. 629-. 1997.

9. Harris, S. J., W. J. Lin, R. D. Hibberd, J. Cobb, R. Middelton, and B. L. Davies, "Experiences with Robotic Systems for Knee Surgery," in *Lecture Notes in Computer Science (LNCS)*, vol. 1205, J. Troccaz, E. Grimson, and R. Mosges, Eds.: Springer, pp. 757-766. 1997.

10. Brandt, G., K. Radermacher, S. Lavallee, H.-W. Staudte, and G. Rau, "A Compact Robot for Image Guided Orthopedic Surgery: Concept and preliminary Results," in *Lecture Notes in Computer Science (LNCS)*, vol. 1205, J. Troccaz, E. Grimson, and R. Mosges, Eds.: Springer, pp. 629-. 1997.

11. Rovetta, A., R. Sala, F. Cosmi, X. Wen, D. Sabbadini, S. Milanesi, A. Togno, L. Angelini, and A. Bejczy, "First experiment in the world of robotic telesurgery for laparoscopy carried out by means of satellites networks and optical fibres networks on 7th July 1993," presented at *IECON Proceedings (Industrial Electronics Conference), Plenary Session: Emerging Technologies, and Factory Automation*, pp. 51-56, 1993.

12. Taylor, R., J. Funda, B. Eldridge, S. Gomory, K. Gurben, D. LaRose, M. Talamini, L. Kavoussi, and J. Anderson, "A Telerobotics Assistant for Laparoscopic Surgery," *IEEE Engineering in Medicine and Biology Magazine*, vol. 14, pp. 279-288, 1995.

13. Finlay, P. A. and M. H. Ornstein, "Controlling the Movement of a Surgical Laparascope," *IEEE Engineering In Medicine and Biology*, pp. 289-291, 1995.

14. Shoham, M., S. Goldberger, M. Roffman, and N. N. Simaan, "Robot Construction for Surgery," presented at First Israeli Symposium on Computer-Aided Surgery, Medical Robotics, and Medical Imaging (ISRACAS'98), Technion City, Haifa, Israel, pp., 1998.

15. Simaan, N. and M. Shoham, "Robot Construction for Surgical Applications," presented at The 1st IFAC Conference on Mechatronic Systems, Darmstadt, Germany, pp. 553-558, 2000.

16. Bunter, S. E. and M. Ghodoussi, "Transforming a Surgical Robot for Human Telesurgery," *IEEE Transactions on Robotics and Automation*, vol. 19, pp. 819-824, 2003.

17. Munoz, V. F., C. Vara-Throbeck, J. G. DeGabriel, J. F. Lozano, E. Sachez-Badahoz, A. Garcia-Cerozo, R. Toscano, and A. Jimenez-Garrido, "A Medical Robotic Assistant for Minimally Invasive Surgery," presented at IEEE International Conference on Robotics and Automation, pp., 2000.

18. Cavusoglu, M. C., M. Cohn, F. Tendick, and S. Sastry, "A Laparascopic telesurgical workstation," *IEEE Transactions on Robotics and Automation*, vol. 15, pp. 728-739, 1999.

19. Madhani, A. J., G. Niemeyer, and K. Salisbury, "The Black Falcon: A Teleoperated Surgical Instrument for Minimally Invasive Surgery," presented at IEEE/RSJ International Conference on Intelligent Robots and Systems (IROS), pp. 936-944, 1998.

20. Lynch, R. C., "Suspension laryngoscopy and its accomplishments," *Ann Otol Rhinol Laryngol*, vol. 24, pp. 429-478, 1915.

21. von-Leden, H., "Microlaryngoscopy: a historical vignette," *J Voice*, vol. 1, pp. 341-346, 1988.

22. Jako, G., "Laryngoscope for microscopic observation, surgery, and photography: the development of an instrument.," *Arch Otolaryngol*, vol. 91, pp. 196-9, 1970.

23. Kleinsasser, O., "*Microlaryngoscopy and endolaryngeal microsurgery*," Stell PM, trans., 1979.

24. Kleinsasser, O., "Microsurgery of the larynx" *Arch Ohren Nasen Kehlkopfheilkd*, vol. 183, pp. 428-3, 1964.

25. Jako, G., "Laser surgery of the vocal cords. An experimental study with carbon dioxide lasers on dogs.," *Laryngoscope*, vol. 82, pp. 2204-16, 1972.

26. Strong, M. and G. Jako, "Laser surgery in the larynx. Early clinical experience with continuous CO 2 laser.," *Ann Otol Rhinol Laryngol*, vol. 81, pp. 791-8., 1972.

27. Myer, C., J. Willging, S. McMurray, and R. Cotton, "Use of a laryngeal micro resector system.," *Laryngoscope*, vol. 109, pp. 1165-6, 1999.

28. Patel, N., M. Rowe, and D. A. O. R. L. Tunkel, "Treatment of recurrent respiratory papillomatosis in children with the microdebrider," vol. 112, pp. 7-10, 2003.

29. Woo, P., J. Casper, B. Griffin, R. Colton, and C. Brewer, "Endoscopic Microsuture Repair of Vocal Fold Defects," *J. Voice*, vol. 9, pp. 332-339, 1995.

30. Plinkert, P. and H. Lowenheim, "Trends and perspectives in minimally invasive surgery in Otorhinolaryngology-Head and Neck Surgery," *Laryngoscope*, vol. 107, pp. 1483-9, 1997.

31. Fleming, D. J., S. McGuff, and C. B. Simpson, "Comparison of Microflap Healing Outcomes with Traditional and Microsuturing Techniques: Initial Results in a Canine Model," *Ann Otol Rhinol Laryngol.*, vol. 110, pp. 707-712, 2001.

32. Charles, S., "Dexterity Enhancement for Surgery," R. H. Taylor, S. Lavallee, G. C. Burdea, and R. Mosges, Eds. Cambridge, MA: MIT Press, pp. 467-472. 1996.

33. Cavusoglu, M., I. Villanueva, and F. Tendick, "Workspace Analysis of Robotics Manipulators for a Teleoperated Suturing Task," presented at IEEE/RSJ International Conference on Intelligent Robots and Systems, Maui, Hl, pp. 2234-2239, 2001.

34. Harada, K., K. Tsubouchi, M. G. Fujie, and T. Chiba, "Micro Manipulators for Intrauterine Fetal Surgery in an Open MRI," presented at IEEE International Conference on Robotics and Automation, pp. 504-509, 2005.

35. Ikuta, K., K. Yamamoto, and K. Sasaki, "Development of Remote Microsurgery Robot and New Surgical Procedure for Deep and Narrow Space," presented at IEEE International Conference on Robotics and Automation, pp. 1103-1108, 2003.

36. Asai, D., S. Katopo, J. Arata, S. i. Warisawa, M. Mitsuishi, A. Morita, S. Sora, T. Kirino, and R. Mochizuki, "Micro-Neurosurgical System in the Deep Surgical Field," presented at MICCAI 2004 (7th International Conference on Medical Image Computing and Computer-Assisted Intervention), pp. 33-40, 2004.

37. Schenker, P. S., E. C. Barlow, C. D. Boswell, H. Das, S. Lee, T. R. Ohm, E. D. Paljug, G. Rodriguez, and S. Charles, "Development of a Telemanipulator for Dexterity Enhanced Microsurgery," presented at 2nd Annual International Symposium on Medical Robotics and Computer Assisted Surgery (MRCAS), pp. 81-88, 1995.

38. Yamashita, H., D. Kim, N. Hata, and T. Dohi, "Multi-Slider Linkage Mechanism for Endoscopic Forceps Manipulator," presented at IEEE International Conference on Intelligent Robots and Systems (IROS), pp. 2577-2582, 2003.

39. Reboulet, C. and S. Durand-Leguay, "Optimal design of redundant parallel mechanism for endoscopic surgery," presented at IEEE International Conference on Intelligent Robots and Systems, pp. 1432-1437, 1999.

40. Piers, J., D. Reynaerts, and H. V. Brussel, "Design of Miniature Parallel Manipulators for Integration in a Self-propelling Endoscope," *Sensors and Actuators*, vol. 85, pp. 409-417, 2000.

41. Merlet, J.-P., "Optimal design for the micro parallel robot MIPS," presented at IEEE International Conference on Robotics and Automation, pp. 1149-1154, 2002.

42. Minor, M. and R. Mukherejee, "A Dexterous Manipulator for Minimally Invasive Surgery," presented at IEEE International Conference on Robotics and Automation, pp. 2057-2064, 1999.

43. Dario, P., C. Paggetti, N. Troisfontaine, E. Papa, T. Ciucci, M. C. Carrozza, and M. Marcacci, "A Miniature Steerable End-Effector for Application in an Integrated System for Computer-Assisted Arthroscopy," presented at IEEE International Conference on Robotics and Automation, pp. 1573-1579, 1997.

44. Dario, P., M. C. Carrozza, A. Pietrabissa, and C. A. Surgery, "Developmnet and In Vitro Testing of a Miniature Robotic System for Comuter-Assisted Clonoscopy," vol. 4, pp. 1-14, 1999.

45. Phee, L., D. Accoto, A. Menciassi, C. Stefanini, M. C. Carrozza, and P. Dario, "Analysis and Development of Locomotion Devices for the Gastrointestinal Tract," *IEEE Transactions on Biomedical Engineering*, vol. 49, pp. 613-616, 2002.

46. Reynaerts, D., J. Peirs, and H. Van Brussel, "Shape memory micro-actuation for a gastro-intesteinal intervention system," *Sensors and Actuators*, vol. 77, pp. 157-166, 1999.

47. Mitsuishi, M., H. Wtanabe, H. Nakanishi, H. Kubota, and Y. IIZUKA, "Dexterity Enhancement for a Tele-micro-surgery System with Multiple Macro-micro Co-located Operation Point Manipulators and Understanding of the Operator's Intention," in *Lecture Notes in Computer Science (LNCS)*, vol. 1205, J. Troccaz, E. Grimson, and R. Mosges, Eds.: Springer, pp. 821-830. 1997.

48. Piers, J., D. Reynaerts, H. Van Brussel, G. De Gersem, and H. T. Tang, "Design of an Advanced Tool Guiding System for Robotic Surgery," presented at IEEE International Conference on Robotics and Automation, pp. 2651-2656, 2003.

49. D'attansio, S., O. Tonet, G. Megali, M. C. Carrozza, and P. Dario, "A Semi-Automatic Handheld Mechatronic Endoscope with Collision-Avoidance Capabilities," presented at IEEE International Conference on Robotics & Aotomation, pp. 1586-1591, 2000.

50. Simaan, N., "High Dexterity Snake-like Robotic Slaves for Minimally Invasive Telesurgery of the Upper Airway," presented at MICCAI 2004 (7th International Conference on Medical Image Computing and Computer-Assisted Intervention), pp. 17-24, 2004.

51. Simaan, N., "Snake-Like Units Using Flexible Backbones and Actuation Redundancy for Enhanced Miniaturization," presented at IEEE International Conference on Robotics and Automation, Barcelona, Spain, pp. In press, 2005.

52. Simaan, N., R. Taylor, and P. Flint, "A Dexterous System for Laryngeal Surgery - Multi-Backbone Bending Snake-like Slaves for Teleoperated Dexterous Surgical Tool Manipulation," presented at IEEE International Conference on Robotics and Automation, New Orleans, pp. 351-357, 2004.

53. Kapoor, A., N. Simaan, and P. Kazanzides, "A System for Speed and Torque Control of DC Motors with Application to Small Snake Robots," presented at IEEE Conference on Mechatronics & Robotics (MECHROB'2004), Aachen, Germany, pp., 2004.

54. Kapoor, A., N. Simaan, and R. Taylor, "Suturing in Confined Spaces: Constrained Motion Control of a Hybrid 8-DoF Robot"; International Conference on Advanced Robotics," International Conference on Advanced Robotics (IACR'2005), pp., 2005.

55. Yamashita, H., N. Hata, M. Hashizume, and T. Dohi, "Handheld Laprascopic Forceps manipulator Using Multi-slider Linkage Mechanisms," presented at MICCAI 2004 (7th International Conference on Medical Image Computing and Computer-Assisted Intervention), pp. 121-128, 2004.

56. Dombre, E., M. Michelin, F. Pierrot, P. Poignet, P. Bidaud, G. Morel, T. Ortmaier, D. Salle, N. Zemiti, P. Gravez, M. Karouia, and N. Bonnet, "MARGE Project: Design, Modelling, and Control of Assistive Devices for Minimally Invasive Surgery," presented at MICCAI 2004 (7th International Conference on Medical Image Computing and Computer-Assisted Intervention), pp. 1-8, 2004.

57. Weinstein, G. S., B. W. O'Malley, and B. G. Hockstein, "Transoral Robotic Surgery: Supraglottic Laryngectomy in a Cnine Model," *The Laryngoscope*, vol. 115, pp. 1315-1319, 2005.

58. Cavusoglu, M. C., W. Williams, F. Tendick, and S. Sastry, "Robotics for Telesurgery: Second Generation Berkley/UCSF Laprascopic Telesurgical Workstation and Looking towards the Future Applications," presented at 39th Allerton Conference on Communication, Control and Computing, Monticello, Italy, pp. Invited Paper, 2001.

59. Faraz, A. and S. Payandeh, "Synthesis and Workspace Study of Endoscopic Extenders with Flexible Stem," (online report) Simon Fraser University, Canada (http://www.ensc.sfu.ca/research/erl/med/), 2003.

60. Adhami, L. and E. C. Maniere, "Optimal Planning for Minimally Invasive Surgical Robots," *IEEE Transactions on Robotics and Automation*, vol. 19, pp. 854-863, 2003.

61. Cost-Maniere, E., L. Adhami, R. Severac-Bastide, A. Lobontie, K. Salisbury, J.-D. Boissonnat, N. Swarup, G. Guthart, E. Mousseaux, and A. Carpentier, "Optimized Port Placement for Totally Endoscopic Coronary Artery Bypass Grafting using the da Vinci Robotic System," in *Lecture Notes in Control and Information Sciences, Experimental Robotics VII*, vol. 271, D. Russ and S. Singh, Eds.: Springer. 2001.

62. Cannon, J. W., J. A. Stoll, S. D. Selha, P. E. Dupont, R. D. Howe, and D. F. Torchiana, "Port Placement Planning in Robot-Assisted Coronary Artery Bypass," *IEEE Transactions on Robotics and Automation*, vol. 19, pp. 912-917, 2003.

63. Hockstein, N., J. Nolan, B. O'Malley, and J. Woo, "Robot-assisted pharyngeal and laryngeal microsurgery: results of robotic cadaver dissections" *Laryngoscope*, vol. 115, pp. 1003-8, 2005.

64. Hockstein, N., J. Nolan, B. O'Malley, and J. Woo, "Robotic microlaryngeal surgery: a technical feasibility study using the daVince surgical robot and an airway mannequin," *Laryngoscope*, vol. 115, pp. 780-5, 2005.

65. McLeod, I. and P. Melder, "Da Vinci robot-assisted excision of a vallecular cyst: a case report.," *Ear Nose Throat J*, vol. 84, pp. 170-2, 2005.

66. Inglis, A., J. Perkins, S. Manning, and J. Mouzakes, " Endoscopic posterior cricoid split and rib grafting in 10 children.," *Laryngoscope*, vol. 113, pp. 2004-9, 2003.

67. Li, M. and R. H. Taylor, "Spatial Motion Constraints in Medical Robot Using Virtual Fixtures Generated by Anatomy," presented at IEEE International Conference on Robotics & Automation, pp. 1270-1275, 2004.

68. Yi, B.-J., R. A. Freeman, and D. Tesar, "Open-loop stiffness control of overconstrained mechanisms/robotic linkage systems," presented at IEEE International Conference on Robotics and Automation, pp. 1340-1345, 1989.

69. Simaan, N. and M. Shoham, "Geometric Interpretation of the Derivatives of parallel Robot's Jacobian Matrix With Application to Stiffness Control," *ASME J. of Mechanical Design*, vol. 125, pp. 33-41, 2003.

70. Yi, B.-J., R. Freeman, and D. Tesar, "Geometric characteristics of antagonistic stiffness in redundantly actuated mechanisms," presented at IEEE International Conference on Robotics and Automation, pp. 654-661, 1993.

71. Shoham, M., M. Burman, E. Zehavi, L. Joskowicz, E. Batkilin, and Y. Kunicher, "Bone-Mounted Miniature Robot for Surgical Procedures: Concept and Clinical Applications," *IEEE Transactions on Robotics and Automation*, vol. 19, pp. 893-901, 2003.

72. Merlet, J.-P., *Parallel Robots*: Kluwer Academic Publishers, 2000.

Chapter 16

FUTURE DEVELOPMENTS IN ROBOTIC SURGERY: AN OUTSIDE-THE-BOX LOOK INTO THE NEXT TEN YEARS

Gregory Auner and Abhilash Pandya
Wayne State University
Detroit, MI USA

Abstract

In this chapter, we give a view of a broader range of medical robotic devices that span nano-robotics (at the sub cellular scale), at the micron range (able to allow laparoscopic microsurgery) and at the macro scale (able to interact with patients and surgeons). We give the current state of medical robotics explaining examples of important research, and give a pragmatic vision of medical robotics in the next decade along with possible avenues of further research.

INTRODUCTION

We foresee that medical robotics will have a significant influence over the next decade. In fact, the power of robots may parallel the importance of imaging technology in medicine today. Robots will enhance the surgeon's senses (e.g. haptics (feel), augmented reality (sight), ultrasound (sound)), motor performance and diagnosis capability. In addition, robots may assist the surgeon and nurses with making rounds, assisting with tools at the operating room and taking care of patients at their bedside. Surgical robots already enhance surgical skills by filtering tremor and scaling motions, but may even be able to automate certain routine tasks to free the surgeon to focus on higher-level tasks. With intelligent interfaces, the robotic system could warn surgeons of incorrect trajectories or restrict the movements of the surgery away from dangerous or critical areas preventing vessel penetration or critical tissue damage. Robotic devices have been used in Cardiac surgery [1-13], Urology [14-16], Fetal Surgery [17, 18], Pediatrics[19-22] Neurosurgery[23, 24], Orthopedics[25, 26] and many other medical disciplines. As with imaging technology, robotics will bring patient care and treatment a leap forward. A good example of the use of robotics is for smaller patients (children) where precision is very important and sometimes not possible due to the small size of the patient, The Children's Hospital of Michigan and Detroit, MI. performs surgery using a robotic system in children [27]. Their experience with their first 60 cases has been positive.

Even with significant technological gains, robotic surgery is still at its infancy. There are some major areas of technological improvement needed for this technology to reach its ultimate potential which include better visualization, tactile sensing, diagnostic sensing, intelligent software and miniaturization[28]. In this article, we give our vision of the future of robotic technology in macro, micro and nano robotics with respect to certain key core technology development in the areas of robotic vision, diagnostic sensors, and sensor fusion. Figure 1 illustrates an overview of the continuum of robots from macro robots which can interact with patients at their bedside and hand tools to surgeons at the operating table to robots built to interact with cells. There can be hybrid robots which have components built at many levels. We conclude with thoughts on the path from the current state-of-art to our envisioned future for medical robots.

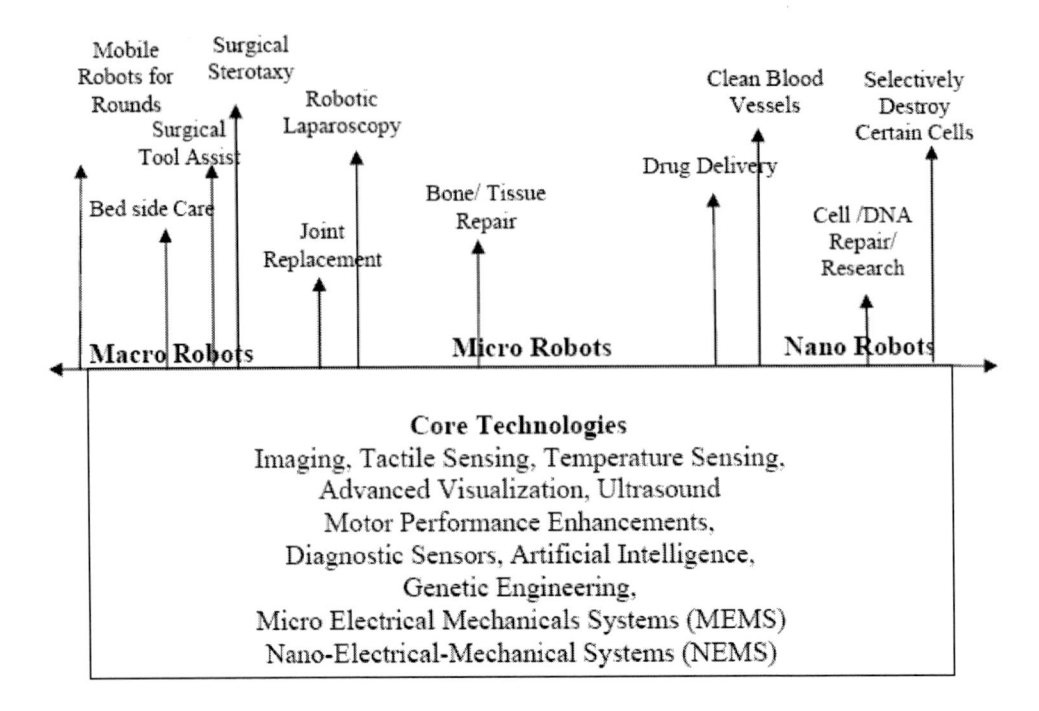

Figure 1: Core technologies and applications for nano, micro and macro robots

MACRO ROBOTS

InTouch Health systems has created the world's first mobile remote presence robot for healthcare. This robot is designed to enable health care assessment, consultation and treatment by a doctor from a remote distance. The idea is that a doctor sitting at a high-tech console can remotely control the robot and "virtually" treat patients. This type of robotic interface will be much more advanced in the near future to allow more complex tasks and can be potentially be made intelligent enough to respond to patient needs autonomously. In fact, a robotic nurse, called Nursebot [29] is already being developed. Nursebot is a collaborative effort by Carnegie Mellon University (CMU), the University of Pittsburgh's nursing department and the University of Michigan computer science program. The robot can remind patients when to take their medication, transport patients to and from asked locations or transmit patient data to a nurse or doctor thereby improving the quality of patient care.

Another robotic device developed at Columbia University, is a surgical technician. Some of the tool sets used in surgery are very complex and need very specialized nurse training. In the case of the Columbia robot, when the surgeon asks for a particular tool a robot hands the instrument to the surgeon and picks it up when he or she is done. In addition, the robot also can anticipate which instrument is needed next and have that tool ready. This robot, which is still under development, is a vision-based artificially-intelligent system. As the shortage with nurses grows, it can be anticipated that this technology will be in use during operations within the next few years and free nurses to do more patient care functions.

Macro robots have distinct high-level use and functionality, robots used that assist surgeons improve their mechanical performance and ease the complex tasks involved in operations take medical robotics to the next level.

MICRO ROBOTS

Aside from the now well-known Zeus and Da Vinci laproscopic robots, there are micro-scale robots that are on the horizon. A new approach to robot-assisted spine and trauma surgery is being developed at Carnegie Mellon University's Robotics Institute[30]. For this approach, a miniature robot is directly mounted on the patient's bony structure near the surgical site. The robot is designed to operate in a semiactive mode to precisely position and orient a drill or a needle in various surgical procedures. Since the robot forms a single rigid body with the anatomy, there is no need for immobilization or motion tracking, which greatly enhances and simplifies the robot's registration to the target anatomy. This robot is called MiniAture Robot for Surgical procedures (MARS). It is a cylindrical 5 x 7 cm3, 200-g, six-degree-of-freedom parallel manipulator. It is developed for two clinical applications surgical tools guiding for spinal pedicle screws placement; and 2) drill guiding for distal locking screws in intramedullary nailing.

Current minimally invasive surgery is performed by long thin endoscopes and laparoscopes which are inserted into natural or surgical orifices in human body. However, they have limited maneuverability and have limited access regions. Many of the gastrointestine (GI) tracks cannot be reached by these tools. IIn an innovative project [31], a highly articulated and modularly designed snake-like robotic mechanism is designed to improve the performance of current minimally invasive surgical tools. This tool is powered by pneumatics. It is self-propelled by sequencing the inflation and deflation of the balloon modules and bellow modules to create inch-worm like motions in the GI tracks. Applications are in inspection of intestines, diagnosis, biopsy, drug delivery, or chemical sampling with specially designed end tools. The surgical tool, also known as the inchworm robot, can be equipped with a fiber-optic camera and inserted through a tiny incision. Once it is inserted, it can walk like an inchworm controlled using a joy stick.

Going even smaller in the micron-range, imagine a microstructure that can interact with red blood cells. Silicon microteeth that open and close like jaws have been developed at Sandia National Laboratories. The microjaws fit in a microchannel about 20 microns wide. When the jaws close, they trap a red blood cell. The jaws, can capture cells, deform them and then release them. The blood cells travel on, regain their former shape and appear unharmed. This group has shown that they can create a micromachine that interacts at the scale of cells. However, autonomous systems have yet to be developed.

NANO ROBOT

Can robots be built below the micron scale? Nanotechnology can be defined as structures and mechanism that extend below 100nm in size. "In nature, nano-scale structures and mechanisms are ubiquitous. Richard Feynman states in his pioneering lecture on nanotechnology[32]..."Nature transforms inexpensive, abundant and inanimate ingredients into, self-repairing, self-aware creatures that walk, wiggle, swim sniff, see, think, and even dream." He poses the question, "What could we humans do if we could assemble the basic ingredients of the material world with a glint of nature's virtuosity?" Pioneering technology in nano and microsystems may lead to this world.

Nano or micro electro mechanical systems (NEMS or MEMS) are truly multidisciplinary fields. They involve solid-state electrical engineers studying the electrical properties of nanostructures, mechanical engineering studying the physical properties of nanostructures and genetic engineers who have come up with methods to study very important nanomachines existing in nature. This section will focus on two avenues of research (1) from the solid-state engineering side—where researchers are trying to use DNA to build nanostructures from DNA molecules and (2) from the genetic engineering side, where researcher are trying to describe the 3D structure and function of molecular machines.

Because this is the newest scale of robotics a few more details are given. In this section, an effort is made to give a greater understanding of the use of one of Nature's most important molecules (DNA) in the field of nanotechnology. DNA in nature functions as an information molecule [33]. It is a "computer program" which dictates what molecular structures should be built, how the molecular machines that are built should function and ultimately, how this living organism should behave. DNA has some amazing properties that allow it to be used for fabrication of nanostructures. This section focuses on DNA and its potential use for nanotechnology. It also provides some ideas for the future imitation of nature for building synthetic/organic hybrid nanomachinery.

It is clear that Nature has built nanomachines that are very functional. The key to Nature's development is a special kind of software that it uses: DNA. DNA's biological importance lies in the specificity of the base pairing that holds the two strands of the double helix together: adenine (A) pairs with thymine (T) and guanine (G) pairs with cytosine (C). The structure that results from these complementary interactions is a linear molecule, that is, it is not branched. However, we have seen that by designing appropriate sequences, it is possible in synthetic systems to produce branched DNA molecules.

DNA is well-known for duplication and storage of genetic information in biology. It has also recently been shown to be highly useful as an engineering material for construction of special purpose computers and micron-scale objects with nanometer-scale feature resolution[34, 35]. Properly designed synthetic DNA can be thought of as a programmable glue which, via specific hybridization of complementary sequences, will reliably self-organize to form desired structures and superstructures. Such engineered structures are inherently information-rich and are suitable for use directly as computers or as templates for imposing specific patterns on various other materials. It is also inherently durable over time.

In theory, DNA can be used to create any desired pattern in two or three dimensions and simultaneously to guide the assembly of a wide variety of other materials into any desired patterned structure. Given diverse mechanical, chemical, catalytic, and electronic properties of these specifically patterned materials, DNA self-assembly techniques hold great promise for bottom-up nanofabrication in a large number of potential applications in wide ranging fields of technology. There is great promise for future applications in fields as diverse as electronics, combinatorial chemistry, nano-robotics, and gene therapy.

The structures and arrays described so far are all static structures. Can a nanomechanical device be produced from DNA? Again, Seeman and LaBean in their article [34, 35] describe a minimal mechanical device using the DNA molecule. This molecule's structure switches between two alternatives in response to an external signal. Seeman's group has developed a two state device predicated on the B–Z transition of DNA. Conventional DNA, known as B-DNA, is a right-handed molecule. However, there is another structure of DNA that is radically different from B-DNA, known as Z-DNA19. Z-DNA is a left-handed molecule. They produced a two-state mechanical device (like a pincer) using a combination of B-DNA and Z-DNA19. The two states are structurally well defined and controllable. Although these steps are significant, they represent the first steps in the evolution of nano-robotic devices.

The unique features of DNA allows it to be used as a building block to created other novel basic structures from which perhaps complex machines can be built. It has also been shown by researchers that DNA nanotechnology can be combined with carbon nanotubes to take advantage of the self-organization properties of DNA. We conjecture that the future will allow for controllable nano and microrobots that can be deployed form medical use for surveillance and perhaps even treatment.

ENABLING TECHNOLOGIES

There are several key technologies which we would like to highlight in this paper. These technologies are well worth researching and should yield results that take medical robotics to the next level.

Diagnostic Sensors

The areas where we feel that sensing systems will most benefit robots are diagnostic sensing. Sensors which can in real-time differentiate between various pathological conditions such as cancer vs. normal tissue would be invaluable. Two such sensors are a Micro Raman probe and a Holographics Ultrasound probe which in the future may both be able to be mounted on the end-effector of a robotic device to provide pathological evaluation.

Cancer treatment, whether with drugs, radiation, or surgery, depends on distinguishing malignant from normal tissue. Visual inspection is seldom adequate for this task. Biopsy with histological evaluation is the gold standard for making this determination. Final results usually require a minimum of 12 to 24 hours, however, and even the more immediate frozen section generally requires at least 20 minutes from the time the tissue is removed until the time an answer is available. The process of evaluating all essential margins and surfaces can be very time-consuming and prone to sampling errors. As the ability to treat cancer improves, the early detection of disease provides an even greater opportunity for intervention resulting in a significant increase in survival.

A very promising sensing system is Raman spectrometer. Raman spectroscopy is a vibrational spectroscopic technique, which originates from inelastic scattering of light by vibrating molecules. This provides detailed information about the bimolecular composition of tissues, which may be used to distinguish between normal and malignant tissues. Raman spectroscopy has been under investigation during the last decade due to its potential application as a molecular-level tool for the diagnosis of cancer[55].

Pathological conditions involve changes in molecular composition or biomarkers of tissue as a result or cause of disease. By measuring Raman marker bands of proteins, lipids or nucleotides, the relative ratios and absolute concentration of each component can be determined and related to pathologic changes. Raman spectroscopy could enable *in vivo* detection of these changes in a minimally invasive, non-destructive manner by using the appropriate excitation laser wavelength and laser power. The Raman spectral data obtained could then be used to guide further clinical action. The importance of Raman spectroscopy lies in its potential *in vivo* application and therefore direct real-time therapeutic intervention based on that information (See Figure 3).

Micro Raman probes can be built to be miniature systems and very specific to a particular pathology. Future robotic system could have on-board sensor systems which include diagnostics capability. These robots will be able to work methodically and perhaps autonomously to remove tissue which it determines to be diseased.

Imagine listing to tissue for abnormalities. The development of novel technology using acoustic holography is within reach for early diagnosis of disease such as cancer due to significant advances in microsystem and signal analysis. Although holography technology has been in existence for over twenty five years, its application in the clinical/diagnostic arena did not come to fruition due to a lack of advanced microsystems and signal analysis technology. What has been missing is a conversion element that can record the ultrasound interference patterns, then reconstruct them with real or synthesized ultrasound interference pattern, and finally reconstruct with real or synthesized ultrasound frequency waves that could be directly

Future Developments in Robotic Surgery 287

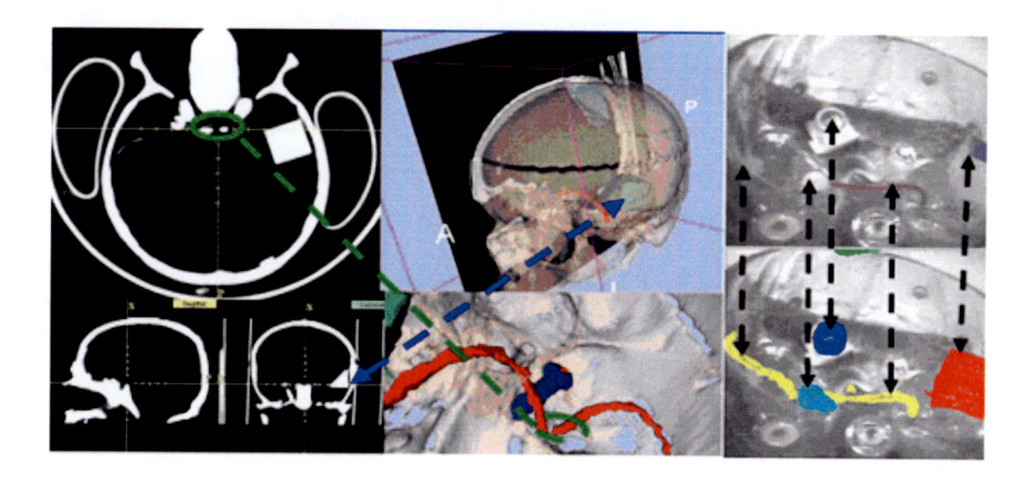

Figure 2: Integration of a Micro Raman Sensor to a Robotic System.

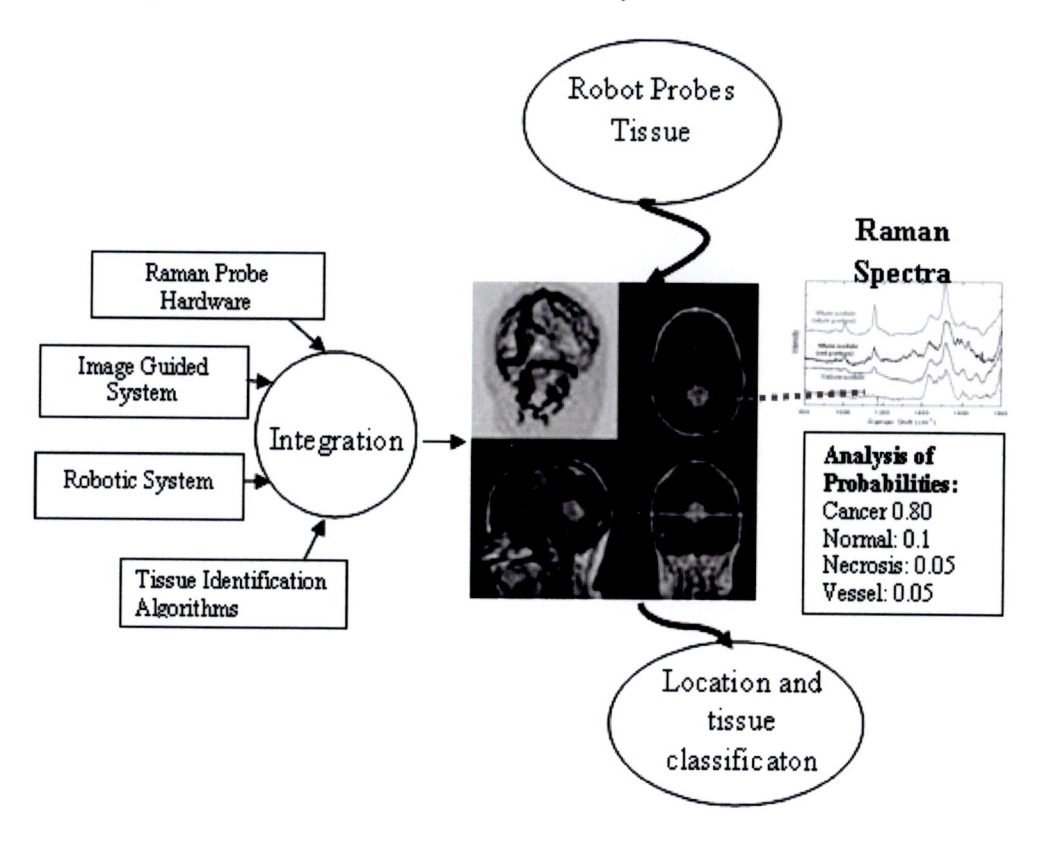

Figure 3: Holographic image created from ultrasound signals

transformed into a visible image. This is now possible using micro-piezoelectric arrays equipped with on chip reconstruction at high spatial and temporal resolution. In addition to 3-D holography imaging, a vital objective of the device is to recover the wave envelope emerging from each pixel. Whereas the hologram requires freezing the waves in time long enough to capture a stable interference pattern with adequate signal-to-noise—typically ten microseconds—the wave envelope itself contains an instantaneous integrated dynamic history of the scattering events along each ray path throughout the volume. If this information is extracted the physical parameters of each resolvable volume element (i.e. ~ 1 cubic mm) in the insonified volume then should enable diagnosis of the nature of the material. In principle, it is possible to distinguish very small tumors from healthy tissues by this method. Preliminary images and phase information are shown in Figure 3.

Robotic Vision (Augmented Reality and Image Guidance)

There have been many studies done to compare and improve the surgical interface and to improve the surgeon's performance[36-39]. However, one of the key problems that robotic surgery poses is that surgeries can become more difficult and can take longer [27]. In robotic surgery the magnification and therefore the size of the field of view changes with the proximity of the endoscope to the objects being viewed [40]. Because of the small incisions and camera view, the surgeon is no longer able to see inside the patient directly. The problem of visualization will be become even more acute with mobile remotely controlled miniature robots. Visualization is critical for systems that use a robotic interface as the surgeon typically operates from a remote location and relies almost entirely on indirect limited field-of-view video of the surgery [28, 40, 41]. Direct linkage of medical robotic systems to patient data and the optimal visualization of that data for the surgical team are important for successful operations.

In their review article on medical robots Cleary and Nguyen [28] state that if medical robots are to reach their full potential, they need to be more integrated systems in which the robots are linked to the imaging modalities or directly to the patient anatomy. They state further that robotics systems need to be developed in an "Image-Compatible" way. Visual information from the patient site needs to be augmented in a way that allows greater situational awareness, accuracy and confidence. That is, these systems must operate within the constraints of various image modalities such as Ultrasound, CT and MRI. This link, they conjecture, is essential if the potential advantages of robots are to be realized in the medical domain.

In addition, surgical planning and information management for these robotic systems is essential for successful operations[28]. Two main problems encountered in robotic surgery are non-optimal port (incisions on the patient's body for the robotic arms) placements and robotic arm collisions. Robotic arm collisions often require manual repositioning of the robotic arms on the operating table that unnecessarily adds to the operative time. Incorrect port placement typically results in robotic arm collisions, can lead to damage to robotic instruments and can also lead to inaccessibility of the operative site. Improved accessibility to the operative site can enhance patient safety[42]. These problems can be avoided in the pre-operative stages given the appropriate visualization tools. For these reasons, it is important that a robust visualization system be built that is linked to patient imaging data that offers the surgeon tools for visualization, robotic system setup and port placement [43].

Computer modeling tools that help visualize the anatomical structures of the patient would greatly aid the surgeon in the pre-operative stage. Visualization tools can help the surgeon determine optimal port placement sites. In addition, these tools will help determine the placement of the robotic arms on the operating table in order to avoid collisions between arms during the procedure while maximizing the range of motion of the instruments. A significant potential exists to impact medical robotics with the pre-operative planning and intra-operative visualization tools[44].

There are two different types of visualization technology that have been used for real-time and pre-operative visualization in the medical domain --Augmented Reality (AR) and Virtual Reality (VR)[45, 46]. These visualization methods are well-suited for Robotic Surgery. Image guidance is an example of Virtual Reality. In Image Guidance Surgery (IGS), the surgeon views a computer-generated world of image data and 3D models after registration. The registration ensures a one-to-one correspondence to the end-effector of the robot and the image coordinates. In contrast, the AR system generates a composite view for the user that includes the live video view fused (registered) with either pre-computed data (e.g., 3D geometry) or other registered sensed data[47]. Augmented Reality is a variation and extension of Virtual Reality and represents a middle ground between computer graphics in a completely synthetically generated world (as in VR) and a normal camera view of the real world[48-52]. The current technique of image guidance does not allow the surgeon to simultaneously use both real and synthetic data[53]. The surgeon can detect anomalies using advanced imaging and sensors and can accurately place their tools within surgical environments with robots. Nevertheless, he also needs his own vision to detect other features that may not be available from the sensor information. This, we conjecture, is one of the advantages of AR[54] (See Figure 2).

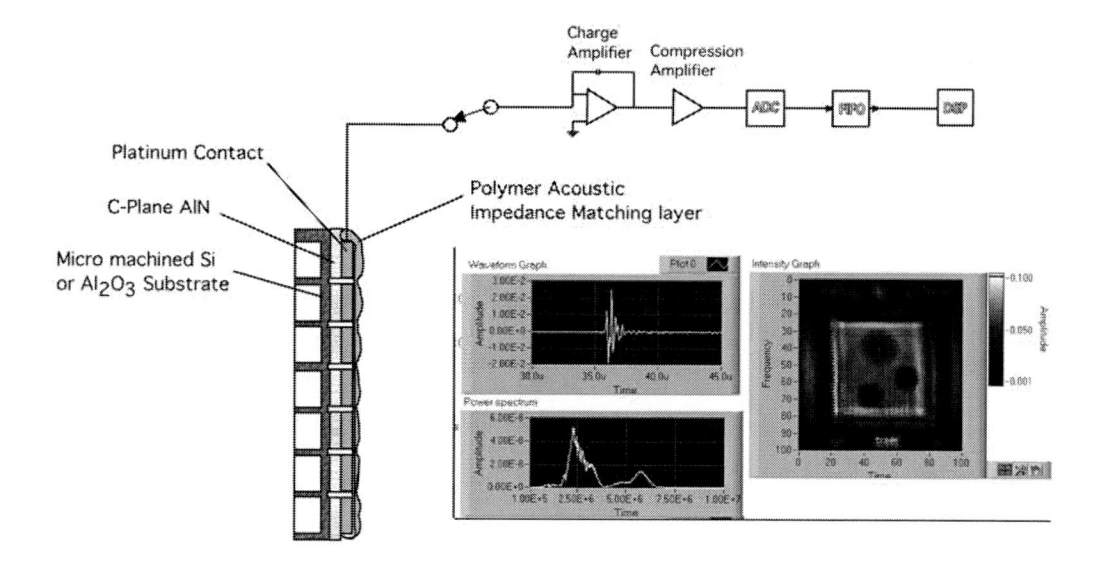

Figure 4. Augmented Reality and Image Guided Visualization

Robotic Touch

Can the sense of hyper touch and temperature be useful for a surgeon? Development of advanced force sensing arrays can advance tactile augmentation on the robot. For example, novel dual mode acoustic wave sensors that can switch between surface acoustic wave and surface transverse wave modes can sense pressure and viscosity in liquid, distinguish force due to liquid or solid interactions and further distinguish between normal and transverse forces (pincing pressure or sliding frictional forces). Since new wide bandgap semiconductor based acoustic sensor arrays have very linear temperature coefficients they can be superb temperature sensors as well. Thus, tactile forces and sensory information on touch and temperature can mimic super human tactile feeling with many orders of magnitude more sensitivity and precision.

CONCLUSIONS

As robots become more autonomous and the surgeries they can assist in performing become more complex, we envision a merging of sensors with robots. Systems such as, pressure sensors, tactile sensors, and temperature sensors will no-doubt become more advanced and will allow the surgeon to perform even more delicate surgeries. In addition, video sensing and imaging sensors will become integrated into robot end-effectors which will give an unprecedented view of the human body in real-time.

Although robots have the potential to improve the precision and capabilities of physicians, the number of robots in clinical use is still very small. First and foremost there needs to be a strong corporation between engineers and clinicians. Engineers need to team with clinicians and biological scientists to understand the needs and build systems which can be truly useful and simple. Building is not enough; these systems need to be tested with surgeon testing to ensure that the performance of the surgeon is positively affected and that the outcome for the patient is enhanced. Clinical trials need to be well organized with results quantified. Only then will these systems be accepted by the medical community.

The merging of sensors with robots is a logical step. Sensors of touch and temperature to enhance the surgeon's haptic sense, imaging sensors to allow greater visualization, and sensors for diagnostics can all be more effective when used in conjunction with robotic devices.

In the realm of nanotechnology, we believe that the future will be melding of two different disciplines—nanotechnology and molecular biology. Molecular biologists have already seen and studied what is possible in the nanotechnology world—they just don't know how to build these systems. Nanotechnologist have show that they can work at these scales and are starting to understand how molecular machines work—some of them are just unaware of what nature has already built. Can DNA be synthesized in a laboratory such that it can carryout assembly instructions for molecular building that we can design? The robot/ machines of this scale could be used to clean vessels, to deliver drugs to specific locations and perhaps seek out and destroy particular types of cells.

In summary, what needs to happen is a melding. A melding of engineers and surgeons, a melding of sensors and robots, a melding of nanotechnologist with microbiologists are all needed for this field to progress.

REFERENCES

1. Ducko CT, Stephenson ER Jr., Sankholkar S., Damiano RJ Jr., Robotically-assisted coronary artery bypass surgery: moving toward a completely endoscopic procedure. *The Heart Surgery Forum* 1999; 2(1): 29-37.

2. Argenziano M, Oz MC, DeRose JJ Jr., Ashton RC Jr., Beck J, Wang F, Chitwood WR, Nifong LW, Dimitui J., Rose EA, Smith CR Jr. Totally endoscopic atrial septal defect repair with robotic assistance. *The Heart Surgery Forum* 2002; 5 (3): 294-300.

3. Ashton RC Jr., McGinnis KM, Connery CP, Swistel DG, Ewing DR, DeRose JJ Jr., Totally endoscopic robotic thymectomy for myasthenia gravis. *The Annals of Thoracic Surgery*, 2003; 75(2): 569-71.

4. Autschbach R, Onnasch JF, Falk V, Walther T, Kruger M., Schilling LO, and Mohr FW, The Leipzig experience with robotic valve surgery. *The Journal of Cardiac Surgery* 2000; 15(1): 82-87.

5. Boehm DH, Detter C, Arnold MB, Deuse T, Reichenspurner H, Robotically assisted coronary artery bypass surgery with the ZEUS telemanipulator system. *Seminars in Thoracic Cardiovascular Surgery 2003*; 15(2): 112-20.

6. Boyd WD, Desai ND, Kiaii B, Rayman R, Menkis AH, McKenzie FN, Novick RJ. A comparison of robot-assisted versus manually constructed endoscopic coronary anastomosis. *The Annals of Thoracic Surgery* 2000;70(3): 839-42; discussion 842-3.

7. Carpentier A, Loulmet D, Aupecle B, Berrebi A, Relland J. Computer-assisted cardiac surgery. *Lancet* 1999; 353(9150): 379-80.

8. Chitwood WR Jr., Nifong LW. Minimally invasive videoscopic mitral valve surgery: the current role of surgical robotics *The Journal Cardiac Surgery* 2000 Jan-Feb;15(1): 61-75.

9. Chitwood WR Jr, Nifong LW, Elbeery JE, Chapman WH, Albrecht R, Kim V, Young JA. Robotic mitral valve repair: trapezoidal resection and prosthetic annuloplasty with the da vinci surgical system.*The Journal of Thoracic and Cardiovascular Surgery* 2000; (6): 1171-1172.

10. Damiano RJ, Jr., Ehrman WJ, Ducko CT, Tabaie HA, Stephenson ER Jr., Kingsley CP, Chambers CE. Initial United States clinical trial of robotically assisted endoscopic coronary artery bypass grafting.*The Journal of Thoracic and Cardiovascular Surgery* 2000; 119(1): 77-82.

11. Kappert U, Schneider J, Cichon R, Gulielmos V, Schade I, Nicolai J, Schueler S, Closed chest totally endoscopic coronary artery bypass surgery: fantasy or reality? *Current Cardiology Reports* 2000; 2(6): 558-63.

12. Nakamura Y, Kishi K. Robotic stabilization that assists cardiac surgery on beating hearts. *Studies in Health Technology and Informatics* 2001;81: 355-61.

13. Nifong LW, Chu VF, Bailey BM, Maziarz DM, Sorrell VL, Holbert D, Chitwood WR Jr. Robotic mitral valve repair: experience with the da Vinci system. *The Annals of Thoracic Surgery* 2003; 75(2): 438-42; discussion 443.

14. Binder J, Jones J, Bentas W. Robot-assisted laparoscopy in urology. Radical prostatectomy and reconstructive retroperitoneal interventions. *Urologe A 2002*; March 41(2): 144-149. German.

15. Hemal AK and Menon M. Laparoscopy, robot, telesurgery and urology: future perspective. *The Journal of Postgraduate Medicine* 2002 Jan-Mar; 48(1): 39-41.

16. Advincula A, Arenas J, Reynolds K. Telerobotic Laparoscopic Genitourinary Case Series. *Surg Endosc*, vol. 17, pp. S293, 2003.

17. Aaronson OS, Tulipan NB, Cywes R, Sundell HW, Davis GH, Bruner JP, Richards WO. Robot-assisted endoscopic intrauterine myelomeningocele repair: a feasibility study. *Pediatric Neurosurgery* 2002. 36 (2): 85-9.

18. Bholat O and Krummel T. Advanced Technologies for Future Fetal Treatment: Surgical Robotics. In: *The Unborn Patient: the Art and Science of Fetal Therapy.* Harrison MR, Adzick NS, Holzgreve W, 3rd edition. Philadelphia: W.B. Saunders, 2001, pp. 681-693.

19. Beals DA, Fletcher JR. Telemedicine and pediatric surgery. *Seminars in Pediatric Surgery* 2000; 9(1) 40-7.

20. Docimo SG, Moore RG, Adams J, Ben-Chaim J, Kavoussi LR. Early experience with telerobotic surgery in children. *The Journal of Telemedicine and Telecare* 1996; 2 suppl 1:48-50.

21. Gutt CN, Markus B, Kim ZG, Meininger D, Brinkmann L, Heller K. Early experiences of robotic surgery in children. *Surgical Endoscopy* 2002, 16; 1083-6.

22. Hollands CM, Dixey LN. Applications of robotic surgery in pediatric patients. *Surgical Laparoscopy Endoscopy Percutaneous Techniques* 2002, 12; 71-6.

23. Li Q, L. Zamorano, Pandya A. The application accuracy of the NeuroMate robot--A quantitative comparison with frameless and frame-based surgical localization systems," *Computer Aided Surgery* 2002, 7; 90-8.

24. Benabid A, Cinquin P, Lavalle S. Computer-driven robot for stereotactic surgery connected to CT scan and magnetic resonance imaging. Technological design and preliminary results.," *Applied Neurophysiology* 1987, 50 (1-6) 153-4.

25. Jakopec M, Harris S, Rodriguez BF. The first clinical application of a "hands-on" robotic knee surgery system. *Computer Aided Surgery* 2001, 6, 329-39.

26. Spencer E, The ROBODOC clinical trial: a robotic assistant for total hip arthroplasty. *Orthopaedic Nursing* 1996, 15, 9-14.

27. Knight C, Cao A, Lorincz A, Gidell K, Langenburg S, Klein M. Application of a Surgical Robot to Open Microsurgery. *Pediatric Endosurgery & Innovative Technique* 2003, 7, 227-232.

28. Cleary K, Nguyen C. State of the Art in Surgical Robotics: Clinical Applications and Technology Challenges. *Computer Aided Surgery* 2001, 6, 312-328.

29. Montemerlo M, Pineau J, Roy N, Thrun S, Verma V. Experiences with a Mobile Robotic Guide for the Elderly, Proceedings of the AAAI National Conference on Artificial Intelligence. 2002.

30. Shoham M, Burman M, Zehavi E, Joskowicz L, Batkilin E, Kunicher Y. Bone-Mounted Miniature Robot for Surgical Procedures: Concept and Clinical Applications. *IEEE Transactions on Robotics and Automation* 2003, 19; 893.

31. Phee L, Ng WS, Chen I-M, Seow FC. Development of new locomotion concepts for use in automation of colonoscopy. presented at 9th International Conference on Biomedical Engineering Society, Singapore, December 1997.

32. Feynman R (Speech), There is Plenty of Room at the Bottom. Presented December 29, 1959 at the annual meeting of the American Physical Society at the California Institute of Technology. Published in: *American Physical Society*, 1960.

33. Drexler KE, *Nanosystems*: Wiley Interscience, 1992.

34. Seeman NC, "DNA Engineering and its applications to Nanotechnology.Review *Trends in Biotechnology* 1999, 17; 437-43.

35. LaBean TH, "Introduction to Self-Assembling DNA Nanostructures for Computation and Nanofabrication. In *Computational Biology and Genome Informatics* (eds. Wang JTL, Wu CH, & Wang PP), ISBN 981-238-257-7 (World Scientific Publishing, Singapore, 2003).

36. Allaf ME, Jackman SV, Schulam PG, Cadeddu JA, Lee BR, Moore RG, Kavoussi LR. Laparoscopic visual field. Voice vs foot pedal interfaces for control of the AESOP robot. *Surgical Endoscopy* 1998, 12 (12); 1415-8.

37. Arezzo A, Ulmer F, Weiss O, Schurr MO, Hamad M, Buess GF. Experimental trial on solo surgery for minimally invasive therapy: comparison of different systems in a phantom model. *Surgical Endoscopy* 2000, 14 (10); 955-9.

38. Jacobs LK, Shayani V, Sackier JM. Determination of the learning curve of the AESOP robot. *Surgical Endoscopy* 1997, 11 (1); 54-5.

39. Kondraske GV, Hamilton EC, Scott DJ, Fischer CA, Tesfay ST, Taneja R, Brown RJ, Jones DB. Surgeon workload and motion efficiency with robot and human laparoscopic camera control. *Surgical Endoscopy* 2002, 16 (11); 1523-7.

40. Burkart A, Debski RE, McMahon PJ, Rudy T, and Musahlv V, Fu FH, van Scyoc A, Woo SL, "Precision of ACL Tunnel Placement Using Traditional and Robotic Techniques," *Computer Aided Surgery* 2001, 6 (5); 270-278.

41. Ayache N, "Medical Computer Vision, Virtual-Reality and Robotics," *Image and Vision Computing* 1995, 13 (4); 295-313.

42. Partin AW, Adams JB, Moore RG, Kavoussi LR, "Complete robot-assisted laparoscopic urologic surgery: a preliminary report," *Journal of the American College of Surgery* 1995, 181 (6); 552-7.

43. Tombropoulos RZ, Adler JR, Latombe JC, "CARABEAMER: a treatment planner for a robotic radiosurgical system with general kinematics," *Medical Image Analysis* 1999, vol. 3 (3); 237–264.

44. R. H. Taylor, P. Dario, and J. Troccaz, "Special issue on medical robotics," *IEEE Transactions on Robotics and Automation* October 2003, 9 (5); 763-764, 2003.

45. Pandya AK, Siadat M, Auner G, Kalash M, Ellis RD, "Development and Human Factors Analysis of Neuronavigation vs. Augmented Reality," presented at *Medicine Meets Virtual Reality*, Newportbeach, CA., 2003.

46. Pandya AK, Siadat M, Zamorano L, Gong J, Li Q, Maida JC, Kakadiaris I, "Tracking Methods for Medical Augmented Reality," presented at *Medical Image Computing and Computer-Assisted Intervention - MICCAI* 2001 (Lecture Notes in Computer Science), Utrecht, The Netherlands, 2001.

47. Pandya A K, Zamorano L (patent authors in alphabetical order), "Augmented Tracking Using Video, Computer Data and/or Sensing Technologies.," In *Application No. 10/101421 Customer Number 26646*. USA: Wayne State University, 2002.

48. Pandya A.K., Siadat M., Maida J., Auner G., Zamorano L., "Robotic Vision Registration and Live-Video Augmentation-- A Prototype for Medical and Space Station Robots," presented at Bioastronautics Investigators Workshop, Galveston, Texas, 2003.

49. Pandya AK, Siadat M, Ye Z, Prasad M, Auner G, Zamorano L, Klein M, "Medical Robot Vision Augmentation--A Prototype," presented at Medicine Meets Virtual Reality, Newport Beach, California, 2003.

50. Pandya AK, Siadat M, Zamorano L, Gong J, Li Q, Maida JC, Kakadiaris I, "Augmented Robotics for Neurosurgery," presented at American Association of Neurological Surgeons, Toronto, Ontario, 2001.

51. Pandya A.K., Zamorano L., Siadat M., Li Q., Gong J., Maida J.C., "Augmented Robotics for Medical and Space Applications," presented at Human Systems 2001, NASA Johnson Space Center, Houston, Tx., 2001.

52. Pandya AK., Siadat M, Gong J, Li Q, Zamorano, L, Maida JC, "Towards Using Augmented Reality for Neurosurgery," presented at Medicine Meets Virtual Reality 9: Outer Space, Inner Space, Virtual Space, Newport Beach, CA, 2001.

53. Azuma R, "A Survey of Augmented Reality," *Presence* 1997, 6; 355-385.

54. Pandya AK, Siadat M, Auner G, "Design, Implementation and Accuracy of a Prototype for Medical Robotic Vision Augmentation," *Computer Aided Surgery* (Accepted for Publication 2005).

55. Wolthuis R, Bakker Schut TC, and C. PJ, "Raman spectroscopic methods for in vitro and in vivo tissue carachterization". In: *Fluorescent and Luminescent Probes for Biological Activity: a practical guide to technology for quantitative real-time analysis,* 2nd edition, Cambridge UK: Academic Press; 1999. 433-455.

ABOUT THE AUTHORS

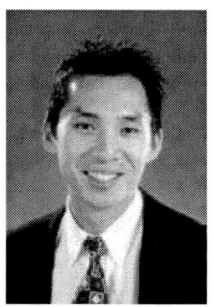

Arnold P. Advincula, M.D.
Assistant Professor
Director of Minimally Invasive
Surgery Program & Fellowship
University of Michigan Medical Center
L 4000 Women's Hospital
1500 East Medical Center Drive
Ann Arbor, Michigan 48109
T: 734-764-8429
F: 734-647-9727
E: aadvincu@umich.edu

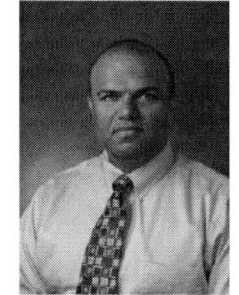

Zilfiqar Ahmed, M.D.
Anesthesia Department
Children's Hospital of Michigan
3901 Beaubien
Detroit, MI 48201
T: 313-745-5535
F: 313-745-5488
E: zahmed@dmc.org

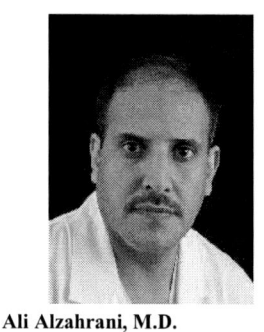

Ali Alzahrani, M.D.
University Louis Pasteur
Founding President IRCAD/EITS
Institute
1 place de l'Hospital – BP426
67091 Strasbourg
France
T: 011-333-88-11-9114
F: 011-333-88-11-9096
E: ali.alzahrani@ircad.u-strasbg.fr

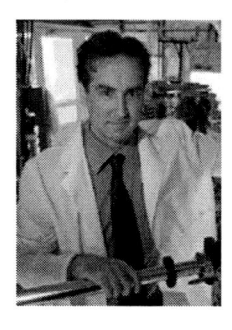

Gregory Auner, Ph.D.
Wayne State University
Engineering Building - #3170
5050 Anthony Wayne Drive
Detroit, Michigan 48201
T: 313-577-3904
F: 313-577-1101
E: gauner@ece.eng.wayne.edu

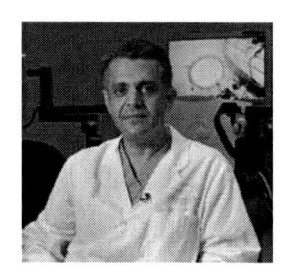

Dr. Mehran Anvari
Dept. of Surgery
St. Joseph's Healthcare
50 Charlton Ave. East
Hamilton, Ontario
Canada L8N 4A6
T: 905-522-2951
F: 905-521-6113

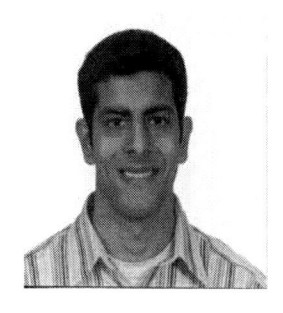

Sumit Bose, Senior Undergraduate
The Whitaker Biomedical
Engineering Institute of Johns
Hopkins
Johns Hopkins University
Clark Hall 316
3400 N. Charles Street
Baltimore, Maryland 21218
T: 410-516-8120
F: 410-516-4771
E: sumitbose@jhu.edu

About the Authors

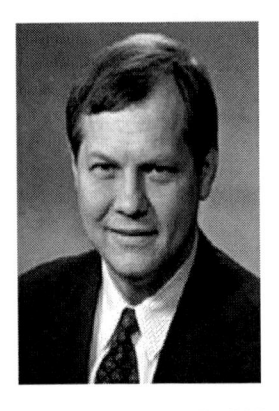

W. Randolph Chitwood, Jr., M.D., FACS, FRCS
Senior Associate Vice Chancellor for Health Sciences
Department of Surgery, Division of Cardiothoracic Surgery
Brody School of Medicine
East Carolina University
600 Moye Boulevard
Greenville, North Carolina 27834
T: 252-744-5080
F: 252-744-5192
E: chitwood@ecu.edu

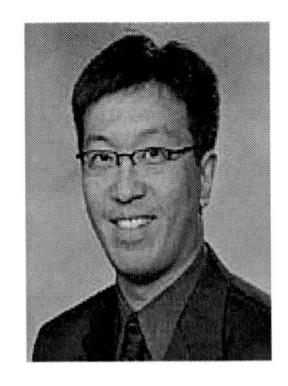

George K. Chow, M.D.
Assistant Professor,
Department of Urology
Mayo Clinic
200 First St. S.W.
Rochester, Minnesota 55905
T: 507-266-4319
F: 507-284-4951
E: chow.george@may.edu

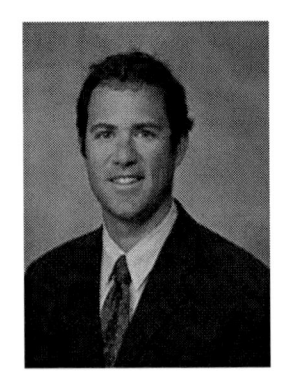

David S. DiMarco, M.D.
Urology Healthcare
2400 Hartman Lane - #200
Springfield, Oregon 97477
T: 541-343-9259
F: 541-485-1957
E: ddimarco@urology
healthcare.org

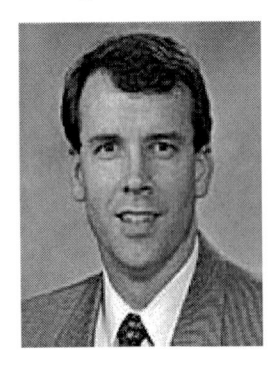

Daniel S. Elliott, M.D.
Associate Professor
Mayo Clinic
Department of Urology
200 First St. S.W.
Rochester, Minnesota 55905
T: 507-266-2518
F: 507-284-4951
E: Elliott.daniel@mayo.edu

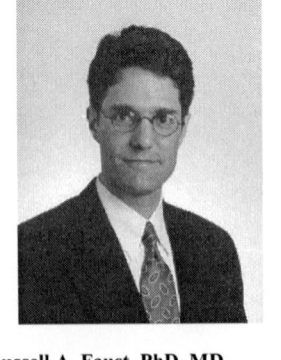

Russell A. Faust, PhD, MD,
Associate Professor, Pediatrics,
Wayne State University
Carls Foundation Endowed Chair in Pediatric Otolaryngology
Children's Hospital of Michigan
3901 Beaubien
Detroit, MI 48201
T: 313-745-5402
F: 313-745-5848
E: faustr@chi.osu.edu
http://www.chmkids.org/chm/ent

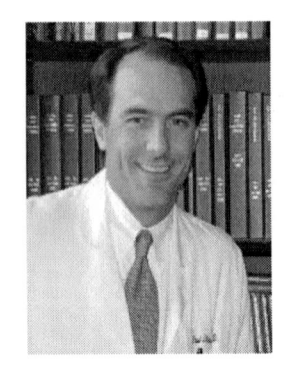

Paul W. Flint, M.D.
Professor, Otolaryngology - Head & Neck Surgery
Director, Center for Laryngeal Voice Disorders
Co-Director, Minimally Invasive Surgical Training Center
Otolaryngology – Head & Neck Surgery
Johns Hopkins School of Medicine
Baltimore, Maryland 21287
T: 410-955-1654
F: 410-955-0035
E: pflint@jhmi.edu

About the Authors

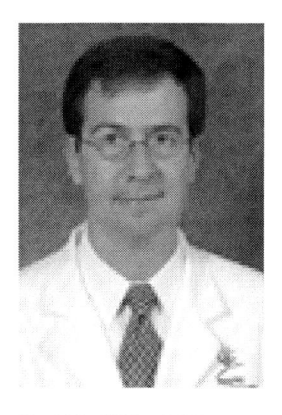

David L. Gibbs, M.D.
Pediatric Surgical Specialists
1310 West Stewart Drive
Suite 308
Orange, California 92868
T: 714-628-8800
F: 714-628-8886
E: pssocdg@sbcglobal.net

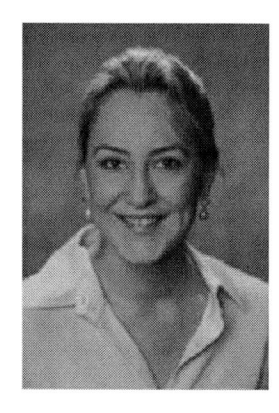

Christine G. Gourin, M.D.
Assistant Professor of
Otolaryngology
Medical College of Georgia
Department of Otolaryngology–
Head and Neck Surgery
1120 Fifteenth Street, BP 4594
Augusta, Georgia 30912
T: 706-721-6100
F: 706-721-0112
E: cgourin@mcg.edu

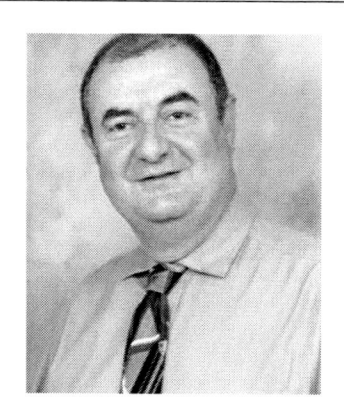

Gabriel Haas, MD
Professor and Chairman
State University of New York
Upstate Medical University
Department of Urology
750 East Adams Street
Syracuse, NY 13210
T: 315-464-6106
F: 315-464-6117
E: haasg@upstate.edu

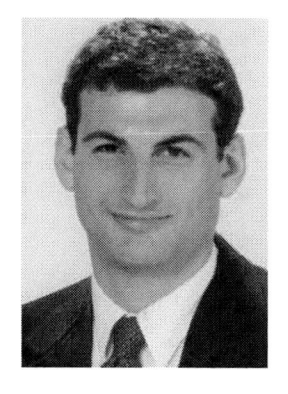

Alecxander Hillel, M.D.
Department of Otolaryngology – Head
and Neck Surgery
Johns Hopkins School of Medicine
JHOC, 6th Floor
601 N. Caroline Street
Baltimore, MD 21287
T: 410-955-1932
F: 410-355-6526
E: ahillel@jhmi.edu

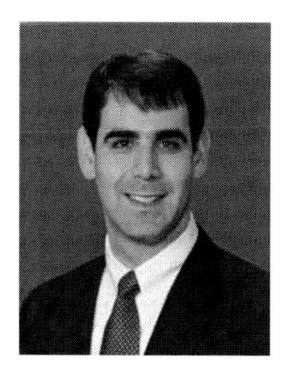

Neil G. Hockstein, M.D.
Family Ear, Nose and Throat
1941 Limestone Road
Suite #210
Wilmington, Delaware 19808
T: 302-998-0300
F: 302-998-5111
E: neilhockstein@verizon.net

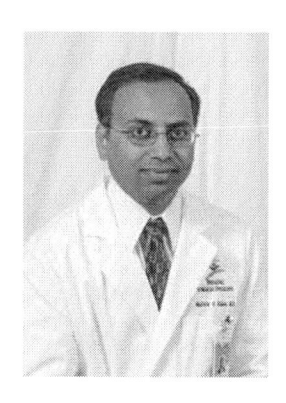

Mustafa H. Kabeer, M.D.
1310 West Stewart Drive
Suite 308
Orange, California 92868
T: 714-628-8800
F: 714-628-8886
E: Kabeer135@hotmail.com

About the Authors

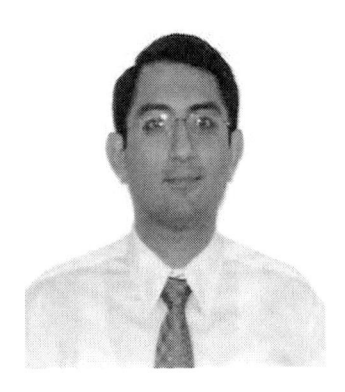

Sanjeev Kaul, M.D., M.Ch.
Robotic Urology Fellow
Vattikuti Urology Institute
Henry Ford Hospital
2700 West Grand Boulevard, K-9
Detroit, MI 48202
T: 313-916-2066
F: 313-916-9962
El: skaul1@hfhs.org

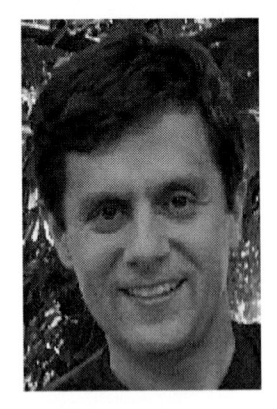

Peter Kazanzides, PhD
Johns Hopkins University
Center for Computer Integrated
Surgical Systems & Technology
B26 New Engineering Building
3400 North Charles Street
Baltimore, MD 21218
T: 410-516-5590
F: 410-516-5553
E: pkaz@cs.jhu.edu
www.cisst.org/~pkaz

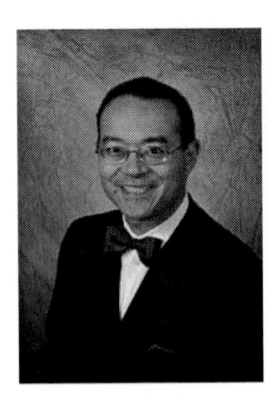

Raymund C. King, MD, JD, FICS
Kings Park Business Center
5700 West Plano Parkway
Suite 1000
Plano, Texas 72093
T: 972-381-2792
F: 972-381-2793
E: rking@rkinglaw.com
www.rkinglaw.com

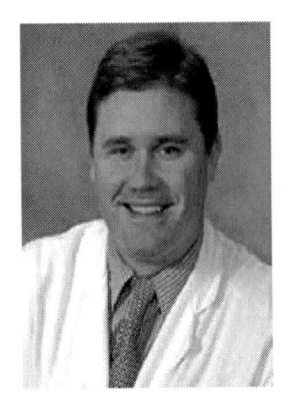

Alan P. Kypson, M.D., F.A.C.S.
Department of Surgery
Division of Cardiothoracic Surgery
Brody School of Medicine
East Carolina University
600 Moye Boulevard
Greenville, North Carolina 27834
T: 252-744-2187
F: 252-744-3618
E: kypsona@ecu.edu

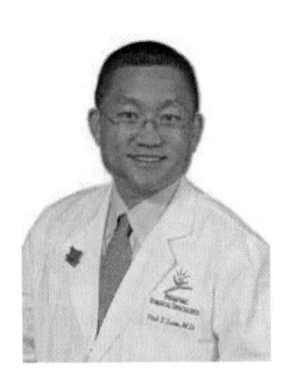

Vinh T. Lam, M.D.
Pediatric Surgical Specialists
1310 West Stewart Drive
Suite 308
Orange, California 92868
T: 714-628-8800
F: 714-628-8886
E: pssocvl@sbcglobal.net

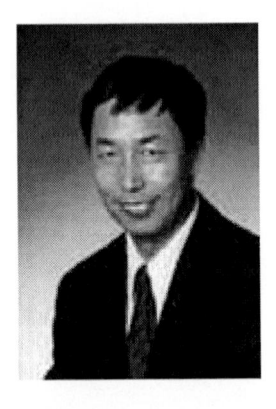

Qinhang Li, M.D., PhD
Assistant Professor
Neurological Surgery Department
Wayne State University
4160 John R.
Suite 930
Detroit, MI 48201
T: 313-745-8225
F: 313-966-0368
E: qli@med.wayne.edu

About the Authors

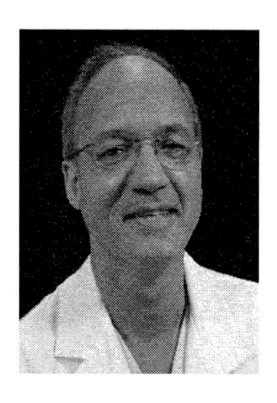

Jacques Marescaux M.D., F.R.C.S.,
Professor, Department of Digestive Surgery
University Louis Pasteur
Founding President IRCAD/EITS Institute
1 place de l'Hospital – BP426
67091 Strasbourg
France
T: 011-333-88-11-9114
F: 011-333-88-11-9096
E: Jacques.marescaux@ircad.u-strasbg.fr

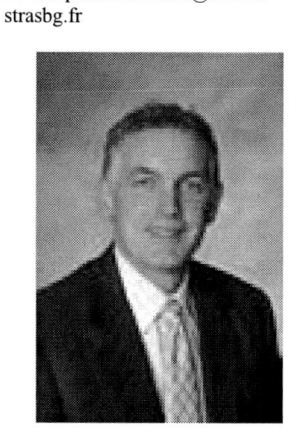

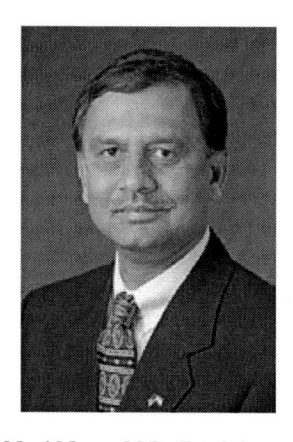

Mani Menon M.D., F.A.C.S.
Raj and Padma Vittikuti Distinguished Chair Director, Vattikuti Urology Institute, Henry Ford Hospital, Detroit, MI
Prof. of Urology, Case Western Reserve University, Cleveland, Ohio
2799 West Grand Boulevard, K-9
Detroit, MI 48201
T: 313-916-2066
F: 313-916-9962
E: mmenon1@hfhs.org

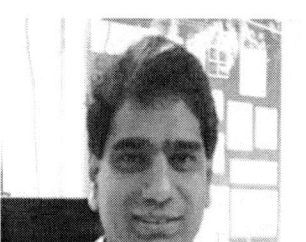

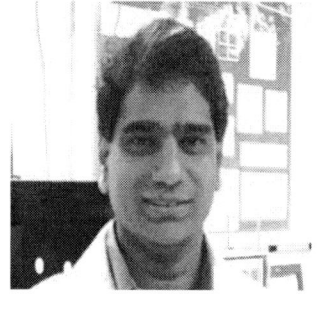

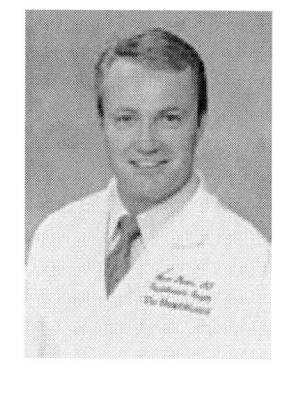

Simon C. Moten, M.B.B.S., F.R.A.C.S.
Department of Surgery
Division of Cardiothoracic Surgery
Brody School of Medicine
East Carolina University
Greenville, North Carolina 27834
T: 252-744-2187
F: 252-744-3542
E: motens@ecu.edu

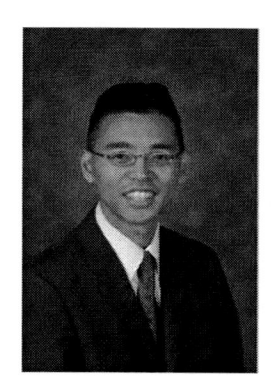

Bert W. O'Malley, M.D.
Gabriel Tucker Professor and Chairman
Department of Otorhinolaryngology
Co-Director, Head and Neck Cancer Center
Co-Director, Center for Cranial Based Surgery
Hospitals of University of Pennsylvania
5 RAVDIN
3400 Spruce Street
Philadelphia, Pennsylvania 19104
T: 215-349-5390
F: 215-615-4334
E: bert.omalley@uphs.upenn.edu

Abilash Pandya, Ph.D.
Wayne State University
Engineering Building #3160
5050 Anthony Wayne Drive
Detroit, Michigan 48201
T: 313-577-9921
F: 313-577-1101
E: apandya@ece.eng.wayne.edu

Richard Rhiew, M.D., PhD
Resident, Neurological Surgery Department
Wayne State University
4160 John R.
Suite 930
Detroit, MI 48201
T: 313-745-8225
F: 313-966-0368
E: rrhiew@med.wayne.edu

About the Authors

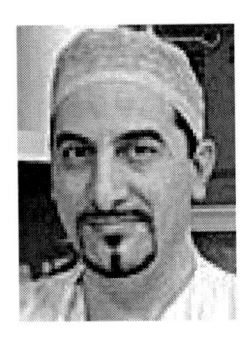

Francesco Rubino, M.D.
IRCAD/EITS Institute
University Louis Pasteur
1 place de l'Hospital – BP426
67091 Strasbourg
France
T: 011-333-88-11-9114
F: 011-333-88-11-9096

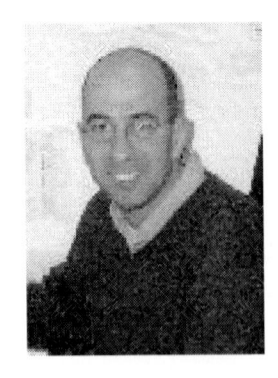

Nabil Simaan, PhD
Director, A.R.M.A . Laboratory
Assistant Professor, Department of
Mechanical Engineering
A.R.M.A. – Advanced Robotics &
Mechanism Applications
Columbia University
500 West 120th Street
New York, NY 10027
T: 212-854-2957
F: 212-854-3304
E: ns2236@columbia.edu

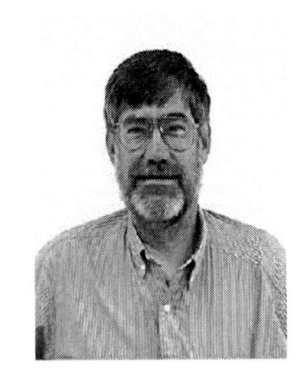

Russell H. Taylor, PhD
Professor of Computer Science
Appointments: Mechanical
 Engineering, Radiology, Surgery
Johns Hopkins University
3400 N. Charles Street
Baltimore, Maryland 21218
T: 410-516-6299
F: 410-516-5553
E: rht@heart.cs.jhu.edu

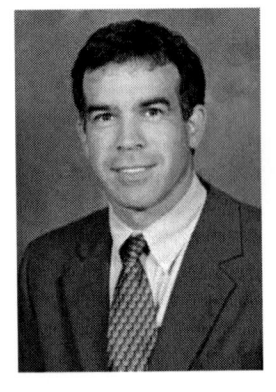

David J. Terris, M.D.
Chairman, Department of
Otolaryngology
Medical College of Georgia
Department of Otolaryngology-Head
and Neck Surgery
1120 15th Street, BP 4109
Augusta, GA 30912
T: 706-721-6100
F: 706-721-0112
E: dterris@mcg.edu
www.mcg.edu/otolaryngology

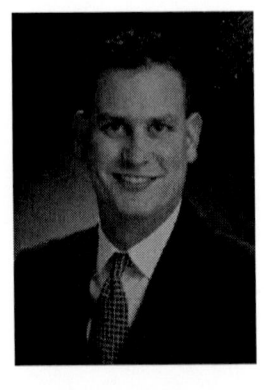

David M. Walters, M.D.
Department of Otolaryngology
Medical College of Georgia
1120 15th Street, BP 4109
Augusta, GA 30912
T: 706-721-6100
F: 706-721-0112
E: dwalters@mcg.edu

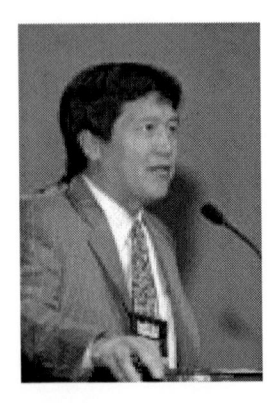

Yulan Wang, Ph.D., CEO
InTouch Health
90 Castilian Drive
Suite 200
Goleta, CA 93117
T: 805-562-8686
F: 805-562-8663
E: ywang@intouchhealth.com
www.intouchhealth.com

About the Authors

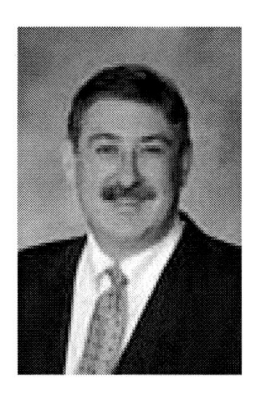

Gregory S. Weinstein, M.D.,
Professor and Vice-Chairman,
Department of Otorhinolaryngology:
Head and Neck Surgery
Co-Director, Center for Head and Neck Cancer
Director Head and Neck Oncology Fellowship
Hospitals of University of Pennsylvania
5 RAVDIN
3400 Spruce Street
Philadelphia, Pennsylvania
T: 215-349-5390
F: 215-349-8953
E: Gregory.weinstein@uphs.upenn.edu

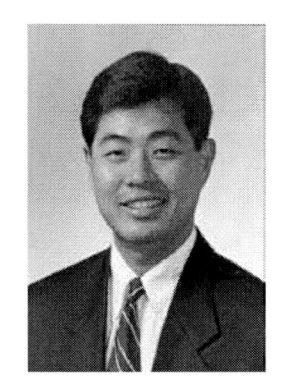

David D. Yuh, M.D.
Associate Professor of Surgery
Director, Minimally Invasive Surgical Program
Johns Hopkins Cardiac Surgery
600 N. Wolfe Street
Blalock 618
Baltimore, Maryland 21287
T: 410-955-9780
F: 410-955-3809
E: dyuh@csurg.jhmi.jhu.edu

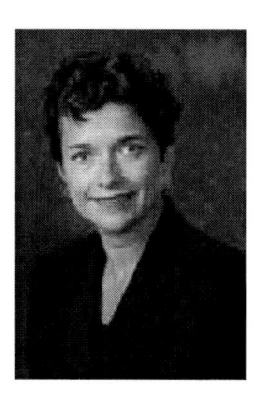

Lucia Zamorano, M.D.
Harper University Hospital
Detroit Medical Center
32841 Middlebelt – Suite 401
Farmington Hills, MI 48334
T: 248-723-2477
Fax: 248-681-3209
lzamoran@dmc.org
www.luciazamorano.com

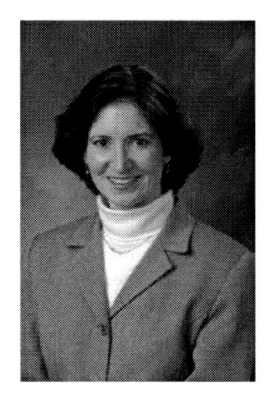

Maria Zestos, M.D., Chief
Anesthesia Department
Children's Hospital of Michigan
3901 Beaubien
Detroit, MI 48201
T: 313-745-5535
F: 313-745-5448
E: mzestos@med.wayne.edu

INDEX

A

accelerator, 154, 156
acetabulum, 62, 67, 68
acidosis, 23
ACL, 67, 69, 294
activation, 8, 179
actuators, 76, 88, 165, 268
adaptability, 151
adaptation, 98, 101
adenine, 132, 284
adenoma, 121
adipose tissue, 109
administrators, xii, 186
adrenal gland, 101
adverse event, 49, 84
aerodigestive tract, 255
age, 22, 28, 29, 33, 42, 43, 137, 138, 142, 143, 154
airways, 262
akinesia, 14
alcoholism, 53
algorithm, 74
alternative, 11, 67, 106, 129, 154, 158, 184, 205, 207, 229, 244, 268, 269, 271
alternatives, 106, 162, 268, 285
alters, 253
amnesia, 14
analgesic, 24, 105, 116
anastomosis, 25, 26, 32, 33, 39, 102, 111, 114, 118, 123, 126, 177, 178, 220, 291
anatomy, 56, 62, 63, 67, 68, 70, 72, 73, 88, 100, 105, 106, 118, 137, 139, 142, 156, 168, 179, 216, 218, 235, 268, 283, 288
anemia, 28
anesthesiologist, xiii, 13, 14, 21, 23, 30, 188, 244, 245
anesthetics, 19
angina, 180
angiography, 178
angioplasty, 178
animals, 26, 49, 249
ankles, 26
anticoagulant, 22
anxiety, 154
aorta, 178, 217
aortic occlusion, 24
appendectomy, 185
applied research, xiv, 162
architecture design, 164
argument, 89
arrest, 24, 176
arterioles, 111, 112
arteriovenous malformation, 159
artery, 11, 22, 24, 25, 95, 118, 122, 125, 173, 176, 177, 178, 184, 216, 217, 226, 248, 250, 291, 292
arthroplasty, 61, 76, 90, 91, 93
arthroscopy, 265
articulation, 10, 187
aspiration, 235, 246, 247, 261
assault, 53
assessment, 22, 26, 27, 177, 203, 255, 283
association, 15, 55, 235
asthma, 139
atelectasis, 20, 30
atrial fibrillation, 173, 182, 184
atrial septal defect, 34, 173, 175, 176, 183, 184, 291
attachment, 61, 83, 217
automation, 5, 101, 293
autonomy, 152
availability, 42, 164, 202
avoidance, 24, 101, 114, 268, 270
awareness, xi, 3, 288
axilla, 179

B

background noise, 38
bandgap, 290
bandwidth, 11, 37, 38, 40, 42, 67, 98, 99
baroreceptor, 18
barriers, xi, 41
basal ganglia, 160
base pair, 284
basic research, 162
behavior, 4
Belgium, 9, 30
bending, 265, 269, 271
benign, 26, 97, 121, 127, 138, 207, 215, 216, 218, 219, 222, 226, 253, 257, 262
benign prostatic hyperplasia, 26
benign tumors, 207
biliary atresia, 200
biomarkers, 286
biomechanics, 64
biopsy, 7, 36, 148, 153, 155, 161, 162, 163, 165, 284
biopsy needle, 161
birth, 28
bladder, 107, 108, 111, 114, 118, 128, 132, 140, 208, 216
bleeding, 20, 24, 42, 118, 127, 143, 188, 207, 246, 247
blood pressure, 19, 21, 24, 26, 28, 29, 227
blood supply, 118
blood transfusion, 188, 215, 246
blood transfusions, 215
blood vessels, 28, 34, 101
body, 15, 16, 17, 21, 24, 25, 28, 29, 30, 49, 88, 106, 167, 186, 188, 189, 206, 244, 246, 263, 283, 288, 290
bowel, 37, 108, 114, 118, 189, 194
bowel obstruction, 37
brachial plexus, 23
bradycardia, 18
brain, 7, 148, 149, 150, 152, 154, 155, 156, 160, 165, 166, 167, 168, 169, 170
brain tumor, 154, 155, 156
breathing, 29
broadband, 36, 39
bronchoscopy, 23, 24
bronchospasm, 16
bronchus, 195
bureaucracy, 50
burn, 53
bypass graft, 32

C

cables, 36, 188
cadaver, 79, 80, 81, 85, 86, 93, 227, 228, 229, 232, 233, 238, 240, 242, 243, 247, 253, 254, 255, 279
caliber, 247
calibration, 78
California, 56, 66, 70, 89, 96, 128, 229, 293, 295
Canada, 37, 77, 92, 98, 279
cancer, 97, 100, 106, 115, 117, 118, 132, 135, 138, 144, 215, 263, 286
candidates, 18, 20, 139
capillary, 24
carbon, 15, 16, 17, 19, 21, 25, 29, 30, 32, 226, 244, 249, 256, 263, 276, 285
carbon dioxide, 15, 16, 17, 19, 21, 25, 29, 30, 32, 226, 244, 249, 256, 263, 276
carbon monoxide, 29
carbon nanotubes, 285
carcinoma, 26, 130, 135, 255, 256, 257
cardiac arrest, 42
cardiac operations, 173, 182
cardiac output, 17, 18, 21, 23, 28, 29
cardiac surgery, 96, 102, 173, 174, 177, 178, 186, 291, 292
cardioplegia, 24, 175, 177, 178
cardiopulmonary bypass, 22, 31, 32, 173, 176, 177, 183, 184
cardiovascular disease, 22
carrier, 36, 157
cartilage, 239, 247, 263
catalyst, 224
catheter, 23, 24, 27, 111, 114, 177, 178, 184, 195, 248
cation, 62
causation, 51
cell, 56, 76, 135, 284
cell phones, 56
cervix, 216
channels, 181, 182, 270
children, 28, 29, 32, 33, 125, 128, 134, 149, 170, 186, 188, 189, 200, 203, 276, 280, 282, 292
cholecystectomy, 185, 187
chronic obstructive pulmonary disease, 17, 22
Civil War, 48
classes, 56, 152
classification, 68, 70, 92, 148, 152, 222, 225
classroom, 37
clinical trials, 7, 10, 61, 82, 83, 90, 228
closure, 34, 114, 177, 207, 212, 214, 216, 264
CO_2, 16, 17, 18, 21, 22, 23, 25, 27, 29, 33, 114, 177, 179, 182, 226, 228, 230, 244, 246, 247, 249, 256
coagulation, 22, 111, 112, 214

cochlear implant, 7
coding, 98
collaboration, 27, 42, 77, 223
collagen, 264
collateral, 118, 156
collateral damage, 156
collisions, 139, 188, 190, 267, 268, 288, 289
colon, 14, 36, 37, 41, 125
colon cancer, 14
colonoscopy, 293
commissure, 238, 250, 257
commitment, xiv
communication, 23, 36, 42, 49, 52, 133
community, 37, 38, 40, 41, 43, 44, 51, 61, 99, 165, 168, 265, 290
compatibility, 168
compensation, 51, 67, 75, 150
competence, 47, 49, 55, 173, 215
complexity, xi, 35, 55, 65, 152, 264
compliance, 16, 18, 29, 34, 50, 54
complications, 16, 18, 22, 24, 30, 34, 36, 37, 39, 40, 41, 44, 63, 64, 82, 84, 99, 116, 137, 146, 173, 175, 177, 183, 187, 207, 221, 226
components, 62, 63, 65, 70, 74, 76, 162, 202, 207, 282
composition, 286
computed tomography, 30, 157
computer systems, 147
computer technology, 167
computing, 56
concentration, 28, 214, 286
concrete, 48
conduct, 52, 268
conduction, 179, 182
confidence, 288
confidentiality, 47, 54
configuration, 38, 41, 108, 163, 164, 238, 267, 269
congenital heart disease, 17
congestive heart failure, 184
conjecture, 285, 288, 289
connective tissue, 263
consensus, xiii, 56, 67
consent, 55, 99
conservation, 207, 214
Constitution, 50
construction, 118, 166, 285
consultants, 9
consumption, 28
contamination, 48
control group, 79, 82, 83, 84
convergence, 47
conversion, 98, 127, 138, 140, 147, 178, 188, 208, 214, 215, 218, 221, 286

conversion rate, 138, 178, 208, 214, 215
cooling, 81, 120
COPD, 22, 139
copper, 36
Copyright, iv
coronary artery bypass graft, 10, 33, 34, 96, 101, 102, 177, 180, 184, 291
coronary artery disease, 22, 177, 178
corporations, 6
cost saving, 88, 161
cost-benefit analysis, 255
costs, 11, 88, 89, 99, 187, 219, 220, 223
cough, 139
counsel, 51
coupling, 185
Court of Appeals, 57
CPB, 22, 24, 25, 177
craniotomy, 159, 161, 163
credentials, 55
critical period, 24
criticism, 86, 87, 117
cryotherapy, 106
CT scan, 27, 63, 66, 70, 72, 80, 84, 85, 86, 87, 149, 169, 293
cues, 42, 183
curiosity, 223
current limit, xiv, 261
curriculum, 56
cutting force, 75
cyberspace, 53
cyst, 39, 159, 185, 189, 234, 242, 246, 256, 266, 280
cystocele, 138, 143
cystoscopy, 39
cytosine, 284

D

damage, 68, 80, 81, 86, 87, 89, 111, 148, 234, 263, 282, 288
data collection, 223
data processing, 167
database, 70
death, 183
decisions, 51, 70
decoding, 98
decomposition, 76
decortication, 185
defects, 145, 146, 264
defibrillator, 23
deficiency, 84
deficit, 21
definition, 52, 53, 54, 68, 126, 148, 152, 200

deflation, 176, 284
deformation, 163, 183
delivery, 17, 24, 28, 43, 154, 177, 178, 179, 180, 220, 261
demand, 153, 161, 163, 240
density, 181
Department of Health and Human Services, 54
deposition, 264
depression, 17, 24
depth perception, 10, 97, 105, 174, 263, 266
desire, 65, 95, 106, 138, 207
destruction, 154, 156
developing nations, 98
deviation, 183
diaphragm, 16
diaphragmatic hernia, 187, 189
diet, 14
disability, 173
discharges, 181
dislocation, 64, 83, 86, 88
displacement, 16, 234
disseminate, 41
dissociation, 28
diversity, 240
division, 38, 110, 111, 190, 238
DNA, 284, 285, 290, 293
dogs, 276
double helix, 284
downsizing, 202
drainage, 19, 39, 177
dream, 284
drug delivery, 284
drugs, 286, 290
ductus arteriosus, 28, 29
duplication, 285
durability, 139, 143, 219
duration, 15, 16, 17, 22, 23, 25, 27, 29, 99, 115

E

earth, 5, 39
eating, 200
ectopic pregnancy, 144
Ecuador, 37
EKG, 21, 23, 26
electrical properties, 284
electrocautery, 29, 36, 109, 112, 177, 214, 216, 230, 244, 247, 249, 256
electrodes, 155
embolism, 18, 22, 29, 226
emergence, 39
emergency physician, 53
emitters, 160

emphysema, 18, 31
encouragement, v
endocrine, 32
endometrial carcinoma, 221
endometriosis, 138, 206
endoscope, 9, 28, 36, 151, 174, 175, 188, 193, 207, 209, 223, 235, 236, 237, 240, 246, 249, 253, 254, 267, 288
endoscopic procedures, xiii, 223, 228, 263
endoscopy, 235
endotracheal intubation, 27, 238
endovascular occlusion, 24
endurance, 13
epiglottis, 238, 251
epilepsy, 160
equipment, xiv, 11, 42, 52, 99, 167, 187, 188
ERD, 21
ergonomics, 77, 97, 161
erosion, 143
esophageal atresia, 200
esophagus, 26, 190, 192, 193
etiology, 130, 207
Europe, 3, 7, 36, 44, 61, 67, 81, 88, 115, 168, 169, 218
European Union, 20
evacuation, 179
evaporation, 26
evidence, 86, 98, 138, 143, 215, 228
evolution, xiv, 32, 96, 206, 224, 285
examinations, 55
excision, 97, 126, 143, 154, 155, 156, 185, 189, 221, 226, 227, 228, 231, 233, 234, 238, 242, 247, 250, 252, 256, 262, 263, 280
excitation, 286
excretion, 29
exercise, 179
experimental design, 234
exposure, 23, 83, 89, 142, 159, 179, 216, 224, 235, 236, 237, 243, 246, 247, 249, 255, 263

F

fabrication, 88, 284
failure, 27, 42, 51, 82, 83, 86, 87, 99, 100, 253
fairness, 52
fallopian tubes, 27
family, 38, 202, 203
fascia, 109, 111, 112, 114, 116, 125, 132, 180
fat, 25, 28, 109, 112
fatigue, 42, 105, 153, 154
FDA, 7, 8, 10, 11, 20, 27, 49, 57, 82, 96, 160, 162, 175, 207, 225, 235
FDA approval, 7, 8, 10, 49, 162, 225, 235

fear, 50, 51
feedback, 8, 42, 67, 70, 78, 89, 98, 140, 149, 165, 167, 173, 182, 183, 184, 187, 214, 220, 229, 234, 263
feet, 26
females, 118, 120
femur, 27, 62, 63, 64, 65, 66, 67, 68, 72, 75, 76, 77, 80, 81, 86, 88
fiber optics, 7
fibrillation, 182
fibroids, 207
fibrous tissue, 85, 207
fidelity, 165, 188, 202
filtration, 14, 28, 243, 244, 249, 250
Finland, 91, 94
fistulas, 266
fixation, 62, 68, 70, 72, 77, 85, 152, 153, 179
flank, 193
flex, 244
flexibility, 15, 54, 139, 151, 268, 271
fluid, 17, 21, 24, 28, 179, 187
Foley catheter, 21, 23, 26, 195, 208, 216, 235
food, 56
foramen, 28
foramen ovale, 28
fractures, 64, 82, 83, 84, 89
France, vii, 7, 11, 39, 77, 91, 92, 95, 98, 169, 224, 225, 268
free will, 5
freedom, 10, 15, 29, 48, 67, 77, 97, 98, 105, 106, 125, 139, 156, 160, 171, 234, 236, 263, 266, 283
freezing, 288
friction, 75
funding, 8, 9, 162, 224

G

gait, 83
gastroesophageal reflux, 21, 203
gene, 285
gene therapy, 285
general anesthesia, 18, 140, 177, 179, 181, 182, 216
General Motors, 5
general surgeon, 7
general surgery, xiii, 95, 96, 97, 100, 101, 186
generation, 68, 265, 266
genetic information, 285
gestures, 5, 95, 100, 101
gland, 226, 227, 228, 230, 231, 232, 233, 241, 242
glasses, 10
glioma, 151
glottis, 253, 268
goals, 14, 89, 99, 234

gold, 118, 120, 127, 129, 286
grades, 183
graph, 231, 232, 233
gravity, 75
growth, 7, 38, 167, 168, 224
growth rate, 167, 168
guanine, 284
guidance, xiv, 7, 24, 27, 36, 37, 41, 68, 70, 152, 153, 158, 159, 160, 161, 163, 171, 202, 235, 289
guidelines, 15, 43, 54

H

habitat, 38
halogen, 205
hands, 7, 8, 9, 68, 73, 87, 140, 167, 186, 193, 206, 214, 235, 293
harm, xiii, 4, 52, 243
harvesting, 22
hazards, 16, 54
healing, 262, 263, 264
health, 38, 43, 47, 50, 52, 54, 103, 283
health care, 43, 47, 52, 283
health information, 54
heart disease, 180
heart failure, 179, 180
heart rate, 25, 28, 29
heat, 28, 93
heating, 28
height, 80, 267
hematocrit, 28
hemoglobin, 28, 143
hemorrhage, 24, 183
hemostasis, 140, 211, 214, 216, 243, 246, 257
Henry Ford, 30, 105, 122
hernia, 14, 37, 200, 227, 228, 230
hernia repair, 37
hiatal hernia, 190, 192, 200
hip, 7, 27, 31, 61, 62, 63, 64, 65, 66, 70, 80, 81, 83, 85, 87, 92, 93, 94, 129, 293
hip arthroplasty, 92, 94, 129, 293
hip joint, 63
hip replacement, 7, 31, 62, 92
hologram, 288
Honda, 5, 6, 12
hormone, 215
hospitalization, 11, 115, 116, 139, 176
hospitals, 27, 40, 53, 67, 88, 99, 187
host, 162
housing, 76, 188
human development, 151
human hand, xiv, 153, 234
human resources, 99, 235

hybrid, 178, 267, 282, 284
hybridization, 285
hydroxyapatite, 62
hypertension, 22
hypothermia, 24
hypothesis, 166
hypoxia, 23, 28, 29
hysterectomy, 10, 32, 138, 143, 144, 146, 205, 206, 207, 215, 216, 218, 219, 220, 221, 222

I

ideas, 28, 284
identification, 118, 149, 154, 155, 159, 169, 178
idiopathic, 179
IL-6, 22
IL-8, 22
illusion, 10
IMA, 24
images, 10, 32, 38, 42, 62, 68, 76, 88, 95, 100, 106, 108, 157, 160, 166, 225, 288
imagination, xiv
imaging modalities, 157, 165, 168, 288
imaging systems, 49
imitation, 284
immobilization, 283
imperforate anus, 185
implementation, 54, 76, 101, 151, 161, 163, 234, 262
in vitro, 49, 295
incidence, 22, 87, 145
incubation period, xi
indexing, 174
indication, 26
induction, 17, 23, 27
industry, xiii, 9, 47
inelastic, 286
infancy, 31, 101, 162, 166, 253, 255, 282
infants, 28, 29, 32, 128
infarction, 24
infection, 22, 83, 162
inferior vena cava, 29, 101, 182
inflation, 216, 230, 284
influence, 165, 281
informed consent, 47, 55, 189
infrastructure, 40
inguinal, 36, 41, 96, 99
inguinal hernia, 41, 96, 99
inguinal hernias, 96
initiation, 187, 216
injury, 5, 13, 18, 23, 24, 29, 51, 83, 101, 114, 125, 127, 140, 151, 173, 182, 183, 186, 187, 228, 247, 253, 254

innovation, 224
input, 66, 70, 153
insertion, 7, 27, 28, 63, 80, 106, 153, 155, 160, 170
insight, xiv, 130
inspiration, v
instability, 86
institutions, 106, 128, 143, 189, 235
instruction, 36, 37, 39
instruments, iv, xiii, xiv, 9, 11, 12, 22, 27, 28, 33, 35, 63, 66, 67, 97, 98, 102, 106, 114, 125, 128, 139, 151, 154, 155, 161, 163, 167, 174, 175, 176, 179, 182, 187, 188, 189, 190, 192, 193, 200, 202, 207, 209, 214, 215, 216, 218, 220, 223, 232, 236, 237, 240, 244, 248, 249, 253, 254, 255, 261, 262, 263, 264, 265, 266, 268, 288, 289
insulation, 21
insurance, 50
integration, 159, 161, 163, 166, 168, 223, 240, 262
integrity, 54, 55, 263
interaction, 36, 51, 152, 201, 202
interactions, 51, 202, 285, 290
interest, 9, 11, 26, 36, 38, 49, 67, 128, 156, 158, 173, 236
interface, 7, 47, 56, 76, 77, 80, 95, 96, 106, 125, 131, 156, 162, 165, 166, 174, 183, 268, 273, 283, 288
interference, 229, 236, 286, 288
interpretation, 52
interval, 85, 215
intervention, 22, 68, 99, 106, 178, 180, 184, 216, 278, 286
interview, 55, 137
intraocular, 18
intraocular pressure, 18
intravenous fluids, 30
intravenously, 24
introitus, 141
investment, 162
IP networks, 42
irradiation, 154
irritability, 23
ischemia, 120, 122
isolation, 101
Israel, 67, 76, 275
Italy, 43, 66, 90, 146, 279

J

Japan, 5, 12, 28, 83, 90, 92, 168, 235
jaundice, 200
joints, 65, 148, 164, 267, 270, 271
judgment, 151
jurisdiction, 53

K

kidney, 39, 120, 122, 133
knee arthroplasty, 34, 61, 91, 94
knees, 81, 84
knowledge, 13, 37, 39, 41, 100, 167
Korea, 67, 69, 85

L

labor, 3, 5
laceration, 182
lactate level, 17
land, 36, 42
language, 3
laparoscope, 36, 114, 206, 207, 232
laparoscopic cholecystectomy, 9, 11, 30, 31, 34, 37, 39, 96, 102, 185, 200, 224, 225, 240
laparoscopy, 18, 22, 32, 33, 34, 44, 95, 96, 97, 98, 100, 125, 128, 131, 138, 140, 143, 144, 186, 187, 194, 203, 205, 206, 207, 208, 214, 215, 219, 220, 262, 264, 265, 275, 292
laparotomy, 26, 37, 118, 206, 207, 208, 214, 215, 218, 219
laproscopic robots, 283
laryngectomy, 239, 242, 249, 250, 251, 256, 262, 265, 273
laryngoscope, xiv, 246, 261, 263, 264, 265, 266, 267, 268, 269, 273
laryngoscopy, 24, 236, 245, 249, 263, 276
larynx, 236, 238, 240, 243, 245, 246, 247, 255, 262, 263, 273, 276
laser ablation, 31, 261
lasers, 256, 263, 276
latency, 38, 39, 42, 44, 98
Latin America, 168
laws, 4, 5, 47, 48, 50, 53, 56
lawyers, 52
lead, 17, 24, 29, 30, 50, 65, 101, 129, 147, 173, 179, 180, 183, 184, 284, 288
leadership, 186
learning, xi, 16, 37, 82, 84, 85, 86, 88, 99, 100, 106, 120, 128, 143, 173, 175, 178, 186, 202, 250, 253, 294
learning process, 100
left ventricle, 181
legal, iv
legislation, iv, 55
leiomyoma, 211, 212, 213
leiomyomata, 207, 214
lens, 108, 109, 112, 142, 150, 188, 235
lesions, 84, 154, 156, 159, 166, 171, 226, 244, 249, 252, 253, 257, 266, 273

levator, 109, 112
liability, iv, 47, 52, 53
lifetime, 138
ligament, 62, 65, 67, 108, 190, 216, 217
likelihood, 52, 68
limitation, 77, 139, 159, 182, 261
linkage, 280, 288
links, 39, 148, 165, 271
lipids, 286
lipoma, 121
litigation, xiii
liver, 100, 101, 127, 190, 191, 193
lobectomy, 185, 196, 241
local anesthetic, 17
localization, 28, 72, 150, 155, 159, 161, 163, 293
location, 8, 9, 11, 15, 17, 20, 21, 35, 36, 53, 64, 65, 95, 98, 99, 100, 155, 207, 214, 215, 224, 225, 228, 265, 267, 288
long distance, 263
longevity, 138
love, v
low risk, 225
lumen, 21, 22, 23, 24, 114, 195
lymph, 109, 118, 128, 135, 217, 219, 226, 227
lymph node, 109, 118, 128, 135, 217, 219, 226, 227

M

macro robots, 282
magnesium, 23
magnetic resonance, 149, 157, 169, 293
magnetic resonance imaging, 149, 157, 169, 293
males, 120
malignancy, 113, 216, 219
malignant growth, 262
management, 13, 85, 127, 130, 134, 135, 144, 205, 206, 207, 220, 221, 236, 243, 244, 249, 250, 255, 288
mandible, 254
manipulation, 7, 25, 35, 44, 95, 101, 114, 129, 155, 158, 161, 163, 164, 170, 174, 183, 185, 186, 194, 224, 236, 261, 264, 265, 267, 268, 270, 271, 273
manufacturing, xiii, 49, 63, 273
market, xiv, 24, 30, 61, 147, 167, 168
market penetration, 61
market segment, 167
market share, 167
marketing, 66
markets, 11, 55, 168
marriage, 5, 14, 166
Mars, 5
marsupialization, 246
mass, 189, 195, 196, 197

MAST, 214
mastery, 246
matrix, 68
measurement, 84
measures, 54, 82, 162, 163, 177, 187, 249
mechanical properties, 80
mechanical ventilation, 26
median, 108, 111, 117, 174, 177, 180, 215, 219
mediastinum, 29, 193
Medicaid, 54
medical robots, 62, 147, 148, 162, 165, 168, 171, 282, 288
Medicare, 54
medication, 143, 283
memory, 151, 158, 265, 278
men, 3, 106, 130
meninges, 155
mental health, 177
mentor, 35, 36, 38
mentoring, 36, 39, 41, 43, 99
mercury, 19
metastasis, 19
micrometer, 153
microscope, 149, 155, 156, 157, 158, 159, 170, 171, 244, 249, 263
Microsoft, 12
microstructure, 284
Middle East, 168
military, 5, 8, 11, 38, 224
miniaturization, xiii, 25, 101, 128, 282
missions, 7, 38
mitral valve, 10, 22, 25, 32, 102, 173, 175, 176, 183, 255, 291, 292
mobility, 264, 266
mode, 39, 66, 68, 70, 73, 75, 78, 151, 160, 166, 234, 246, 254, 262, 267, 271, 283, 290
modeling, 227, 289
models, xiv, 62, 100, 183, 200, 225, 227, 236, 240, 289
modules, 28, 67, 284
molecular biology, 290
molecular structure, 284
molecules, 284, 285, 286
momentum, 240
money, 235
monitoring, 16, 23, 26, 30, 44, 48, 83, 100, 102, 177, 268
morbidity, 22, 96, 99, 103, 106, 137, 138, 139, 143, 215, 224
mortality, 97, 103, 176, 224, 227
mortality rate, 176, 227
motion, 8, 10, 14, 15, 27, 28, 37, 65, 67, 72, 73, 75, 77, 81, 84, 85, 87, 97, 98, 148, 150, 151, 152, 153, 154, 157, 164, 168, 174, 183, 187, 206, 207, 236, 237, 244, 249, 268, 269, 271, 283, 289, 294
motivation, 62, 65, 81, 95
motor control, 76, 268
movement, 8, 10, 11, 25, 29, 97, 105, 150, 151, 153, 159, 161, 185, 186, 187, 189, 206, 207, 235, 244, 254, 256, 266
MRI, 156, 157, 158, 159, 160, 165, 166, 170, 277, 288
mucosa, 250, 252, 253
multimedia, 56
muscle relaxant, 21
muscle relaxation, 16
muscles, 17, 83, 86, 250
mutuality, 51
myasthenia gravis, 291
myelomeningocele, 204, 292
myocardial ischemia, 24
myocardium, 25

N

nanofabrication, 285
nanomachines, 284
nanostructures, 284
nanotechnology, 284, 285, 290
nasogastric tube, 140, 216
National Aeronautics and Space Administration, 7, 224
National Institutes of Health, 56, 224, 274
navigation system, 62, 65, 67, 68, 69, 70, 73, 77, 147, 150, 152, 155, 163, 166, 167, 169
necrosis, 80
needs, 23, 27, 30, 56, 73, 75, 86, 164, 165, 202, 264, 283, 288, 289, 290
negative attitudes, 200
neonates, 28
nephrectomy, 120, 122, 133
nerve, 13, 18, 80, 81, 83, 84, 87, 97, 106, 109, 112, 116, 129, 132, 150, 179, 181, 182, 217, 218
nerve fibers, 132
nervous system, 19
Netherlands, 294
network, 38, 39, 40, 98, 99, 100
neurosurgery, 34, 148, 149, 150, 151, 153, 155, 157, 160, 161, 163, 164, 168, 169, 170, 171, 265
next generation, 42
nicotinamide, 132
Nissen fundoplication, 10, 36, 37, 41, 97, 99, 185, 189, 190, 191, 193
nodes, 109, 118, 217
nucleotides, 286
nurses, 53, 282, 283

nursing, 283

O

obesity, 97, 138, 144
obligate, 28
observations, 145
obstruction, 125, 126, 234
obstructive sleep apnea, 243
occlusion, 23, 25, 31, 177
omentum, 217
operating system, 164
operator, 9, 42, 48, 100, 263
opioids, 21, 26
optical fiber, 98
optimal performance, 42, 265
optimism, 200
optimization, 13, 14, 72, 268
optimization method, 72
oral antibiotic, 138, 143
orbit, 254
organ, 13, 14, 26, 31, 100, 106, 145, 152, 262
organism, 284
organizations, 56
orientation, 66, 77, 87, 148, 156, 159, 161, 163, 182, 217, 265, 269
orthopedic surgeon, 27
outline, 71, 262
output, 29
ovarian tumor, 221
oxygen, 17, 24, 28, 32, 34
oxygen consumption, 32

P

Pacific, 168
pacing, 23, 25, 179, 180, 184
pain, 13, 14, 18, 23, 26, 27, 64, 72, 81, 82, 83, 84, 86, 87, 93, 105, 116, 126, 143, 173, 174, 175, 177, 185, 187, 200, 206, 207, 262
pain management, 13, 14
paradigm shift, 148, 240
parallel platform, 271
paralysis, 19, 24, 26, 27, 262
parameter, 68, 75
parathyroid, 226
parathyroidectomy, 226, 241
parenchyma, 27
partnership, 162
passive, 7, 68, 69, 70, 72, 73, 75, 77, 148, 152, 161, 223, 225, 240, 268, 269
patella, 65, 76
patent ductus arteriosus, 203

patents, 9
pathology, 97, 159, 205, 207, 209, 215, 219, 220, 226, 240, 286
pathways, 182
pedal, 174, 294
pelvic relaxation, 145
pelvis, 97, 114, 125, 126, 176, 214
perforation, 19
perfusion, 16, 17, 18, 23, 29, 30, 177
pericardium, 176, 179, 182
periosteum, 141
peritoneal cavity, 16, 17
peritoneum, 122, 137, 142, 216, 217
permit, 42, 174
perseverance, xiv
perspective, xiii, 62, 157, 158, 161, 163, 246, 292
PET, 157
pH, 227
pharynx, 236, 238, 240, 243, 244, 245, 246, 247, 255, 262
photographs, 48, 89
physical interaction, 147
physical properties, 284
physiology, 13, 14, 16, 18, 22, 28, 29
pigs, 33, 126, 200
pilot study, 32, 33, 102, 132, 220
pitch, 70, 74, 106
pituitary tumors, 242
planning, 62, 66, 73, 74, 76, 80, 81, 86, 88, 100, 101, 153, 157, 158, 159, 160, 161, 166, 168, 288, 289
pleasure, xi
pleura, 195
plexus, 111
pneumonia, 20
pneumothorax, 16, 18, 19, 21, 23, 227
polypropylene, 137, 141, 178, 183
population, 30, 79, 187, 203
port of entry, 195
portal vein, 100
ports, 48, 108, 114, 125, 126, 127, 128, 137, 139, 140, 176, 177, 179, 188, 189, 191, 193, 194, 195, 197, 210, 216, 244, 262, 265
positive end expiratory pressure, 23
positron, 157
positron emission tomography, 157
postoperative outcome, 177
potassium, 150
power, 49, 50, 76, 244, 268, 281, 286
preference, 106
pregnancy, 53, 207, 219
preparation, iv, 24, 63, 64, 65, 67, 77, 80, 81, 86, 93, 123

pre-planning, 167
presbyopia, 28
pressure, 16, 17, 18, 19, 21, 22, 23, 24, 25, 29, 110, 132, 139, 207, 214, 216, 228, 230, 290
prevention, 13, 49, 114, 130, 142, 246
primary brain tumor, 159
primary hyperparathyroidism, 241
principle, 162, 249, 265, 288
privacy, 47, 54
probe, 157, 160, 181, 182, 286
production, 5, 28, 56, 264, 270
production costs, 56, 270
professions, 47
program, 15, 38, 40, 97, 186, 222, 283, 284
programming, 9
prolapse, 135, 137, 138, 139, 142, 143, 144, 145, 146, 207, 219, 220
proliferation, 105, 235
prophylaxis, 214
prostate, 11, 26, 106, 108, 109, 111, 112, 129, 130, 132, 255
prostate cancer, 106, 129, 130
prostatectomy, 10, 26, 106, 107, 115, 116, 117, 118, 119, 129, 130, 131, 132, 186, 247, 255, 256, 292
prostheses, 62, 63, 64, 65, 66, 70, 81, 83, 86, 88
prosthesis, 7, 27, 30, 62, 63, 64, 65, 66, 70, 72, 73, 74, 75, 77, 78, 80, 81, 82, 84, 85, 86, 87
proteins, 286
protocol, 23, 24
prototype, 7, 67, 68, 76, 77, 78, 151, 154, 164, 166, 175, 181, 224, 271
public interest, 3
pulmonary artery pressure, 23
pulmonary embolism, 83, 87, 94
pulmonary hypertension, 22
pulmonary vascular resistance, 17, 23
pulse, 21, 23, 26, 181
PUMA, 27, 148, 154, 155, 163, 165
pyloric stenosis, 21
pyloroplasty, 189

Q

QRS complex, 179
qualifications, 55
quality of life, 106, 176, 177, 179, 184
quality of service, 98

R

radiation, 106, 154, 286
radiation therapy, 106
radical cystectomy, 132

radio, 82
radiotherapy, 154, 219
Raman spectra, 286
Raman spectroscopy, 286
range, 9, 27, 36, 39, 48, 84, 96, 97, 120, 162, 187, 207, 214, 215, 237, 281, 284, 289
real time, 11
reality, 5, 7, 8, 9, 15, 44, 48, 100, 101, 103, 148, 161, 164, 167, 202, 224, 240, 281, 292
recall, 24
reciprocity, 50
recognition, 157, 167, 183, 235, 242
reconstruction, 62, 65, 67, 91, 92, 100, 118, 134, 135, 146, 156, 261, 262, 264, 265, 273, 287
recovery, xiii, 5, 24, 73, 75, 88, 96, 105, 106, 129, 143, 164, 185, 187, 200, 206, 263
rectocele, 138, 143
rectosigmoid, 208
rectum, 112
recurrence, 14, 117
red blood cells, 284
reduction, 16, 36, 61, 62, 88, 215, 224, 235, 265
redundancy, 40, 270, 271
reflection, 140, 151
regulation, xiii, 49
regulations, 53, 54, 55
regulatory oversight, xiv
relationship, 47, 50, 51, 52, 56, 64, 97
relationships, 30, 51
reliability, 87, 95, 98
renal cell carcinoma, 121
repair, 10, 24, 25, 62, 64, 126, 127, 128, 135, 137, 138, 139, 142, 143, 144, 146, 173, 175, 176, 177, 183, 184, 185, 187, 189, 190, 192, 200, 203, 204, 207, 255, 263, 266, 273, 291, 292
repetitions, 183
replacement, 7, 25, 27, 33, 64, 70, 76, 91, 94, 187
resection, 14, 19, 26, 65, 67, 68, 74, 99, 101, 112, 113, 121, 129, 149, 155, 156, 159, 161, 163, 170, 176, 189, 196, 198, 214, 226, 227, 228, 232, 233, 238, 241, 242, 253, 254, 255, 256, 266, 273, 291
resistance, 17, 55, 63, 179, 180, 254
resolution, 160, 185, 271, 285, 287
resources, 50, 56
respiratory, 17, 18, 29, 34, 150, 168, 248, 276
response time, 78
responsibility, iv, 14, 225, 240
responsiveness, 234
retention, 38
retrieval, iv, 112
right ventricle, 179
rights, iv, 9, 11, 50, 54
rings, 210

risk, 16, 24, 29, 52, 54, 83, 86, 125, 138, 139, 162, 164, 182, 183, 186, 209, 214, 215, 221, 224, 225, 235, 253, 254
risk benefit, 16
risk factors, 138
robot hand, 148, 174, 283
robotic vision, xiv, 282
robotics, xiii, 4, 5, 11, 12, 13, 48, 66, 68, 89, 95, 97, 99, 101, 138, 143, 144, 147, 148, 149, 151, 152, 160, 161, 162, 163, 164, 165, 166, 167, 168, 169, 170, 174, 175, 186, 188, 189, 200, 202, 205, 207, 214, 215, 219, 222, 225, 240, 249, 253, 262, 281, 282, 283, 284, 285, 288, 289, 291, 294
rotations, 70
rubber, 268
rural areas, 38

S

sacrum, 138, 142
safety, 15, 16, 36, 42, 49, 50, 70, 72, 82, 87, 96, 98, 133, 147, 148, 152, 154, 161, 162, 164, 167, 168, 171, 174, 182, 223, 245, 249, 253, 255, 257, 288
sales, 167, 168
sample, xiv
sampling, 234, 284, 286
sampling error, 286
satellite, 36, 42, 48
satellite technology, 42
satisfaction, 11, 137, 138, 223
saturation, 17
savings, 99
scaling, 10, 28, 97, 98, 108, 109, 112, 153, 174, 187, 234, 244, 249, 266, 282
scapula, 195
scar tissue, 262, 264
scattering, 286, 288
school, 52, 56, 225
scientific knowledge, 47, 56
scoliosis, 22
scores, 82, 83, 84, 87
search, 70, 72, 126, 138, 200
security, 40, 47, 54, 117
selecting, 64, 70, 158, 240
self, 3, 7, 284, 285
self-assembly, 285
self-organization, 285
self-repair, 284
semiconductor, 290
seminal vesicle, 111
sensation, 7, 25, 42
sensing, 163, 165, 262, 268, 282, 286, 290
sensitivity, 48, 290

sensors, xiv, 8, 162, 163, 235, 268, 282, 286, 289, 290
separation, 187, 193, 202
septum, 176
sequencing, 284
series, 36, 37, 40, 115, 116, 117, 118, 120, 126, 127, 183, 200, 215, 218, 219, 229, 232, 249
services, iv, 42, 48, 50, 53, 57
shape, 16, 62, 64, 65, 73, 78, 79, 265, 284
shaping, 161, 163
sheep, 204
shock, 29
shortage, 283
shoulders, 14, 217
sickle cell, 21
sigmoid colon, 108
signals, 42, 48, 153, 174, 183, 287
simulation, iv, 38, 100, 101, 173
Singapore, 240, 293, 294
sinus, 179, 235, 242, 267
sinuses, 182, 235, 240
sites, 36, 52, 98, 99, 100, 166, 189, 190, 191, 193, 194, 253, 289
skills, xiv, 37, 41, 99, 100, 131, 143, 183, 185, 206, 219, 282
skin, 15, 22, 25, 100, 106, 114, 142, 155, 253
skin cancer, 106
smooth muscle, 207
Socrates, 11
sodium, 21, 28
software, 49, 68, 72, 73, 76, 80, 83, 85, 87, 97, 156, 158, 160, 161, 162, 164, 165, 166, 168, 282, 284
spectroscopy, 286
spectrum, 226, 240
speculation, 175
speed, 48, 76, 78, 98, 156, 249
spin, 78
spine, 19, 61, 62, 75, 108, 170, 253, 254, 283
spleen, 125, 193, 194
stability, 65, 80, 81, 84, 86, 93
stabilization, 178, 292
stabilizers, 25
stages, 16, 61, 168, 182, 262, 268, 288
standard deviation, 81, 163
standardization, 101
standards, 52, 54, 164, 168, 182
stapes, 234, 242
Star Wars, 5
statistics, 129
sterile, 188, 189
sternocleidomastoid, 232
stochastic model, 183
stomach, 21, 26, 216

storage, 285
strategies, 246
strength, 139, 151
stress, 13, 16, 29, 42, 55, 64, 83, 142
stroke, 19, 20
stroke volume, 19, 20
students, 56
subcutaneous emphysema, 17, 21, 226
substitution, 183, 238
success rate, 125, 137, 138, 139
Sudan, 132
summaries, 221
superior vena cava, 24, 182
superiority, 151
supervision, 15
supply, 199, 271
support staff, 41
suprapubic, 26
Supreme Court, 50
surface area, 28, 189
surgical intervention, 148, 152, 223, 262
surgical resection, 162
surveillance, 221, 285
survival, 103, 106, 180, 203, 240, 286
survivors, 200
susceptibility, 151
suture, 109, 111, 114, 128, 140, 177, 178, 179, 183, 200, 209, 214, 216, 219, 263, 266, 273

T

tachycardia, 24
targets, 154, 158, 160
taxonomy, 224, 225
teaching, 11, 35, 36, 40, 41, 98, 99, 100
technician, 283
technological advancement, 206
technological change, 186
teeth, 248, 253, 254
tele surgical systems, 152
telecommunications, 35, 36, 38, 39, 42, 47, 98
tele-mentoring, xiii
telephone, 37, 48, 51
tele-presence medicine, xiii
television, 186, 187
temperature, 13, 24, 28, 81, 290
tension, 23, 85, 114, 126, 142, 183
testicular cancer, 135
theory, 87, 157, 285
therapeutics, xi
therapy, 106, 130, 138, 143, 243, 294
thermal properties, 247
thoracoscopy, 18, 22, 32, 186, 187, 265

thoracotomy, 20, 25, 26, 175, 177, 179, 180
threats, 54
threshold, 87, 179, 180
thrombosis, 28, 84
thymine, 284
thymus, 227
thyroid, 226, 233, 239, 241, 242
tibia, 65, 68, 75
tissue, 11, 65, 68, 80, 85, 101, 105, 108, 113, 129, 139, 140, 149, 151, 153, 154, 155, 163, 169, 173, 183, 185, 209, 213, 214, 216, 227, 234, 247, 255, 261, 263, 264, 265, 267, 273, 282, 286, 295
titanium, 27, 72
tonsillectomy, 250
topology, 152
trachea, 24
tracheoesophageal fistula, 185, 200
tracheostomy, 263
tracking, 67, 76, 78, 154, 163, 262, 283
trainees, 100, 173, 183
training, xiv, 11, 35, 37, 39, 43, 44, 56, 99, 100, 143, 162, 175, 187, 206, 215, 219, 222, 283
trajectory, 151, 153, 155, 157, 158, 159, 160, 162, 244
transection, 107, 111, 216, 247, 249, 253
transformation, 72
transfusion, 13, 20, 115, 215
transition, 187, 226, 285
translation, 39, 86, 131
transmission, 42, 48, 54, 99, 265
transparency, 100
transplantation, 122, 123, 133
transport, 98, 283
transurethral resection, 26
transverse colon, 217
trauma, 27, 167, 177, 228, 262, 263, 283
tremor, 10, 14, 28, 67, 77, 95, 98, 102, 139, 151, 153, 174, 185, 186, 187, 234, 235, 243, 244, 249, 250, 253, 263, 266, 282
trend, 67, 88, 215
trial, 31, 79, 82, 83, 94, 101, 129, 291, 293, 294
trochanter, 83, 86
tubal ligation, 96, 207
tumor, 14, 25, 26, 120, 155, 156, 159, 160, 166, 209, 221
tumors, 19, 101, 120, 127, 159, 207, 241, 249, 250, 288

U

UK, 7, 74, 295
ultrasound, 25, 39, 154, 156, 160, 165, 166, 235, 281, 286, 287

uncertainty, 81
uniform, 64, 151, 186
United States, 7, 36, 38, 44, 49, 53, 57, 101, 105, 138, 162, 175, 176, 207, 215, 220, 221, 225, 291
upper airways, 261, 262, 264
urban centres, 38, 40
ureter, 122
ureteropelvic junction obstruction, 134
ureters, 216, 217
urethra, 109, 110, 112, 114, 205
urine, 28
urologist, 106
uterine fibroids, 207, 221
uterine prolapse, 128
uterus, 27, 118, 132, 207, 209, 210, 214, 216

V

vagina, 132, 138, 140, 142, 143, 216
valgus, 86
validation, 268
values, 22, 80, 81
variability, 86, 103
variable, 16, 21, 29, 48, 126, 157
variables, 82
variation, 289
varus, 86
vascular surgery, 96
vasculature, 125
vasoconstriction, 19, 28
vasodilation, 24
vasopressin, 17, 214
vasopressin level, 17
vein, 28, 31, 36, 84, 101, 106, 109, 122, 125, 176, 177, 182, 217
velocity, 75, 92, 268
ventilation, 15, 16, 17, 19, 20, 22, 23, 25, 28, 29, 30, 31, 32, 176, 177, 179, 181, 182
ventricle, 249
vessels, 23, 25, 29, 31, 32, 109, 118, 120, 122, 123, 125, 174, 178, 179, 190, 194, 195, 217, 244, 247, 253, 255, 290

virtual reality (VR), 100
viscosity, 290
vision, 7, 8, 9, 11, 14, 18, 22, 25, 29, 100, 106, 107, 108, 112, 139, 140, 185, 187, 202, 206, 207, 248, 263, 281, 282, 283, 289
visual field, 294
visualization, 15, 19, 25, 35, 73, 105, 108, 111, 118, 129, 158, 159, 160, 163, 164, 166, 182, 186, 187, 189, 194, 195, 206, 216, 229, 235, 246, 261, 264, 282, 288, 289, 290
voice, 8, 150, 155, 157, 158, 166, 170, 175, 206, 220, 235, 242, 243, 250, 262, 264

W

water, 28
weakness, 39
webpages, 56
websites, 52, 55
weight ratio, 271
wells, 7
wires, 76, 270, 271
women, 138, 143, 144, 145, 207, 221
work, xiii, xiv, 3, 11, 16, 19, 29, 41, 48, 54, 66, 73, 105, 148, 149, 152, 164, 165, 167, 168, 171, 187, 224, 226, 229, 235, 236, 245, 246, 249, 264, 273, 286, 290
workers, 5
workload, 294
workstation, 8, 10, 66, 80, 86, 157, 158, 275
wound healing, 256
wrists, 265
writing, 51

X

xenon, 157, 205

Y

yield, 241, 285

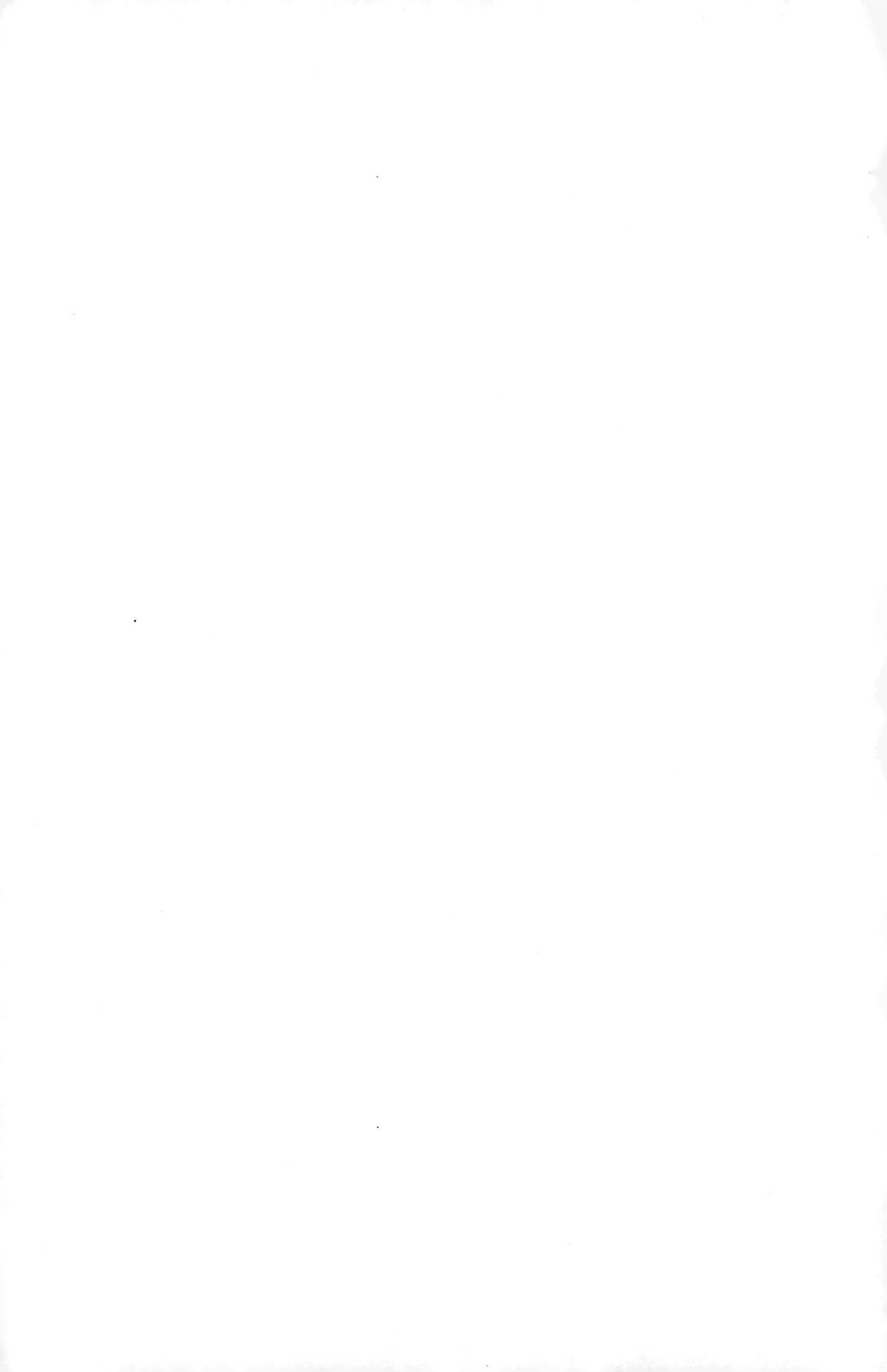